ALTERNATIVE
MEDICINE

Recent Titles in
Health and Medical Issues Today

Obesity
Evelyn B. Kelly

Organ Transplantation
David Petechuk

Stem Cells
Evelyn B. Kelly

ALTERNATIVE MEDICINE

Christine A. Larson

Health and Medical Issues Today

GREENWOOD PRESS
Westport, Connecticut • London

Library of Congress Cataloging-in-Publication Data

Larson, Christine A., 1953–
    Alternative medicine / Christine A. Larson.
      p. cm.—(Health and medical issues today, ISSN 1558–7592)
    Includes bibliographical references and index.
    ISBN 0–313–33718–7 (alk. paper)
    1. Alternative medicine. I. Title. II. Series.
    [DNLM: 1. Complementary Therapies. WB 890 L334a 2006]
  R733.L37   2007
  610—dc22   2006029482

British Library Cataloguing in Publication Data is available.

Library of Congress Catalog Card Number: 2006029482
ISBN: 0–313–33718–7
ISSN: 1558–7592

First published in 2007

Greenwood Press, 88 Post Road West, Westport, CT 06881
An imprint of Greenwood Publishing Group, Inc.
www.greenwood.com

Printed in the United States of America

The paper used in this book complies with the
Permanent Paper Standard issued by the National
Information Standards Organization (Z39.48–1984).

10 9 8 7 6 5 4 3 2 1

Science is a search for the truth. The effort to understand the world involves the rejection of bias, dogma, of revelation but not the rejection of morality. One way in which scientists work is by observing the world, making note of phenomena and analyzing them.

Linus Pauling, Ph.D.

This book is dedicated to Dr. Linus Pauling, the only recipient of two unshared Nobel Prizes for his work. Dr. Pauling received his bachelor's degree from Oregon Agricultural College, now Oregon State University, in chemical engineering and his doctorate in chemistry and mathematical physics. He is considered one of the greatest scientific minds of the twentieth century. Pauling coined the term *orthomolecular medicine* in 1968, describing it as "the right molecules in the right concentration." Although I did not know Dr. Pauling, nor was I familiar with his research at the time, I applied orthomolecular medicine in the process of restoring my health.

Dr. Pauling died on August 19, 1994, but his work on micronutrients continues at the Linus Pauling Institute at Oregon State University in Corvallis, Oregon. This book is dedicated to medical mavericks like Dr. Linus Pauling, whose work contributes to the understanding of disease, as well as its resolution through natural approaches. The Linus Pauling Institute is listed as one of the first two Centers of Excellence for Research in Complementary and Alternative Medicine in the United States by NCCAM of the National Institutes of Health (NIH).

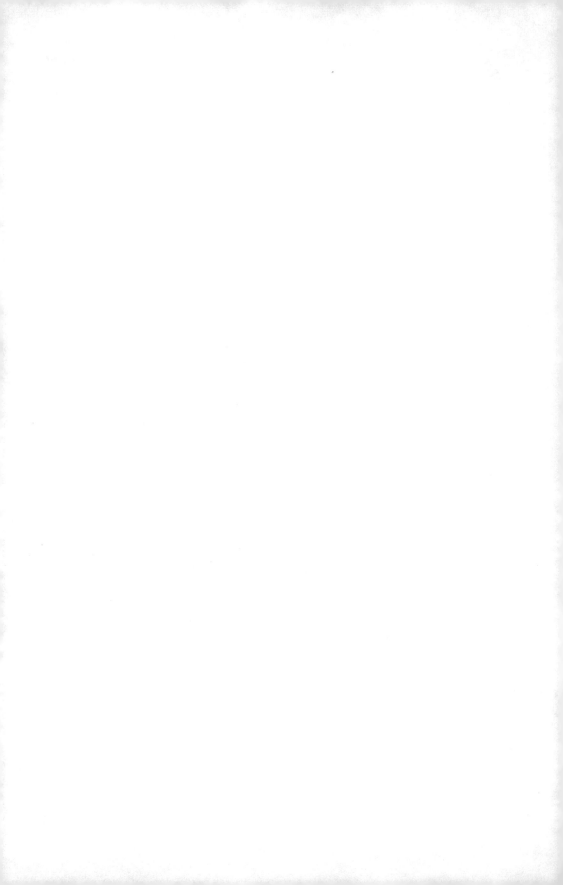

CONTENTS

Section Three   References and Resources

SERIES FOREWORD

Every day, the public is bombarded with information on developments in medicine and health care. Whether it is on the latest techniques in treatments or research, or on concerns over public health threats, this information directly impacts the lives of people more than almost any other issue. Although there are many sources for understanding these topics—from Web sites and blogs to newspapers and magazines—students and ordinary citizens often need one resource that makes sense of the complex health and medical issues affecting their daily lives.

The *Health and Medical Issues Today* series provides just such a one-stop resource for obtaining a solid overview of the most controversial areas of health care today. Each volume addresses one topic and provides a balanced summary of what is known. These volumes provide an excellent first step for students and lay people interested in understanding how health care works in our society today.

Each volume is broken into several sections to provide readers and researchers with easy access to the information they need:

- Section I provides overview chapters on background information—including chapters on such areas as the historical, scientific, medical, social, and legal issues involved—that a citizen needs to intelligently understand the topic.
- Section II provides capsule examinations of the most heated contemporary issues and debates, and analyzes in a balanced manner the viewpoints held by various advocates in the debates.

- Section III provides a selection of reference material, including annotated primary source documents, a timeline of important events, and an annotated bibliography of useful print and electronic resources that serve as the best next step in learning about the topic at hand.

The *Health and Medical Issues Today* series strives to provide readers with all the information needed to begin making sense of some of the most important debates going on in the world today. The series will include volumes on such topics as stem-cell research, obesity, gene therapy, alternative medicine, organ transplantation, mental health, and more.

PREFACE

Alternative medicine is a term that causes confusion for most people. What is alternative medicine? How does it compare with conventional medicine? What is integrative medicine? Is integrative medicine the same as alternative medicine? How does alternative medicine compare with holistic health? What do all of these practices have in common, and what are their differences? Do they work? Are they safe?

The reason most consumers choose to explore alternative approaches to healing is a very simple one: what they're currently doing isn't working. The intent of this book is to provide what I refer to as "The Savvy Consumer's Guide to Healthcare." It is the culmination of a journey that began several years ago, when I experienced health problems. The restoration of my health and what I learned in the process underlies much of the material in this book. It also served as the basis for my doctoral work in evidence-based medicine at the University of Kentucky.

There is a mystique surrounding medicine in which the doctor is seen as God. As much as I respect science and the men and women who have gone through the academic process to become clinicians and researchers, they are not gods. This book strips away the mystique to examine the science underlying medicine. Science is about seeking the truth, which in medicine equates to knowing what works and what doesn't. Medicine, in its true form, is about problem solving—not merely treating the symptoms, but understanding causal factors that underlie the disease process and, as a result of that understanding, reversing or eliminating the causal factors, leading to health restoration.

Depending on the statistics one draws from, roughly 20–50 percent of medicine is science based. That means that 50–80 percent of what we refer to as medicine is a virtual unknown: we do not know what works and what doesn't work. These statistics may be startling, but they are very useful statistics. If you have a condition that is troubling, limiting, and maybe even life-threatening, these statistics can provide you with the hope and encouragement to lead you to explore a variety of approaches to healing.

One of the myths surrounding alternative medicine concerns its novelty. Many alternative approaches date back some 3000–5000 years, with their origins in Chinese medicine or ayurvedic medicine. If you pray or take vitamins, which many people do, you are practicing alternative medicine. If you exercise, modify your diet, or limit your intake of sugars and refined carbohydrates, you're practicing alternative medicine. This book will debunk some of the myths that surround alternative medicine.

Many alternative therapies have not been evaluated for their efficacy. Some are dangerous, some are a waste of money, and some may compound your health problems. However, there are also many therapies used in conventional medical practice that have not been evaluated for their efficacy either. Many are dangerous, some are a waste of money, and some may compound your health problems. Those are the facts.

This book is written for consumers, novices to the concept of alternative medicine; it is not written for the scientific community, although I have relied heavily on the scientific studies that are available on complementary and alternative medicine. The book's intent is to provide a broad overview of alternative medicine, the controversies surrounding it, and the science underlying it.

There are some 4000 books on alternative medicine. I have attempted to focus on the scientific sources and to distill that research into a comprehensible form for you, the consumer. Toward that end I have focused on the six categories of complementary and alternative forms of medicine designated by the National Institutes of Health's official governing body, the National Center for Complementary and Alternative Medicine (NCCAM), as an organizational tool for presenting this information. NCCAM is the regulatory arm charged with the evaluation of complementary and alternative medicine for the United States. For consumers not familiar with the National Institutes of Health (NIH), it is the hub of medical research, funding, and evaluation for the United States. NCCAM is to CAM (complementary and alternative medicine) what the FDA is to prescription drug evaluation.

The content of the book, which is part of the series "Health and Medical Issues Today," consists of four overview chapters, which provide grounding in the key content, six chapters on "controversies," which explore the critical issues that surround alternative medicine, and a section of annotated source material that includes seminal scientific work in the arena of complementary and alternative therapies.

The book is intended to provide basic knowledge and scientific grounding. If it helps you to understand the realities of healthcare and the limits of what is currently known, it will have accomplished part of its task. If it provides you with hope and makes you eager to learn more, it will have accomplished part of its task. If you come away from the book understanding the limits of science as well as its merits, you will emerge a savvy consumer, which is the ultimate purpose of the book.

Chapters 1–4 describe the origins of alternative medicine, the theories underlying alternative medicine, the business of alternative medicine, and the consumers who seek alternative therapies. Chapter 1, "The Origins of Alternative Medicine," introduces the ten principles of holistic medical practice, established jointly by the American Board of Holistic Medicine (ABHM) and the American Holistic Medical Association (AHMA), using highlights of both scientific studies and sources by leading authors in the trade press to illustrate the main concepts.

Chapter 2, "The Theories Underlying Alternative Medicine," provides information on the thinking that underlies the various complementary and alternative forms of medicine along with their origins. Chapter 3, "The Business of Alternative Medicine," gives the most recent data on dollars spent on complementary and alternative forms of medical therapies, and the most popular forms of therapy utilized. It also provides data on who the consumers of these therapies are.

Chapter 4, "Why Consumers Seek Alternative Treatments," provides a detailed analysis, based on the most recent data available, of the reasons behind the growth of the $47 billion industry called complementary and alternative medicine and what is fueling that growth.

Chapters 5–10 describe the controversies in the field, looking at critical issues facing healthcare today, from skyrocketing costs to the emergence of prescription drug use as the fourth leading cause of death in the United States; from issues of efficacy and safety in the use of alternative therapies to regulatory issues in the arena of complementary and alternative therapies; from issues of culture and its impact on health to errors in medicine and the benefits and drawbacks of prescription drugs versus alternative therapies.

Chapter 5, "Do Alternative Therapies Work?" focuses on issues of efficacy, the science underlying the use of complementary and alternative medicine. Included in this chapter are the scientific criticisms of CAM therapies, as well as references to the Institute of Medicine reports *Crossing the Quality Chasm* and *To Err Is Human*, two documents that are included in their entirety in Appendix A. These are recommended reading for anyone accessing the healthcare system.

Chapter 6, "Should Alternative Medicine Be Regulated by the Government?" looks at safety and efficacy concerns in the use of complementary and alternative forms of medicine. From a scientific standpoint, medical therapies should have an established track record, data available to verify its efficacy. Many alternative therapies do not have the support of substantive randomized, controlled trials, which underlie good science. This chapter looks at the issues surrounding that controversy. The critical objectives should be protection of the consumer from exploitation and ensuring the safety and efficacy of products or regimens for the consumer. However, consumers need to be aware that the fact that a product has FDA approval does not necessarily mean that the drug is safe and effective for all consumers taking it, as illustrated by the case of Vioxx, which is chronicled in the chapter.

Chapter 7, "Should Managed Care Provide Coverage for Alternative Therapies?" looks at the necessity to shift from the "disease model," where consumers do not access the healthcare system until they are diseased, to a preventive model, where consumers utilize tools at their command, primarily diet and exercise, to maintain health and prevent disease. You may discover that the best HMO available is yourself.

Chapter 8, "Pharmaceuticals versus Alternative Therapies," uses scientific data to evaluate safety and efficacy issues surrounding the use of alternative therapies and prescription drugs. In this area, I have highlighted the work of the Institute of Medicine and their seminal works *To Err Is Human* and *Crossing the Quality Chasm*, primarily because they provide a dispassionate, scientific view of the realities of healthcare and the unvarnished, raw data that consumers need to become familiar with.

Chapter 9, "Culture and Health: Who Bears Responsibility for Health and Healthcare?" looks at the basic relationship between culture and health and the responsibilities surrounding healthcare. The United States currently spends more on healthcare than any other industrialized nation, and yet our population is less healthy, with higher incidences of chronic diseases and reduced life expectancy, than our peer nations. As Barlett and Steele (2004, p. 13) point out, "Americans pay for a Hummer but get a Ford Escort." Or, as various scientific studies that I include report, "we're spending more but getting less." This chapter sheds light on these cultural issues.

Chapter 10, "The Future of Health and Healthcare," looks at some of the critical challenges in healthcare today, such as the escalating costs and use of prescription drugs. One interesting statistic is that there are more deaths due to prescription drug use than deaths due to motor vehicle accidents, AIDS, and breast cancer combined.

Appendix A consists of the annotated documents that serve as the grounding for the book itself. These reports are considered fundamental within the scientific community; however, the typical consumer is not familiar with their content. It is my belief that you need to be, as they will prepare you for some of the realities of navigating the health care system.

These documents include the Institute of Medicine's *To Err Is Human: Building a Safer Health System* and *Crossing the Quality Chasm: A New Health System for the 21st Century*, two of the most informative documents on U.S. healthcare available.

NCCAM's *Advance Data from Vital and Health Statistics: Complementary and Alternative Medicine Use among Adults: United States, 2002* provides the raw data on this growing phenomenon called complementary and alternative medicine. *Important Events in NCCAM History* presents the timeline of events that led to the development of NCCAM at NIH.

The next document, *Get the Facts: 10 Things to Know about Evaluating Medical Resources on the Web*, provides the consumer with cautions regarding information available on the Internet. Keep in mind that the availability of information on the Internet in no way speaks to its legitimacy. Be cautious about what you read on the Internet. The final document, *Executive Summary: Complementary and Alternative Medicine in the United States*, prepared by the Committee on the Use of Complementary and Alternative Medicine by the American Public, is self-explanatory.

Although the title of this book is *Alternative Medicine*, the content of the book is better described as: *The Savvy Consumer's Guide to Healthcare*. It is recommended reading for anyone accessing the healthcare system in search of medical solutions. When illness strikes, it will cause you to readjust your expectations of conventional medicine and place higher expectations on yourself. It is said that upwards of 85 percent of health conditions are self-limiting, meaning that we contribute to the creation of our health problems. If we contribute to the creation of illness, then we are the ultimate architects of its resolution.

INTRODUCTION: WHAT IS ALTERNATIVE MEDICINE?

Alternative medicine is any form of healing therapy outside the confines of allopathic or traditional medicine (which uses pharmaceuticals, radiation, chemotherapy, and surgical procedures). Alternative medicine includes all forms of therapy from acupuncture to Zen Buddhism as potential pathways to health.

The National Center for Complementary and Alternative Medicine, an arm of the National Institutes of Health, notes five categories of alternative and complementary medicine that are outside the realm of traditional medicine: alternative medical systems, such as Chinese medicine; mind–body integration, such as cognitive therapies; biologically based therapies, such as nutritional supplements; manipulation and body-based methods, such as yoga; and energy therapies, such as qi gong. Chapter 1 explores these various types of alternative and complementary forms of medicine.

SECTION ONE

Overview

CHAPTER 1

The Origins of Alternative Medicine

This chapter discusses the origins of alternative medicine, which, in large part, is a return to a more holistic and natural approach to healing. Often, what's old becomes new again. Such is the case with alternative medicine. Many of the healing therapies utilized in the current practice of alternative medicine incorporate energy therapies, such as qi gong, which has been an ancient tradition of Chinese culture for 3000 years and was first published in the *Yellow Emperor's Classic of Internal Medicine*. Ayurvedic medicine, considered another type of alternative medical system integrating the mind, body, and spirit, had its origins in India and has been practiced for some 5000 years. The theme of this chapter is "revisiting the past," and the chapter explores the ancient healing traditions that are classified as alternative and complementary forms of healthcare.

Alternative medicine, to many people, connotes foreign, novel, and unique therapies, somehow quite removed from the mainstream. There are alternative therapies that do include innovative procedures, such as chelation therapy; however, what many consumers may be surprised to learn is that if you pray, exercise, or take vitamins, you are practicing forms of alternative medicine. The term *alternative* literally means making a choice between options available. Knowing what available options are is critical in making that decision. This chapter discusses those options.

As stated in the introduction, the National Center for Complementary and Alternative Medicine (NCCAM), an official arm of the National Institutes of Health, notes five categories of alternative and complementary medicine that are outside the realm of allopathic medicine (traditional Western medicine): alternative medical systems; mind–body integration;

biologically based therapies; manipulation and body-based methods; and energy therapies.

ALTERNATIVE MEDICAL SYSTEMS

Alternative medical systems, according to NCCAM, include Chinese medicine, ayurvedic medicine, naturopathy, and homeopathy.

Chinese Medicine

Traditional Chinese medicine focuses on two opposing life energies, the *yin* and the *yang*. Disease is caused by blockage in this life energy, resulting in either pain or illness. Some of the treatment methods include acupuncture, body therapies, nutrition, and herbal medicines (NCCAM 2004).

Ayurvedic Medicine

Ayurvedic medicine is an ancient medical system originating in India several thousand years ago and emphasizes integration of the mind, body, and spirit and the ability to restore health through that integration. According to ayurvedic medicine, a person's constitution, which embodies both physical and psychological aspects, determines the body's optimal functioning. There are body types, known as *doshas*, which are divided into three categories: *vata*, *pitta*, and *kapha*. Each of these body types is thought to be characterized by personality types and tendencies toward certain health problems. Various imbalances in the *doshas* can occur as a result of a number of factors, namely, unhealthy diet; insufficient exercise; and lack of proper protection from the elements, germs, or various chemicals (NCCAM 2005).

William Collinge attributes ayurveda's growing popularity in the United States to the success of Deepak Chopra, M.D., an endocrinologist by training and former chief of staff at New Memorial Hospital in Stoneham, Massachusetts. As a result of Chopra's success and visibility in the field of holistic health, ayurvedic medicine has become much more widely known.

Some of the treatment options included with ayurvedic medicine, according to the NCCAM, include "detoxification of impurities; yoga; stretching; breathing exercises; meditation; herbal remedies; specific dietary changes; amounts of metal or mineral preparations; and massage therapy" (NCCAM 2005, p. 4).

Naturopathy

Naturopathy had its origins in Europe, specifically Germany. Benedict Lust, who migrated to the United States in 1892 to introduce hydrotherapy methods, is attributed with its introduction in the United States and the founding of the first school of naturopathic medicine in New York City, which graduated its first class of students in 1902. The focus of naturopathic medicine, according to Lust (Collinge 1987, p. 98), includes the following.

> The natural system for curing disease is based on a return to nature in regulating the diet, breathing, exercising, bathing and the employment of various forces to eliminate the poisonous products in the system, and so raise the vitality of the patient to a proper standard of health.

The six basic principles of naturopathy, according to the NCCAM (2004), include "the healing power of nature; identification and treatment of the cause of disease; the concept of first do no harm; the doctor as teacher; treatment of the whole person; and prevention." If we look at the six principles of naturopathy in more depth, how do they compare with conventional medical practices?

The Healing Power of Nature   The concept of the "healing power of nature" refers to connecting with nature, or the life force, which is constant, although ever changing. Connecting with nature involves getting outside yourself, getting beyond whatever health limitations are concerning you. Further, the "healing power of nature" involves a connection with this life force, taking some action, either through exercise or an activity such as gardening, that connects us with life. Naturopathy involves taking an active role in your own health, becoming your own health maintenance organization, as opposed to conventional medicine's traditional approach of prescription drugs.

Identification and Treatment of the Cause of Disease   The second concept of naturopathy, "identification and treatment of the cause of disease," focuses on addressing the root cause (i.e., eliminating the problem that is resulting in the illness). Consider a common ailment, high blood pressure, and its treatment through conventional medicine. Diuretics are the most common treatment. If the root cause is obesity and sedentary lifestyle, then the use of diuretics but failure to address those contributing factors will have the end result of treating symptoms but not correcting the root problem.

First Doing No Harm   The third concept of naturopathy, that of "first do no harm," is also the basis of the Hippocratic Oath, which is taken by allopathic physicians as well and refers to, at the very least, not creating a more serious problem than you're attempting to correct. In business, it's referred to as the risk–benefit analysis, ensuring that the benefits of the action taken outweigh the risks that will be incurred. In healthcare it means that you choose the intervention that offers the maximum benefit and the lowest risk. Another way of looking at it is to say that treatments or interventions should start with the least invasive, most conservative intervention first, and if positive outcomes do not result, then you move upward to more aggressive, more invasive treatments, with the primary focus being resolution of the underlying health problem.

The Doctor as Teacher   The fourth concept of naturopathy, that of "doctor as teacher," is a critical one. In naturopathy, the doctor is seen as a guide and not a God, a person who has specialized clinical training and credentials that provide a foundation for advising the patient on what steps are necessary to restore health. Naturopathy involves patients' interest in and commitment to their own health, which is a prerequisite to health restoration. In conventional medicine, there is more likely to be an unquestioned reliance on the physician as a type of God-like figure who somehow is capable of providing the "magic bullet" that will resolve health problems without any corrective actions on the part of the patient.

Treatment of the Whole Person   The fifth naturopathic concept, that of "treatment of the whole person," connotes that a global assessment of the patient be done rather than one based solely on presenting symptoms. The "whole person" concept refers to the mental state of the patient, the physical state of the patient, and the spiritual state of the patient and how the three states interact to provide the global assessment of the patient's health. Conventional medicine, in contrast, is based on the "disease model," which evaluates the presenting physical symptoms almost exclusively, with treatments following the assessment.

Prevention   The sixth concept, that of "prevention," involves a focus on what patients can do for themselves to restore and maintain health. The focus is on changing patterns of behavior (e.g., diet, exercise, and reduction of stress) to assist in health restoration and, ideally, to alter the old patterns of behavior that led to illness. In contrast, conventional medicine has its primary focus on the "disease state," meaning that patients do not interact with the healthcare system until they are symptomatic. The symptomatology drives the treatment, whereas the underlying causal factors may continue, with treatment focused on symptoms exclusively.

Homeopathy

Homeopathy had its origins with Samuel Christian Hahnemann (1755–1843), who developed the "law of similars," meaning that one could choose therapies on the basis of how well symptoms produced by remedies were a match for the symptoms of the disease. Homeopathic treatments are felt to remedy the underlying cause of the problem by providing diluted concentrations of raw mineral or plant preparations.

HOLISTIC HEALTH

A more global foundation for this book includes referencing alternative and complementary forms of healthcare under the umbrella of holistic health. Setting the stage for a better understanding of this arena is the American Holistic Medical Association's definition of holistic health, as well as its ten principles of holistic health. The ten principles will be outlined, as well as references to current literature and examples of the principles themselves.

Definition of Holistic Health

The definition and foundational beliefs of the specialty of Integrative Holistic Medicine, as outlined jointly by the American Board of Holistic Medicine (ABHM) and the American Holistic Medical Association (AHMA)—which, according to Dr. Robert Ivker, former president of the association, has certified over 800 physicians, M.D.'s, and D.O.'s in the art, science, and practice of Integrative Holistic Medicine (AHMA 2005)—are as follows:

> Integrative Holistic Medicine is the art and science of healing that addresses care of the whole person—body, mind and spirit. The practice of holistic medicine integrates conventional and complementary therapies to promote optimal health and to prevent and treat disease by addressing contributing factors.

The Ten Principles of Integrative Holistic Medicine

Integrative Holistic Medicine comprises ten principles, which are discussed at length in this section.

(Principle 1) Optimal Health as the Primary Goal

> It is the conscious pursuit of the highest level of functioning and balance of the physical, environmental, mental, emotional, social and spiritual aspects of human experience, resulting in a dynamic state of being fully alive. This creates a condition of well-being regardless of the presence or absence of disease. (AHMA 2005)

If we look at traditional, or allopathic, medicine as offering four primary approaches to dealing with disease—prescription medication, diagnostic tests and procedures, radiation, and surgery—an alternative approach, using noninvasive and natural methods of diet, exercise, and counseling, can prove to be more effective in addressing the underlying conditions and restoring the patient to health. The following example may shed light on its impacts on one area of healthcare: coronary heart disease.

In 1990, Dean Ornish, M.D., published his ground-breaking research, *Dr. Dean Ornish's Program for Reversing Heart Disease*. His book introduced a scientifically proven program to reverse coronary heart disease without cholesterol-lowering drugs or surgical interventions. The program involved four simple components: a diet low in fat and cholesterol, stress reduction, routine exercise, and support groups. His interest in this new approach stemmed from his training in medical school at Baylor College of Medicine, where he worked side by side with Dr. Michael DeBakey, a renowned cardiologist and transplant surgeon. The frequent bypass surgeries that he observed served as a metaphor for what he viewed as "bypassing the core problems of coronary heart disease" and treating the results of the problem versus the problem itself, such as sedentary lifestyle, poor diet, and inability to manage stress.

To test his assumption that by focusing on the core problems that caused coronary heart disease, the result could be altered, or perhaps reversed, Ornish conducted a double-blind study. In that study, coronary heart disease patients were randomly assigned to one of two groups. Patients in the treatment group were to follow the Ornish protocol, incorporating a low-fat, low-cholesterol diet with exercise and group support. Patients in the control group had the "standard treatment protocol" for coronary heart disease. The result was that 82 percent of the patients in the treatment group had "some measure of reversal of their coronary artery blockage, whereas the control group, who followed doctor's orders became measurably worse, according to cardiac PET scans that measured blood flow to the heart" (Ornish 1990, p. 19).

In this study, conventional medical wisdom and gold standard protocols were, in fact, worsening the health of patients under physicians' care. The alternative approach, Ornish's questioning of conventional wisdom, was in fact the beginning of a holistic approach to treating coronary heart disease with a focus on diet, exercise, and support that has since become widely accepted. An update to Ornish's pioneering research in the field continues with a 2004 article in *Forbes* magazine entitled "Just Say No," referring to the backlash against the costs, risks, and side effects of prescription medication.

Robert Langreth's article (2004), which follows the *Forbes* cover story "Pharma's New Enemy: Clean Living," profiles case studies of patients and medications used, as well as alternative approaches to the resolution of patients' healthcare problems. The lead story profiles Wesley Miller, a 65-year-old hospital food service director from West Virginia. Mr. Miller had undergone a triple-bypass procedure in 1994.

In 2001, Miller was taking sixteen different medications, among them Lipitor for cholesterol, Glucotrol for diabetes, and three diuretics to lower blood pressure. The blockages had returned and, because Miller was a high-risk patient, surgery wasn't advised. Fortunately, Miller discovered Ornish's "low-tech" diet of low fat, daily exercise, stress reduction, and group support. The outcome was that Miller's angina lessened, he lost 49 pounds in eight months, his cholesterol levels decreased from 243 to 110, and his blood sugar fell into the normal range. His comment about the transformation: "It has totally changed my life and given me reason to live again."

The downside of the holistic approach is that patients must have a commitment to their own health and be willing to do what's necessary to address their health issues. In healthcare, there are very few "quick fixes" in terms of sustained weight loss and restoration of health. Even bariatric surgical procedures, which have become popular now that obesity is classified as a medical condition and managed care companies are providing coverage for such procedures, come with certain risks. Without significant changes in diet and exercise the weight returns over time, along with the health problems that typically coincide with morbid obesity, such as high blood pressure, elevated cholesterol levels, and prediabetic or diabetic conditions.

Further, recent news reports indicate that plastic surgeries, such as "tummy-tucks" to eliminate abdominal weight gain, primarily in women, are, in the long term, unsuccessful unless the individual addresses diet and exercise to reduce weight gain; without this proactive patient approach, in time the abdominal fat tissue returns.

Granted, all of these procedures, when warranted, can be advantageous, even life saving. However, they do come with their risks, particularly for patients who are morbidly obese, who are considered "at risk" for highly invasive procedures, and who typically have co-morbidities, such as high blood pressure, coronary heart disease, high cholesterol, and diabetes. Additionally, given the poor condition of these patients' health, highly invasive major surgical procedures do not come without substantial risk. Many patients, all too eager to eliminate the weight, may not be fully aware of the risks involved. In short, there are no "quick fixes," even with procedures touted as safe and effective.

(Principle 2) "The Healing Power of Love"

> Holistic medical practitioners strive to meet the patient with grace, kindness, acceptance and spirit without condition as love is life's most powerful healer.

The ability to express honest emotion is not only necessary for psychological health, but is essential for physical health as well. Gary Null, Ph.D., a nutrition and fitness specialist, pointed out at an American Academy of Anti-Aging conference in Chicago (2005b) that the "mind–body relationship can't be healthy unless you're happy."

A second panelist, Stephen Sinatra, M.D., a metabolic cardiologist and former Chief of Cardiology at Manchester Memorial Hospital in Manchester, Connecticut, stated that falling in love is one way to ensure good health. He also pointed out that expressing emotions has a physiological impact on health. In a study that he conducted with men and women concerning the health effects of the ability to express emotions, he found that women tended to express emotions freely, whereas men tended to repress emotions.

The result of these differences was that the men had a 90 percent rate of coronary heart disease, whereas women, who were able to express emotions more readily, did not show evidence of coronary heart disease. In his book *Heartbreak and Heart Disease* (1996a, p. 174) Sinatra points out that acquiring the ability to cry and release tensions in the body has a positive impact on health. At the Chicago conference, Sinatra encouraged audience members to acquire the ability and willingness to cry, as it has proven health benefits.

Numerous authors have written about the effects of attitudes on healing. Norman Cousins, a former adjunct professor of the University of California–Los Angeles (UCLA) and author of *Head First: The Biology of Hope and the Healing Power of the Human Spirit* (1989), chronicled how positive emotions helped him combat personal health problems. He pointed out that positive emotions are not just something felt by the individual but rather are "biochemical realities" that play a significant role in health restoration.

More recently, Candace Pert, M.D., a cellular biologist from the National Institutes of Health, noted that each of us holds intelligence at the cellular level that is responsive to the external environment. Her book *Molecules of Emotion* provides further evidence that we are grounded in our external environment and responsive to it at the most basic level. Her fundamental message is that our bodies hold intelligence that makes us sensitive to our environment in ways heretofore not recognized. We are part and parcel of the external environment, and our ability to work within that environment and to master its challenges is paramount to health. Inability to address those challenges effectively will ultimately take its toll on our bodies.

Gabor Mate, M.D., a French-Canadian physician, in his book *When the Body Says No: Understanding the Stress–Disease Connection* (2003) not only details the connection between stress and illness but goes a step further to detail different disease states associated with the repression of emotions. His work involves research that connects a person's coping style to the illnesses he or she develops. "When we have been prevented from learning to say no, our bodies may end up saying it for us" (2003, p. 15). While serving as medical coordinator of the Palliative Care Unit at Vancouver Hospital, Mate saw similarities in coping mechanisms among patients suffering from degenerative neurological diseases, such as amyotrophic lateral sclerosis (ALS), multiple sclerosis, ulcerative colitis, Crohn's disease, fibromyalgia, and skin disorders. The inability to say no in words took its toll physically, and patients' bodies began to speak for them in a painful and sometimes fatal way.

An example Mate provides in his book was a study done in 1984 with three groups of patients: one group who had cancer, one group with heart disease, and a control group without serious illness. The study involved showing slides with vulgar or disturbing phrases attached. A dermograph was attached to each participant to assess the body's electrical skin reactions, along with the person's verbal response for the level of distress felt with each slide. The result was that all three groups had identical physical responses; however, the patients with malignant melanoma displayed coping mechanisms characterized as "repressive." The cardiovascular patients were characterized as having the least inhibited response. Mate's conclusion: "The study demonstrated that people can experience emotional stresses with measurable physical effects on their systems while managing to sequester their feelings in a place completely beyond conscious awareness" (2003, p. 42). Mate points out an important lesson in healing, frequently cited in self-help literature: "You can't heal when you can't feel."

(Principle 3) The Whole Person

Holistic medical practitioners view people as the unity of body, mind and spirit and the systems in which they live.

Carolyn Myss, Ph.D., and C. Norman Shealy, M.D., in their book *The Creation of Health: The Emotional, Psychological and Spiritual Responses*

That Promote Health and Healing (1993), point out that individuals who develop illness exhibit one of eight different dysfunctional patterns in addressing stress:

> Unresolved or deeply consuming emotional, psychological or spiritual stress in one's life; degrees of control that negative belief patterns have upon a person's reality; inability to give and receive love; lack of humor or the ability to distinguish minor versus major stressors and adapt one's energy level accordingly; how effectively one exercises power of choice, in holding dominion over movement and the activities in one's life; how well a person attends to the needs of the physical body itself; suffering that accompanies the absence or loss of meaning in one's life; and a tendency toward denial. (1993, pp. 8–10)

Much has been written by Hans Selye (1978) and other authors about the "flight or fight" response to stressors. In the animal kingdom, the ability to assess the nature of the threat (i.e., to fight or flee) determines whether the animal lives or dies. The transfer of the "fight or flight" syndrome to modern-day human challenges, however, breaks down in its effectiveness. There are many things that are not under the control of employees in postmodern life (technology breakdowns, cybercrime, traffic flow, political decisions, and so on), so the coping style of "fight or flight" is frequently not applicable. The inability to apply the template to resolve the problem results in increased stress levels and offers little recourse for a solution. Learning to "live with the challenges" and develop a more appropriate "stress reduction template" is required.

Erik Erikson, a developmental psychologist by training, has pointed out (1980) that we all go through challenges in life, and the stages of transition are the same for all. Whether we rise to those challenges or admit defeat and go under is the challenge posed to us daily. Numerous self-help groups speak to the value of relying on spiritual guidance for transcendence of the common human condition and navigation of critical challenges in life. Within that power rests the solution. The spiritual solution that many draw on is always present, always available, and of tremendous strength, particularly during times of transition and loss.

(Principle 4) Prevention and Treatment

> Holistic medical practitioners promote health, prevent illness and help raise awareness of disease in our lives rather than merely managing symptoms. A holistic approach relieves symptoms, modifies contributing factors, and enhances the patient's life system to optimize future well-being.

What does it mean to "promote health, prevent illness, and help raise awareness of disease in our lives?" Given that there are 4000+ books on the topic of alternative medicine, it means a wide range of things to a wide range of people.

There are many books written about fitness and taking charge of one's life. George Sheehan, M.D., author of *Running and Being: The Total Experience* (1978), dubbed by *Sports Illustrated* as "perhaps our most important philosopher of sport," provides one illustration of what exercise did for him. Sheehan was a cardiologist who took up fitness, specifically long-distance running, at midlife. His comment about taking up exercise is that "one day [an individual] will wake up and discover that somewhere along the way he has begun to see the order and law and love and truth that makes men free."

What exercise did for Sheehan was transformative. His transformation began through running, something he had participated in competitively in his youth. Running let him view himself in an entirely new light, psychologically as well as physically.

Deepak Chopra addresses the need to challenge old assumptions held about the "aging process" and suggests that when we think differently, we will begin to act differently, and our world will change. He points out that change is often made not by studying the "norm" but rather by studying the exceptions to the norm, as was the case with Galileo, Copernicus, Newton, and Einstein. They studied the anomalies, the exceptions to the norm, and, by doing so, transformed the thinking of that time. "These and other great scientists paid attention to anomalies and sought to understand the mechanism that explains them. When something doesn't fit the paradigm, doesn't fit the pattern, doesn't fit the theory, it forces us to examine the model we are using. It compels us to expand or change the theory to incorporate the exceptional situation" (Chopra 2001, p. 15).

In science, looking at the anomalies can lead us in an entirely different direction and, perhaps, to a solution, as was the case of Drs. Barry J. Marshall and J. Robin Warren in their 2005 Nobel Prize–winning discovery of *Helicobacter pylori*, the causal factor in peptic ulcers.

Marshall, an internist, and Warren, a pathologist, epitomize the value of "looking at things with a new perspective." Instead of merely replicating what researchers for decades had believed—that peptic ulcers were the result of spicy food and excessive gastric juices—they looked in the opposite direction. Much like pioneer medical researchers early on, Marshall offered himself up as a human guinea pig, ingesting the bacteria *Helicobacter pylori* and undergoing endoscopies prior to the ingestion, several days after the ingestion, and then after an antibiotic was taken to address the bacterial infection. The endoscopies provided a type of "time-lapse photography" proving their point. Two researchers challenged old assumptions and treatment protocols by looking in the opposite direction, and they found the cure.

Andrew Weil, M.D., a Harvard-trained physician who tired of traditional medicine at midlife and traveled to South America to study the healing arts in tribal culture, returned a different man. He emerged from that experience more fit and healthy than he had been in some time and wrote several *New York Times* bestsellers, one of which was *8 Weeks to Optimum Health*. In that book, much of the advice given appears to resemble good, old-fashioned medicine. Some of the suggestions Weil provides are as follows: Toss out all foods that contain preservatives; place plants or flowers in your home; take a fast from the 11:00 PM news, if you have insomnia; stock your kitchen with healthy foods; drink plenty of healthy fluids; and get moderate exercise.

Alternative solutions? Yes. Unusual? Not particularly. In fact, they make perfect sense. Further, it is well within our ability to do these things, and the advantages of doing them can benefit our health. Weil has since begun even more significant work within the heart of traditional medicine at the academic health center at the University of Arizona–Tucson, incorporating much of what he has learned and practiced into the curriculum; doing so will benefit thousands of patients throughout the United States, as medical students graduate and begin putting into practice what they've learned.

One of the critical points in the focus on prevention is the role that the person plays in his or her own health. No physician can demand allegiance to health or make individuals exercise or take good care of their bodies. The model that is at the core of traditional medicine is the disease model, which utilizes prescription medications, radiation, and surgical procedures in its arsenal. If you're interested in something beyond those three approaches, then it is wise to look elsewhere. Traditional practitioners are going to practice what they were taught to practice: that which draws from their experience and is provided in guidelines established in their professional association specialties through diagnostic and treatment protocols.

(Principle 5) Innate Healing Power

All people have innate powers of healing in their bodies, minds, and spirits. Holistic medical practitioners evoke and help patients utilize these powers to affect the healing process.

It is impossible to read literature on health and illness without coming across the intersection of books on spirituality. If it's true that "dis-ease" is an uneasiness within the body that ultimately takes the form of illness, then to understand the root cause of the disease, one must travel inward to understand and address that uneasiness. Some authors in alternative health speak to the issue of the mind–body–spirit connection and its importance in bringing about harmony and wholeness within the body.

There are many different approaches taken to bring that union of mind–body–spirit back into focus, from walking and getting in touch with nature, to tai chi—an ancient and gentle form of martial arts—to yoga (which means "union"), to spirituality and all its various forms.

Thyroid disease is one of many conditions that is impacted by stress. The ability to moderate stressors in life and address them in a healthy way is paramount to maintaining thyroid health. One book on addressing thyroid dysfunction and restoring health was written by a physician and his nurse-practitioner wife, Dr. Richard and Kara Lee Shames's *Thyroid Power: Ten Steps to Thyroid Health.* That book provides an authoritative overview of thyroid disease and steps for the patient to take in order to restore and maintain thyroid health. One of the most useful suggestions in the book stemmed from the support groups that Kara Lee leads for individuals suffering from thyroid disease. Her suggestion is to ask the thyroid what it is trying to convey. The thyroid, in holistic literature, refers to the "voice" of the individual. Allowing that part of the body to say what it wants to say, allowing it to have its voice, according to the authors, may help in correcting the problem.

Allowing release of that energy from that particular site is a freeing up of toxic energy. Expressing anger appropriately has been found to be healthy for the heart and other organs, and the same may be true for the thyroid gland. Many authors in the field of holistic health suggest that the site of the disease is symbolic of the nature of the problem. The example of coronary heart disease and the proverbial "type A personality" is a case in point illustrating that those prone to coronary heart disease are those who are quick to anger and have difficulty dealing with frustration. If we apply a comparable analysis to thyroid disease, then difficulty expressing oneself or finding one's voice could be a contributory factor to thyroid disease.

What many authors have written about in the area of spontaneous healing and other books of that sort are the inexplicable and extraordinary ways in which some people are able to heal from a seemingly terminal illness. What brings about that phenomenon? No one is quite sure. Science, certainly, is not. But if we look a bit closer at science, in a 2003 presentation to the Disease Management Congress, Samuel Nussbaum, M.D., chief medical officer of a large managed care company in the United States, pointed out that 50 percent of medicine is science based. In other words, 50 percent of what we've come to know as medicine does *not* have as its basis the rigors of solid scientific grounding. That is, 50 percent is unknown, yet to be discovered, yet to be proven.

This makes these seemingly "miraculous recoveries" perhaps more plausible. It may even shed light on new ways of looking at disease, as authors such as Chopra have pointed out. By studying the anomalies in science, the exceptions to the norm, we can perhaps better understand the condition itself, what led to the condition, and perhaps the avenue that leads to a cure.

If all of us have within us a type of internal wisdom, then it may be wise to begin tapping into that internal wisdom through faith, exercise, and wholeness, uniting the body, mind, and spirit.

(Principle 6) Integration of Healing Systems

> Holistic medical practitioners embrace a lifetime of learning about all safe and effective options in diagnosis and treatment. These options come from a variety of traditions, and are selected in order to best meet the unique needs of the patient. The realm of choices may include lifestyle modification and complementary approaches as well as conventional drugs and surgery.

Weil, in one of his early books, *Health and Healing: Understanding Conventional & Alternative Medicine* (1983, p. 83), suggests guidelines for the use of various healing systems, whether allopathic or alternative medicine, when he states the following:

> Regular medicine is the most effective system I know for dealing with many common and serious problems, among them acute trauma; acute infections associated with bacteria, protozoa, some fungi, parasites and a few other organisms; acute medical emergencies; and acute surgical emergencies. . . . I would look elsewhere than conventional medicine for help if I contracted a severe viral disease, like hepatitis or polio, or a metabolic disease like diabetes. I would not seek allopathic treatment for cancer, except for a few varieties, or for such chronic ailments as arthritis, asthma, hypertension (high blood pressure), multiple sclerosis, or for many other chronic diseases of the digestive, circulatory, musculoskeletal, and nervous systems. Although allopaths give lip service to the concept of preventive medicine, for practical purposes they are unable to prevent most of the diseases that disable and kill people today.

If you're the victim of a motor vehicle accident or a burn victim, Western medicine has significant advantages over all other forms of care. It is life saving. However, most medical cases are not acute cases but rather chronic conditions for which conventional medicine typically cannot provide the cure. In chronic conditions, allopathic medicine can alleviate pain, but medications come with risks as well.

Arthur Jores, M.D., in *Medicine in the Crisis of Our Times* (1961), points out, "In many cases, medical science prevents the patient from dying without restoring him to health. It is thus the primary cause of chronic illness. Modern medicine, in comparison to the healing arts of the old-fashioned general practitioner, primarily benefits those who hardly ever get sick."

In short, it is key that consumers know where to look and for what remedy. Allopathic medicine, as mentioned earlier, is limited to invasive procedures—a wide variety of "technological gadgetry," as Weil refers to it in *Health and Healing* (1983, p. 115)—and prescription medication has its side effects and limitations.

The recent situation with Vioxx is a case in point. Vioxx was a drug for arthritis, made by Merck. An astute data analyst at the insurance company Kaiser Permanente noticed a spike in sudden cardiac deaths among clients in their database. Further research indicated that the common denominator appeared to be the drug Vioxx. As a result, the company alerted the U.S. Food and Drug Administration (FDA). The FDA, in turn, forced Merck to pull Vioxx. A news report by Rita Rubin (2004, p. 1) in *USA Today*, which chronicled the events that led to the recall, noted that in the clinical trials with Vioxx the drug showed evidence of cardiac effects. However, because the information was proprietary (that is, it belonged to Merck), the lead researcher was prohibited from publishing the adverse effects, and Vioxx was released onto the market.

An interesting area of exploration, insulin resistance and its relevance to coronary heart disease, appeared recently in the literature. Drs. Rachel F. and Richard F. Heller and Fredric Vagnini's book *The Carbohydrate Addict's Healthy Heart Program: Break Your Carbo-Insulin Connection to Heart Disease* (1999) discusses the carbohydrate-insulin connection to heart disease and sheds light on millions of individuals who struggle with obesity, heart disease, and diabetes. Vagnini, a cardiologist and staunch proponent of the link between carbohydrates and coronary heart disease, points out in the book's foreword that "traditional medicine was not exactly failing my patients but it wasn't helping them to succeed either."

Vagnini's own health problems and his excess weight, coupled with the negative lab tests he received, served as the "wake-up call" for him to explore insulin resistance and its modification through diet. The result was that he lost 90 pounds and his risk factors for coronary heart disease were virtually eliminated.

Vagnini has since become a proponent of the diet proposed by the Hellers, as well as of nutritional supplements to support metabolism and stable functioning. His comments regarding their dietary program are as follows:

> The Hellers' insulin-balancing program made good sense, good science and good medicine. It explained and complemented what I already knew about preventive medicine and added a further key component of insulin balance and reduction of insulin resistance. Their eating program literally changed my life and, of paramount importance to me, it has also done the same for many of my patients. (1999, p. 26)

In the book, the Hellers point out that "hyperinsulinemia plays a crucial role in the three critical changes that lead to the development of heart disease" (1999, p. 92). Extensive research from around the world is linking heart disease and excess insulin levels. Understanding that link and reducing insulin levels appears to be the answer to maintenance of a strong and healthy heart.

Insulin resistance is beginning to be referenced in women's health literature, as a result of the frequency of bilateral oophorectomies (removal of both ovaries), which can compound metabolic changes and result in insulin resistance. In a recent publication by William Parker, M.D., and colleagues (2005, pp. 219–226) on ovarian conservation, he points out that 55 percent of hysterectomies are done in conjunction with bilateral oophorectomies, with fewer than 5 percent having the clinical markers for cancer. What this means to women undergoing these procedures without scientific justification is that such procedures may be reducing the life span of women undergoing them and increasing their incidence of coronary heart disease.

(Principle 7) Relationship-Centered Care

> The ideal practitioner–patient relationship is a partnership which encourages patient autonomy and values the needs and insights of both parties. The quality of this relationship is an essential contributor to the healing process.

This particular tenet of holistic health is critical in the partnership of healing. Seeing clinicians as guides and not gods should be a fundamental building block of the interactions surrounding the healing process. Talcott Parsons, often referred to as the "Father of Medical Sociology" and author of *The Social System*, (1951), a book that looks at institutions within society and their interdependencies, includes in that book a definitive analysis outlining the doctor–patient relationship entitled "The Sick-Role Adaptation." In "The Sick Role Adaptation," he clearly defined the responsibilities of the patient and the clinician and saw the doctor–patient relationship as involving well-defined roles that were acted out on the "stage of healthcare." Parsons saw the resumption of normal responsibilities on the part of the patient as paramount to the healthy functioning of society. Healthy individuals make for a productive society.

The "Sick-Role Adaptation," like any work, was a product of its cultural and historical context. Writing in the 1950s, Parsons attempted to make sense of what he saw in medicine at that time. In the 1950s, the skills of the physician and the diagnostic and treatment protocols were unquestioned. The relationship was clearly a dependent one, wherein the physician was a pseudo–parent figure and the patient was viewed as inexperienced and childlike. Further, the recommendations of the physician, if followed, were presumed to return the patient to full functioning, without exception. In many instances, the physicians were probably correct. However, in today's world, the old adage "We're not in Kansas anymore" is the byline. Healthcare systems have changed, protocols are under question, and errors in medicine are frequently cited in the news. With the Institute of Medicine's recent announcement that the fourth leading cause of death in the United States is prescription drugs, clearly one senses that the "Marcus Welby, M.D." days of the 1960s and 1970s have given way to new realities in healthcare.

So what is the new model of holistic health, and what role does the patient play? Construction of the new model starts with an assumption that both individuals (doctor and patient) are adults and that the patient participates fully in the healing pathway. The clinician is viewed as an expert in the clinical role, a specialist with advanced knowledge and training. However, one must also realize that clinicians will practice the diagnostic and treatment procedures they have been taught. Consequently, there is wide variation in the skills and knowledge base of clinicians nationally, in general practice, as well as in specialty areas. Not everyone is practicing "state-of-the-art" medicine, as is evidenced by the tremendous geographic variation in a wide range of diagnostic and treatment protocols in virtually all areas of medicine.

In short, physicians are not gods but guides, and patients would serve themselves well by recognizing this. Physicians are men and women who are subject to the limitations of their skill and knowledge. Further, they are bound by the protocols taught during their medical education, many of which have not changed significantly since their development, decades earlier, in the 1940s and 1950s. A case in point follows with a specific niche of healthcare, the diagnosis and treatment of symptomatic uterine fibroids.

Personal experience in addressing a health issue is a powerful teacher. After undergoing a surgical procedure for symptomatic fibroids, my health declined precipitously, with weight gain, high blood pressure, high cholesterol, and increasingly debilitating fatigue. My attempts to understand and address these health conditions involved consultations with generalists, nutritionists, and specialists. The diagnosis was severe thyroid toxicosis, unspecified. The treatment recommendation was a thyroidectomy with radiation, requiring a lifetime prescription for thyroid hormone.

Although my thyroid was not functioning normally, it appeared to make sense to understand the underlying cause of the problem and assist the thyroid to normalize rather than remove and radiate it, thus destroying it entirely. The option of a second surgical procedure, with radiation, did not seem like an attractive solution, so I took it upon myself to understand and address the problem. The underlying problem that was contributing to the weight gain, high cholesterol, fatigue, and a prediabetic condition was simply insulin resistance, my inability to metabolize refined carbohydrates and sugar as I had once been able to do.

With a clear understanding of the underlying problem, I was able to research the appropriate dietary changes I needed to make, along with nutritional supplements that I required, and was able to eliminate the weight gain and normalize cholesterol, blood pressure, and glucose levels. As those issues were addressed, thyroid levels normalized. These experiences provided insight and knowledge that were powerful, and I learned firsthand some of the limitations of modern medicine, as well as its reliance on invasive procedures to remedy health problems.

Further research that I conducted, which became my doctoral work, confirmed that bilateral oophorectomies, common with hysterectomies in 55 percent of women being treated for fibroids, can contribute to insulin resistance in many women, which, if left untreated, can contribute to high blood pressure, high cholesterol, and coronary heart disease.

Recent research by William Parker et al. (2005) on ovarian conservation illustrates that without long-term health outcome data available, we simply don't know the impacts of various invasive procedures such as oophorectomies on long-term health. In their article, Parker and his team question the "gold standard" treatment of bilateral oophorectomies in the absence of significant clinical markers for cancer. The team's research indicated that less than 5 percent of women undergoing these procedures have the clinical indications for cancer, meaning that the remaining 50 percent are undergoing this invasive procedure without clinical justification. Parker's team of researchers recommend that long-term, quality-of-life studies be conducted to explore these findings further.

An additional factor that is important to recognize in this healthcare niche of treatment for symptomatic uterine fibroids is that the traditional "gold standard" treatment for women undergoing these procedures postoperatively is long-term hormone replacement therapy (HRT). Hormone replacement therapy was the "treatment of choice" for decades for menopausal and postmenopausal women, until the Women's Health Initiative (2002) study results were published. The protocol literally went unquestioned, and millions of women took HRT religiously for decades. The Women's Health Initiative (2002) study results found that rather than HRT having a "heart-protective effect," as researchers had hoped to find, HRT *increased* the risk of heart disease, cancer, and stroke in women taking the drug.

These study results and lack of science underlying many procedures thought to be scientifically "sound" provide insight that medicine is fallible, and clearly there is much about many areas of healthcare that is neither understood nor supported with good science. As a result, clinicians operate out of the protocols they were taught in medical school, and once protocols become accepted as the gold standard, they become institutionalized.

Once institutionalized, the gold standard treatments become unquestioned standards. Jerry Avorn, M.D., Chief of Pharmacoepidemiology at Brigham & Women's, in his book *Powerful Medicines: The Benefits, Risks and Costs of Prescription Drugs* (2004, pp. 33–36), provides the most thorough background on the events that led up to the WHI study results.

"How could we be so wrong for so long?" is the question Avorn poses regarding the HRT debacle. Some of the answers involve the typically short-term (6 to 8 weeks) basis of clinical trials; subjects enrolled typically tend to be young (perhaps college students); and rarely do drugs prescribed, even if they are problematic long term, show evidence of toxic effects in a 6- to 8-week time period.

These issues and examples are pointed out here to illustrate that Parsons's "Sick-Role Adaptation" and his unquestioned allegiance and reliance on the "expert" opinion provided by the clinician, in this instance, underscore the problems inherent in that role definition in the cultural context of healthcare in 2006. These fallacies do not amount to criticism of the clinician or of Parsons, for that matter; rather, they point to the need for better science underlying existing protocols, as well as the need to periodically reassess what are considered gold standard treatments to determine whether they still hold up to the rigors of scientific testing.

Kenneth R. Pelletier, M.D. (2000, p. 51) points out that "as much as 20 to 50 percent of conventional care, and virtually all surgery, has not been evaluated by RCTs" (randomized controlled trials). According to Dr. Richard Smith, editor of the *British Medical Journal*, "Only about 15 percent of medical interventions are supported by solid scientific evidence. . . . This is partly because only 1 percent of the articles in medical journals are scientifically sound, and partly because many treatments have never been assessed at all" (Pelletier 2000, p. 51).

Those are important statistics to keep in mind when health issues, after repeated diagnosis and treatment, bring no resolution. Pelletier (2000, p. 51) goes on to say, ". . . the United States Office of Technology Assessment reported in 1978 and again in 1990 that only an estimated 10 to 20 percent of all conventional medical interventions have been empirically proven. That figure still remains accurate today."

(Principle 8) Individuality

Holistic medical practitioners focus patient care on the unique needs and nature of the person who has the illness rather than the illness that has the person.

There is a case study referenced by Chopra (2001, pp. 25–26) when he was a resident on a coronary care unit. He had a feeling that all of the patients had a specific explanation as to why they suffered heart attacks at the particular point in time they did. So he asked them that very question: "Why did you suffer a heart attack at this particular point in time?" Each had an explanation. One had received a promotion but his wife did not want to relocate. A second was upset because his son didn't want to go to law school. All of them offered explanations as to why they had the "attack" at that particular point in life.

What compelled Chopra to ask the question was that in reviewing the positron emission tomography (PET) scans of the coronary arteries, he noticed that all of the men had shown significant coronary artery blockage for some time, decades earlier for some. Why hadn't they succumbed to a heart attack earlier in their lives; why wait until their mid-fifties? How had they been able to ward off the "attack" for decades, only to succumb to it later in life? Chopra found that there were specific factors that took on a cumulative effect, the "straw that broke the camel's back," so to speak. When we focus on the person who has the illness rather than the illness that has the person, we begin to look at external events in the patient's life (e.g., marital status and health, work life) as well as the patient's emotional resilience and ability to handle life's stressors.

Norman Cousins refers to the need to be "in control" of one's destiny as critical to health. When he encountered health problems and was asked to take a "stress test," he initially failed it. He requested a second one, and he brought music to calm him. He also asked to rearrange the exercise equipment in order to increase his comfort level with the test. The result was that he passed the stress test. He attributes his ability to exert control over the testing environment as contributing to the different results obtained in the second test. As humans, the ability to have control over health outcomes is a critical element in health. Cousins's recommendation to anyone with a debilitating illness is "Don't defy the diagnosis, try to defy the verdict."

Weil (1983, pp. 52–62) lists nine principles regarding the nature of health and healing that underscore the importance of taking into account the unique needs and nature of the person who has the illness as opposed to the illness alone. These principles are as follows:

1. "Perfect health is not attainable."
2. "It is all right to be sick—healing is a dynamic equilibrium that changes in response to new conditions. An illness is a necessary complement to health."
3. "The body has innate healing abilities—cure comes from inside not outside."
4. "Agents of disease are not the causes of disease—the underlying causes of disease are nonmaterial."
5. "All illness is psychosomatic—the mind and the body are interdependent and together can cause or prevent sickness."
6. "Subtle manifestations of illness precede gross ones—learn to recognize the signals."
7. "Everybody is different."
8. "Everybody has a weak point—which is yours?"
9. "Blood is the principal carrier of healing energy—a healthy circulatory system is the keystone of healing."

If we take each one of these principles and elaborate on it, the result is a new perspective on the entire arena of health and illness. The first principle views health as a static state, ever changing. Perfect health that never changes is unrealistic. As living organisms, we are subject to the ups and downs of everyday existence. Health is to be viewed as a dynamic process rather than a static one. We all have days when we feel at our best, just as we have days when we don't.

The second principle views illness as a part of life. Instead of criticizing illness as an undesirable state to be avoided at all costs, we need to view health and illness as flip sides of the same coin, a type of balancing act or equilibrium that we strive to attain. An illustration of this balance is an unrelenting stressful job, with extensive travel and projects that are without reprieve. As there are no opportunities for vacation time because each project has a pressing deadline, the employee becomes ill and requires time off. Is illness viewed, in this example, as a negative? Perhaps the body is attempting to speak the person's mind, or the body is overriding the person's inability to ask for vacation time.

In the third principle, "The body has innate healing abilities—cure comes from inside not outside," what is suggested is certainly not the norm in allopathic medicine. Allopathic or traditional medicine focuses on the "magic bullet" approach, the cure coming from someone (the physician) and something (prescription medication, radiation, surgery) outside the individual. To understand Weil's point, if we look at another of his principles, namely that the "underlying causes of disease are nonmaterial," then the underlying causes of disease come from another arena than where we typically think they originate; they come, for example, from our thoughts and beliefs.

Weil's fourth principle, "Agents of disease are not the causes of disease—the causes of disease are nonmaterial," refers to the fact that we're exposed to germs and bacteria on a daily basis, but our immune systems are generally strong enough to protect us against illness. If you think about the last time you became ill or caught a "cold," chances are that you were under stress; perhaps you hadn't slept well in several nights and were under emotional strain. Those factors can have a cumulative effect. We all experience, as Lynn Payer writes in *Medicine and Culture* (1988, p. 61) "outside insults" to the body. Disease occurs as the body's response to those "insults." Most of the time, if our immune systems are healthy, we slough off those insults without effort. However, if the immune system is not functioning well, due to lack of adequate rest or "burning the candle at both ends," then illness may be the result.

The fifth principle, "All illness is psychosomatic—the mind and the body are interdependent and together can cause or prevent sickness," illustrates the impact of the mind and its "state" on the body. Much has been written in the literature on the mind–body connection. Larry Dossey, M.D., in his book *Healing Beyond the Body: Medicine and the Infinite Reach of the Mind* (2001a, p. 53), provides an example of a healthcare scare where he had been invited to give a lecture on healthcare and was suddenly and unexpectedly stricken ill.

> Feverish and faint, I had to struggle during the final moments of my talk to remain on my feet. Even though I felt horrible, I recall being amused by the irony that I, the visiting physician-expert, had become ill while lecturing on

health. Was this a cosmic lesson in humility? Within minutes I was shaken with the severest chills I have ever experienced, and I had a high fever. I knew I might be septic and that I should consider emergency medical treatment. But for reasons I will explain later, I chose to remain where I was.

Two holistic practitioners who had invited him to present at the conference—Dr. Jeanne Achterberg, senior editor of *Alternative Therapies*, and Dr. Frank Lewis of the *Alternative Therapies* advisory board—were asked by Dossey's wife to come to the aid of her husband. The ritual performed on Dossey was that of "the eating papers," a treatment that Jakob Walter, a foot soldier in Napoleon's Grande Armée, had undergone successfully in 1812: swallowing a small piece of paper with healing words written on it.

Obviously, Dossey not only survived but saw fit to use the example in his book. He refers to "eating your words" as *Esszettel*, a custom that has its origins in the consumption of written prayers. He suggests that the success of "the eating prayers" may result from the placebo response or from the "empathetic intentions of the person administering them" (p. 53).

Much of Dossey's work in his books *Prayer Is Good Medicine* and *Healing Words: The Power of Prayer and the Practice of Medicine* speaks to the value of prayer for the individual afflicted with illness, as well as "intercessory prayer," the power of individuals praying on behalf of the afflicted. The conclusion that the body and mind are interdependent and together can cause or prevent disease is an important one to ponder, as it entails viewing health and illness in an entirely new way.

Weil's sixth principle, "Subtle manifestations of illness precede gross ones—learn to recognize the signals," indicates that the genesis of the illness that manifests itself physically is in the incubation stage for quite some time, giving subtle cues that something is amiss and it is necessary to take corrective action. Ignoring the cues that the body is giving us will ultimately take its toll physically. Indicators of the body's breaking down in response to stress, for example, are present long before the breakdown manifests itself physically.

Thoughts and their impact on health are powerful, as is evidenced by the "placebo" effect and the "nocebo" effect. Chopra (2001, pp. 26–27) provides two examples to illustrate his point. First is the case of patients with asthma being given salt water and being told that the salt water would alleviate their symptoms. The result was that they tended to breathe better as a result of their belief that that outcome would occur. This is known in science as the "placebo effect." The opposite effect was found as well, where patients given the salt water but told there would be a negative effect tended to experience the negative outcome, otherwise known as the "nocebo effect." All of this underscores the importance of attitude in relation to one's health and the impact of strongly held beliefs on the body.

The seventh, eighth, and ninth principles, according to Weil (1983, pp. 52–62), "Everybody is different," "Every body has a weak point—which is yours?" and "Blood is the principal carrier of healing energy—a healthy circulatory system is the keystone of healing," are all important to remember in understanding health and illness. Knowing your particular anatomy and its strengths and weaknesses is critical to being able to provide the nutrition, exercise, and care needed to maintain health. Achilles tendons, for example, are different for each of us. Being cognizant of that fact and providing the self-care necessary to address it is critical to one's individual health maintenance program.

(Principle 9) Teaching by Example

> Holistic medical practitioners continually work toward the personal incorporation of the principles of holistic health, which then profoundly influence the quality of the healing relationship.

If we're cognizant of what traditional medicine has to offer, namely medications, procedures, surgery, and radiation, then we will not be disappointed. Clearly, these can be life saving and are to thousands of people each year. However, there are limitations to each of those, and each is highly dependent on accurate diagnosis and treatment and solid scientific underpinnings for the protocols. There are clearly many alternative treatments that have not been proven to be effective, but it is wise to keep in mind that many of the current pharmaceutical products on the market do not come without some measure of risk.

It's important to know what you're seeking and to make wise choices regarding the clinician with whom you develop a partnership. The best consumer is an informed consumer, and being informed requires a willingness to take responsibility for one's health and healthcare and an interest in developing a partnership with the clinician. If the clinician appears not to be open to exploring avenues that you suggest and is closed-minded about the prospects of complementary medicine, then perhaps it is wise to seek someone who is more agreeable or, at the very least, someone willing to work with you to explore alternative and complementary solutions to the problem.

Dossey (2001a, pp. 53–55) points out the value of an open mind on the part of the clinician when he comments that "in one five-year study, researchers found that only one-third of women with breast cancer who used alternative medicine in addition to conventional treatment told their personal physicians they had done so. The women's three reasons were a belief that their doctors weren't interested, would respond negatively and criticize them, or had inadequate training in alternative medicine or were biased against it." To the women, conventional medicine was viewed "as a potentially helpful system, but also a potentially uncaring, intimidating, biased and closed-minded one."

(Principle 10) Learning Opportunities

All life experiences, including birth, joy, suffering, and the dying process, are profound learning opportunities for both patients and health care practitioners.

If, as Weil concludes, the disease process is at work for a considerable amount of time in the body before it manifests itself outwardly, before the illness takes form there is a type of imbalance of energy within the body. Chinese medicine references energy imbalances, and one of the more prominent authors in the field of energy medicine is Carolyn Myss, Ph.D., a best-selling author and medical intuitive. According to energy medicine, illness takes form as a result of some type of imbalance with the body itself. Myss takes that further by saying that the type of illness a person gets and where in the body it lodges is as important to understanding and addressing it as the type of illness itself (1998, pp.1–10).

An interesting look at the origin of illness is Myss's use of the seven chakras, a body concept from India, alongside the developmental stages of life described by Erik Erikson. In her book *Anatomy of the Spirit: The Seven Stages of Power and Healing* (1996), Myss applies Erikson's developmental stages to "lessons in mastery" with the chakra locations, to provide the representation of what each chakra means and what must be mastered with each chakra in movement toward wholeness.

As with any illness, these approaches are templates for understanding, with no scientific guarantees of effectiveness. However, having control over one's destiny and health, even if it means coming to peace with the disease and learning from it, is valuable. Viktor Frankl, survivor of the Nazi concentration camps and author of the book *Man's Search for Meaning* (2000), commented that there is one thing that no person can control or take from you, and that is your ability to think, your free will. In the case of illness, that is a critical element to remember and honor. It gives the person who is suffering from the illness a positive focus, something to use as a tool for gaining meaning from the experience.

There are numerous books by practitioners that speak to the issue of spontaneous healing, of patients who have undergone inexplicable recoveries from serious illness. The billions spent annually on alternative and complementary medicine underscore the desire for individuals to seek a different pathway to health. Not all of those remedies are scientifically proven, but, in reality, neither are many aspects of traditional medicine. There is much yet to be learned.

In conclusion, the arena of alternative and complementary medicine opens up avenues for healing that are available to everyone, regardless of healthcare coverage, avenues that provide a new pathway toward health and healing. Critical for consumers in this journey is to know exactly what conventional medicine offers, its risks and benefits, as well as what alternative and complementary medicine offers, its risks and benefits, and to make their choices accordingly.

CHAPTER 2

The Theories Underlying Alternative Medicine

A number of theories are used in alternative medicine, depending on the avenue for healing that you take, but a central theme of alternative medicine is to galvanize the healing forces within your own body to bring about health. According to energy medicine, disease occurs when there is an imbalance in the energy centers in the body, and by releasing this blocked energy, you can work toward restoring your health.

Ayurvedic medicine, with its origins in India, focuses on integration of the mind, body, and spirit into a well-balanced whole. Without that balance, the theory is that one is incapable of living a healthy life. The National Center for Complementary and Alternative Medicine (2002) lists five categories of alternative and complementary medicine: alternative medical systems (e.g., Chinese medicine), mind–body integration (e.g., cognitive therapies), biologically based therapies (e.g., nutritional supplements), manipulation and body-based methods (e.g., yoga), and energy therapies, such as therapeutic touch.

This chapter provides overviews of these five categories and examples of each in practice, as popularized in the current literature, as well as scientific studies by Nobel Prize winners, holistic practitioners, metabolic cardiologists, and a number of authors in the field who have done extensive work in these areas.

CHINESE MEDICINE

The first alternative medical system is Chinese medicine. Chinese medicine, rather than being something new to the healthcare field, was first referenced some 3000 years ago in the *Yellow Emperor's Classic of Internal Medicine*, a comprehensive series of texts that systematically outlined the theoretical origins and practical applications of traditional Chinese medicine. It involves a focus of life energy, or "chi," with illness being a type of blockage of that life energy. According to Credit et al. (2003), types of Chinese medicine include forms of acupuncture, herbal remedies, and exercise, such as tai chi and qi gong.

The theory behind Chinese medicine is that life energy flows along meridians in the body, and forms of intervention, such as those listed in the preceding paragraph, are avenues to dislodge the blockage and allow the life energy to flow once again. Chinese medicine also incorporates two opposing forces, the yin and the yang, and the challenges imposed by regulating the balance of these two vital forces. The yin and the yang are thought to be complementary but opposing forces that coexist—for example, night and day, dark and light, summer and winter, male and female. In healthcare, they can represent remedies, such as cold versus hot treatments for various ailments.

The theoretical basis of traditional Chinese medicine involves the Eight Principles, according to William Collinge, M.PH., Ph.D., which include "four pairs of complementary opposites that describe the patterns of disharmony within the person." According to Collinge, these patterns of disharmony are as follows:

> Interior/exterior, referring to the location of disharmony in the body (internal organs versus skin or bones); hot/cold, referring to qualities of the disease pattern, such as fever or thirst versus chilliness or desire to drink warm liquids; full/empty, referring to whether the condition is acute or chronic and whether the body's responses are strong or weak; and the balance of yin/yang, which adds further to the description of the other six principles. (1987, pp. 20–21)

AYURVEDIC MEDICINE

A second type of alternative medical system is ayurvedic medicine, which originated in India roughly 5000 years ago and was recently popularized by Deepak Chopra, M.D., author of a number of bestsellers on a wide range of healthcare topics. According to NCCAM, the purpose of this type of medical system is to both "integrate and balance the body, mind and spirit." The term *ayurvedic* comes from the root *ayur*, meaning "life," and *veda*, meaning "science." Ayurvedic medicine has its origins in Hinduism, an ancient religion, and focuses on several fundamental beliefs regarding health and wholeness. Some of the major beliefs of ayurvedic medicine, according to Chopra (2001), are that we are all part of the whole and are born into perfection, into total alignment with the universe. Separation from this alignment, be it physical, spiritual, or emotional, creates disruption, resulting in disease. This state of "dis-ease" is a direct result of imbalance with universal principles. Health, on the other hand, represents alignment with the universe, harmony with life principles, and the pursuit of positive goals.

Additionally, ayurvedic medicine has an elaborate diagnostic and treatment method, depending on one's particular "constitution" and body type. Just as in conventional medicine, it is felt that there are certain persons prone to coronary heart disease, such as "type A" personalities. According to the ayurvedic belief system, disease occurs as a result of the person's constitution, or emotional and physical state, as well as the person's particular body type, or *prakriti*, and the effect of imbalances due to a sedentary lifestyle and improper diet.

The three body types, known as *vata*, *pitta*, and *kapha*, are defined as follows. The *vata dosha* is considered responsible for respiration, blood circulation, and healthy functioning of the nervous system; the *pitta dosha* is responsible for "processing nutrients, air and water in the body," and the *kapha dosha* is responsible for immune system function (Chopra 2000, p. 35). It is felt that each of these doshas has specific health problems associated with it.

MIND–BODY INTEGRATION

Mind–body integration is another category of alternative and complementary medicine, with an emphasis on the mind in the healing proposition. NCAAM includes several therapies under this particular heading: "hypnosis; visual imagery; meditation; yoga; biofeedback; tai chi; qi gong; cognitive behavioral group support; autogenic training; and spirituality."

Dr. Herbert Benson, of the Harvard Medical School, popularized this brand of alternative medicine in the 1970s with the development of the "relaxation response" (Benson 2000). Focused relaxation and meditation were found to have a positive impact in dealing with hypertension, coronary heart disease, and other serious health conditions. Fundamental to this way of thought is Johannes Schultz's (1969) "autogenic training," developed in the 1930s, which is a type of relaxation response that focuses intention on a particular area of the body, with the use of repeated statements or mantras that are believed to help reduce tension and result in a relaxed state.

In the mind–body approach to health, the mental state of the patient is seen as contributing to the illness or disease state, and a dramatic shift in thinking can bring about an improvement in health. Much has been written in the field of health about the importance of a patient's positive attitude and outlook in combating illness. Attitudinal factors appear to be the most difficult to change but are at the core of health and wellness.

Gary Null, Ph.D., a nutrition advocate and the author of several *New York Times* best-selling books on the topic, including *The Complete Encyclopedia of Natural Healing* (2005a), addressed the 2005 American Academy on Anti-Aging and stated that you cannot be healthy unless you are happy. Attitude affects health in a direct way. In his book *The Power of Your Subconscious Mind*, Joseph Murphy (2000) states that health is the "natural state" of being, and illness is a literal type of "dis-ease" in some facet of one's life. The approach to health, then, lies in the affirmations we give ourselves, our ability to see ourselves as healthy in our mind's eye and to work toward that vision until we attain health.

Mind–body techniques are an avenue to wellness and are not new strategies. The separation of mind from body is a Western notion in which the body is seen as mechanical, and diagnosis and treatment of various ailments as separate and apart from the whole. Historically, mind and body were seen as one. If we look at the mind–body focus realistically, then, it is a return to an earlier model in which the body and the mind formed an integral whole and could not be treated separately from one another.

Whether you're talking about hypnosis, relaxation, visual imagery, yoga, biofeedback, tai chi, qi gong, group support, autogenic training, or spirituality, belief plays a significant role. The importance of visual imagery has been written about by numerous authors, such as Wayne Dyer, Ph.D., whose book *You'll See It When You Believe It* (1969) discusses the power of faith, the power of belief, and the power of visualization. A second book by Dyer, *Manifest Your Destiny: The Nine Spiritual Principles for Getting Anything You Want* (1999), underscores the importance of union with self (no disharmony) and alignment with our "higher self" as critical to manifesting our deepest desires. Without a deep belief in our personal goals and our capacity to make them a reality, manifesting them is not a possibility.

A prerequisite for manifesting, or bringing about, our deepest desires is the ability to look into the world unseen, as that is where creation occurs. Any great creation or discovery, any innovation was, in the initial stages, a mere thought in someone's mind. An architect first envisions the edifice that is to be, then creates it. The CEO first envisions the company that is to be, then creates it. The winning coach first envisions the team and then creates it. The ability to believe before you see is the ability to visualize, or to see in your "mind's eye," the destination you're seeking before you actually arrive. This does not mean that your goal consists of a dream; quite the contrary. What it means is that you take meaningful action toward the image you hold in your mind, and the image will then have a tendency to take form in the real world.

In the case of obesity, for example, merely sitting on the sofa wishing you were thin will not bring you a svelte, attractive body. However, holding a svelte, attractive body as your goal and then taking meaningful action toward that goal—for example, exercise and diet modification—will help you arrive at your desired destination. As Deepak Chopra writes, "Belief creates biology" (2001, p. 26). If we believe that we co-create our reality with our thoughts and beliefs, then to change our reality, we must first look at the thoughts and beliefs we hold and be willing to change them.

Various types of meditation, yoga, and other stretching exercises, which focus our thoughts on releasing tension, are believed to have positive results in eliciting healing mechanisms. If you are tense and focused excessively on a certain issue, it is thought that setting aside the issue and focusing on something more positive provides a new perspective and may lead to solutions. Tension does not promote a relaxed posture with which to generate solutions. A relaxed state, however, often is conducive to problem solving.

BIOLOGICALLY BASED THERAPIES

Orthomolecular medicine falls in the category of biologically based therapies. Orthomolecular medicine approaches disease as an imbalance in the body, which causes either an overproduction of unnecessary chemicals or a deficiency of necessary chemicals. As a result of this imbalance, various health issues may surface. Weight gain caused by insulin resistance represents the body's inability to metabolize carbohydrates and sugar. The solution is to eliminate sugar and refined carbohydrates from the diet and to develop a nutrition and exercise plan to restore balance.

The term *orthomolecular medicine* was coined by Linus Pauling, Ph.D., a molecular biologist and the only recipient of two unshared Nobel Prizes, and refers to "the practice of preventing and treating disease by providing the body with optimal amounts of substances which are natural to the body" (Pauling 2004). Pauling states that "orthomolecular therapy consists in the prevention and treatment of disease by varying the concentrations in the human body of substances that are normally present" (Orthomolecular Medicine Hall of Fame 2006). The article in which Pauling introduced the term *orthomolecular medicine* was published in 1968 in the journal *Science* and was titled "Orthomolecular Psychiatry."

Volumes have been written by many authors in the genre of biologically based therapies. They focus on health, in general, but also typically address specific health issues. In one of his early books, *Dr. Atkins' Nutrition Breakthrough: How to Treat Your Medical Condition Without Drugs* (1981), Robert Atkins, M.D., who developed the Atkins diet, discussed the importance of nutrition and exercise in the alleviation of symptoms associated with many conditions and, in many instances, in the elimination of the disease.

One example that Atkins provides, and there are many, is insulin resistance. Insulin resistance is a condition where the individual is no longer able to metabolize refined carbohydrates or sugar. A number of books and articles have been written on the subject, including *Syndrome X: The Complete Nutritional Guide to Prevent and Reverse Insulin Resistance,* by Challem, Berkson, and Smith (2000), and "Psychological Factors and Metabolic Control of Insulin-Dependent Mellitus" (Stenstrom 1997), which provide scientific explanations for the development of insulin resistance.

However, instead of merely pointing out the problem—which typically is characterized by weight gain, increased levels of cholesterol, elevated blood pressure, and sometimes fluctuating thyroid levels—Atkins, in his early work, outlined a solution, namely the virtual elimination from the diet of refined carbohydrates; cataloging carbohydrate intake on a daily basis; reading the labels on all prepared foods one ingests (including soft drinks, gum, and candy), providing a type of intake inventory to help with dietary modification; and introducing a well-balanced diet that focuses on a balance of proteins and complex carbohydrates.

Dr. Stephen Sinatra's work with coronary heart disease is another example of the benefits of orthomolecular medicine as a type of biologically based therapy, essentially a natural approach to health that focuses on diet, exercise, and nutritional supplements (when needed). I heard Dr. Sinatra speak at the 2005 Conference of the American Academy on Anti-Aging in Chicago, and I interviewed him in 2006 for this book. I was curious as to how he came to embrace the holistic and complementary approaches to health and healing.

Dr. Sinatra is a board-certified cardiologist, a certified bioenergenic psychotherapist, and a certified nutrition and anti-aging specialist. He practices in Manchester, Connecticut, and has written several books, including *Optimum Health, Heartbreak and Heart Disease, Heart Sense for Women, Lower Your Blood Pressure in Eight Weeks*, and *The Sinatra Solution: Metabolic Cardiology*. In 1994 he was part of a team of twelve doctors who lectured widely throughout the United States on the value of nutritionals as a useful adjunct therapy in treating cardiology patients. (Nutritionals are supplements that offset deficiencies of natural substances that are not being produced at optimal levels to ensure healthy functioning. For example, scurvy is thought to be an example of vitamin C deficiency, the "cure" for which is vitamin C supplementation.) There were 2000 doctors in the audience, and apparently they liked what they heard, as he was subsequently asked to address the American Academy of Anti-Aging Medicine.

What piqued Dr. Sinatra's interest in the use of nutritionals as an adjunct to traditional medicine in the treatment of cardiology patents was his meeting with a man by the name of Jacob Rinse in 1978, who was 91 at the time and a Dutch chemist. Rinse told Dr. Sinatra that he had the cure for atherosclerosis, which consisted of a "concoction of nutriceuticals that he had developed." Rinse had refused a coronary bypass procedure in the 1970s and had used nutriceuticals and stress reduction to treat his coronary heart disease.

One of the things that made Sinatra curious was why individuals who had previously undergone coronary bypass procedures would return to his office several years later with the same condition. Why was the problem recurring? Sinatra felt that much of the research in cardiology failed to include a focus on energy depletion. His own research into the antioxidants used by a personal friend, and the attendant health the friend enjoyed, led Sinatra to explore their application to cardiovascular disease. He began thinking about the oxygenation process and the heart. Through his research he developed what he refers to as the "triad of cardiac health—Coenzyme Q10, L-carnitine, and D-ribose" (Sinatra 2005, pp. 22–23).

James Roberts, M.D., a colleague of Dr. Sinatra, asks in the foreword to the book *The Sinatra Solution: Metabolic Cardiology,* why doesn't this information become widely known and used? Roberts states, "The orthodox medical community is ten years behind in this research, and most Americans may have to wait for their current physicians to get old, retire and be replaced by the next generation of physicians, who are now being taught these basics to a much greater degree" (Sinatra 2005, p. 4).

Roberts points out that nutrition can provide answers to many questions in medicine and that although pharmaceuticals can contribute to health, they are not the final solution. Roberts continues: "A better answer is for physicians and patients to learn more about the biology of disease and the biochemical keys to energy production. This knowledge provides the insight needed to support the heart and recovery of our health, well beyond what drug and surgical therapies can provide" (Sinatra 2005, p. 4).

The results of this new approach, in Dr. Roberts's words, are as follows:

> Now twelve years out from being the number one emergency room admitter in my primary hospital, I don't have a single patient in the hospital the majority of the time. My heart failure admission rate is nearly zero (and I haven't had to get out of bed in the middle of the night to see a sick patient for over a year). I believe it's the Coenzyme Q10, L-carnitine and D-ribose that have kept my patients out of the hospital. Getting to the metabolic cause and effect of heart disease has helped their hearts get better and improved their quality of life. (Sinatra 2005, p. 4)

The Orthomolecular Hall of Fame is sponsored by the International Society of Orthomolecular Medicine (ISOM), which also publishes the trade publication *Journal of Orthomolecular Medicine.* Notables who were inducted into the 2005 Orthomolecular Hall of Fame for their research in the area of orthomolecular medicine include the following (Saul 2005):

- Max Gerson, M.D., who developed a regimen for the treatment of oncology patients through detoxification and the use of nutriceuticals. Apparently, for 70 years his work was proven to both increase the life span and improve the quality of life for patients severely impacted by cancer.
- Albert Szent-Gyorgyi, Ph.D., who in 1933 coined the term *ascorbic acid*, which Szent-Gyorgyi believed would prevent scurvy. In 1937 Szent-Gyorgyi won the Nobel Prize for discovering vitamin C (i.e., ascorbic acid) and for being the first to predict that ascorbic acid would be used to treat cancer.
- Cornelius Moerman, M.D., who was a staunch advocate of using nutriceuticals to treat cancer. Moerman believed that cancer resulted from a type of deterioration of the body. The goal in therapy is not to radiate but rather to strengthen the immune system, and nutriceuticals play a critical role in this process.
- Fredrick Klenner, M.D., whose work focused on the therapeutic effects of megadoses of ascorbic acid and who used himself as the first guinea pig in his research. Abram Hoffer pointed out that Dr. Klenner's work with polio patients given vitamin C resulted in their suffering "no residual effects from the polio." Results of a controlled study of seventy children in England, 50 percent treated with ascorbic acid and 50 percent with placebo, in which none treated with ascorbic acid developed paralysis whereas 20 percent of the placebo group did, were never published; however; the Salk vaccine had by then been developed, and no one was interested in vitamins.

- Josef Issels, M.D., who practiced in Germany, dealt with detoxification and a nutriceutical regimen for treatment of patients with terminal cancer. His thinking was that cancer and tumors caused by cancer were the result of immune system damage and that the appropriate approach to correcting the problem was simple detoxification, along with good nutrition. Dr. Gert Schuitemaker (2005), president of the International Society of Orthomolecular Medicine (ISOM) writes that Dr. Issels's clinic was ordered closed by the "Kriminalpolizei" at the instigation of medical opponents, and that reports of his 17 percent success rate with 252 terminal cancer patients who had survived for five years (a disproportionately high rate) went unnoticed.
- Emanuel Cheraskin, M.D., D.M.D., who received the Orthomolecular Medicine Physician of the Year award from the International Society of Orthomolecular Medicine in 1996 for his work, believed that oral health is a template for the overall health of the individual. Cheraskin once referred to modern healthcare as "the fastest-growing failing business in Western civilization" (Orthomolecular Medicine Hall of Fame 2006).
- David Horrobin, M.D., Ph.D., who studied the use of fatty acids in treating human disease. His study explored the role of "fatty acids, schizophrenia, and its role in evolution," which formed the basis for his book *The Madness of Adam and Eve: How Schizophrenia Shaped Society* (2001).
- Hugh Desaix Riordan, M.D., who was considered another medical maverick and was a staunch believer in the value of orthomolecular medicine. Abram Hoffer pointed out that Riordan was one of the first to demonstrate the therapeutic effects of high doses of vitamin C in treating cancer. Riordan's primary work focused on treatment of the schizophrenic syndrome and cancer through megadoses of vitamin C.

The work of all these individuals was significant, and the impact of their research and publications on the health of various populations is well documented. Why, then, has their research, some of it done in the 1950s, not been adopted or explored further in Western medicine? Fredrick Klenner, M.D., put it this way: "Some physicians would stand by and see their patient die rather than use ascorbic acid because, in their finite minds, it exists as only a vitamin" (Orthomolecular Medicine Hall of Fame 2006). Klenner's work has been consistently rejected by orthodox medicine.

Of the eight men included in the Orthomolecular Medicine Hall of Fame for 2005, Max Gerson was described by Albert Schweitzer, M.D.

and Nobel Prize laureate, as "one of the most eminent geniuses in medical history" (Orthomolecular Medicine Hall of Fame 2006). Albert Szent-Gyorgyi won the Nobel Prize in 1937, and others published scientific papers and books documenting their successful approaches to treating disease with nutriceuticals, but today many of them are virtual unknowns within the field of traditional medicine.

The rejection of their ideas, it would appear, reflects the inability of traditional medicine to entertain a different approach to healthcare. Perhaps the economics involved in traditional medicine serves as a barrier to orthomolecular medicine. Looking at healthcare through a new set of eyes appears to be what is necessary. Albert Szent-Gyorgyi put it this way: "Discovery consists of seeing what everybody has seen, and thinking what nobody has thought" (Orthomolecular Medicine Hall of Fame 2006).

MANIPULATION AND BODY-BASED METHODS

A fourth category of alternative and complementary medicine is manipulation and body-based methods, which include various types of massage therapy, bodywork, and "healing touch." There are various types of yoga, as well as a number of different types of massage, including Swedish massage, neuromuscular massage, and deep tissue massage. Craniosacral therapy and reflexology are examples of integrative methods used in bodywork.

The principles behind various types of bodywork, according to Collinge (1987, pp. 268–71), include

> movement of lymphatic fluid, thought to rid the body of . . . waste, toxins and pathogens; release of toxins, due to stored tension or trauma and restoration through hands-on techniques; release of tensions due to stress, injury or trauma. Structure and function are interdependent with attention paid to the musculoskeletal system thought to be the framework for healthy functioning; enhancement of all bodily functions; mind-body integration; reduction of stress; and energy flow.

ENERGY THERAPIES

The fifth type of alternative and complementary medicine consists of energy therapies. Energy therapies focus on the major energy centers within the body, known as the chakras, beginning with the root chakra, at the spine, and moving upward through the body to the crown of the head. Those who have written extensively about energy medicine have utilized the seven chakras and their locations in the body as representative of Erik Erikson's developmental stages; this requires the individual to revisit those developmental stages and address the challenges they represent as an avenue to healing. These and other core theories underlying alternative medicine are explored in this section.

Carolyn Myss, Ph.D. and author of the book *Anatomy of the Spirit: The Seven Stages of Power and Healing* (1996, pp. 61–78), sees the chakras and where they are housed anatomically as being in alignment with certain developmental challenges that every human being faces in life. She refers to them in her book as the "Seven Power Centers or Chakras of the Kundalini System."

The first chakra, known as *Muladhara* in Indian terms, is housed at the root of the spinal cord. Myss refers to it as "root support," connecting the individual to earth energy and rooted at the core of every being. The second chakra, known as *Svadisthana*, or "Her Special Abode," is housed in the genital area. The third chakra, referred to in the Kundalini system as the *Maipura*, is housed in the gut and is also called the "City of the Shining Jewel." The fourth chakra, referred to in Kundalini as *Anahata*, is housed in the chest and is also called "Not Struck—the pure sound of creation." The fifth chakra, referred to in the Kundalini system as *Vishudda*, or "Purified," is housed in the throat. The sixth chakra, known as *Ajna*, is housed in the forehead and is also called "Command" or "The Qualified Absolute." The seventh chakra, known as *Sahasrara*, is also called the "Thousand Petaled" or "The Unqualified Absolute" and is housed in the crown of the head.

Myss goes a step further in applying the knowledge of chakras and the ten *sefirot,* or the "ten qualities of divine nature," taken from the Kabbalah's "Tree of Life" (Myss 1996, p. 72), to understanding and addressing illness by using a type of template for addressing and resolving health issues that is grounded in divine guidance.

The ten sefirot, from the root chakra to the crown, include the following: *Shekhinah*, "the energy of the mystical community of humanity"; *Yesod*, "the procreative force of God"; *Nezah*, the "energy of the endurance of God"; *Hod*, the "energy of the majesty of God"; *Tif'eret*, the "energy of compassion, harmony and beauty"; *Hesed*, the "energy of love and the mercy of God"; *Gevurah*, the "energy of the power of judgment"; *Hokmah*, "the energy of wisdom and the contact point between the Divine and human thought"; *Binah*, "the energy of the Divine mother, symbolic of the understanding and intelligence of God"; and *Keter*, the "energy of the Divine that flows into physical manifestation" (Myss 1996, p. 73).

In her book *Anatomy of the Spirit: The Seven Stages of Power and Healing* (1996, p. 73), Myss looks at the seven sacraments of Catholicism and applies them to the seven chakras. She refers to the linking of the sacraments and chakras as a type of "script for the development of our consciousness and a symbolic life map of the inevitable challenges of our healing process."

The script, according to the chakras, includes developmental stages, each with its own challenge to be mastered: (1) merging the energy of the tribal chakra, the sacrament of baptism, and the sefirah of Shekhinah, drawing from the "Tree of Life" in the Kabbalah, with the divine message that "all is one"; (2) merging the partnership chakra, the sacrament of communion, and the sefirah of Yesod with the divine message of "honor one another"; (3) merging the personal power chakra, the sacrament of confirmation, and the sefirot of Hod and Nezah with the divine message of "honor oneself"; (4) merging the chakra of emotional power, the sacrament of marriage, and the sefirah of Tiferet with the divine message of "love is divine power"; (5) merging the chakra of willpower, the sacrament of confession, and the sefirot of Hesed and Gevurah with the divine message of "surrender personal will to divine will"; (6) merging the chakra of the mind, the sacrament of ordination, and the sefirot of Binah and Hokhmah with the divine message of "seek only the truth"; and (7) merging the chakra of the spirit, the sacrament of extreme unction, and the sefirah of Keter with the divine message of "live in the present moment."

Myss, a medical intuitive who began her work under the direction of neurologist Dr. Norm Shealey, believes that in the field of energy medicine, several common truths serve as the foundation of medical intuition. They all have to do with where we place our life energy; where there may be blockages; and what we as individuals can do to release these blockages, understand our illness, and work to resolve the conditions that created the illness. These are the "truths" that she espouses:

> Misdirecting the power of one's spirit will generate negative consequences to one's body and life. Every human being will encounter a series of challenges that tests one's allegiance to heaven. These tests will come in the form of disintegration of one's physical power base; the inevitable loss of wealth, family, health or worldly power. The loss will activate a crisis of faith, forcing one to ask, "What is it, or who is it, that I have faith in?" Or, "into whose hands have I commended my spirit?" (Myss 1996, p. 78)

To heal from the misdirection of one's spirit, one has to be willing to release the past, cleanse one's spirit, and return to the present moment. "Believe as if it were true now" is a spiritual command from the Book of

Daniel that individuals can use to visualize or pray in the present time (Myss 1996, p. 78).

Although some readers of this book may question the value of energy therapies, much of energy medicine draws on 3000 years of tradition, with origins in Chinese medicine, which focuses on the imbalance of energy centers within the body and the required removal of various blockages of one's chi, or life energy. What Myss has provided is a modern update of the theme of energy medicine, with a spiritual foundation. To shift our way of thinking from being a "victim" of disease to being a participant in the creation of health is an entirely different approach. It positions the individual as an "active participant" in the task at hand, not a "passive recipient" at the mercy of the healthcare system. For individuals who want to take an active role in creating health, it represents a useful template for change. Lessons can be and often are learned from the worst of circumstances. In that sense, illness can provide us with growth and perhaps a deeper, more meaningful life than we would have had otherwise. At the very least, it will provide us with an opportunity to bring meaning to our experience, which, in and of itself, is a worthwhile objective. If we can somehow make sense of our experience, through whatever means, we can make peace with it and move forward.

Other types of energy medicine include various forms of martial arts, such as qi gong and tai chi. Both tai chi and qi gong are ancient forms of martial arts, a gentle form of self-defense. They also provide a type of fitness training that focuses one's energy on various parts of the body, centering that energy to accomplish certain tasks. Focused energy is attained through the process of aligning one's "chi" or life energy appropriately. An example is the ability of focused individuals to walk barefoot across a bed of hot coals and not burn their flesh. This action springs from focused intent. Belief is a powerful thing and, when harnessed with focused intent, can be very powerful.

CONCLUSION

The theories underlying the various general forms of alternative medicine are as diverse as the various types of conventional medical practices. The critical point to remember in reviewing these forms of therapy is their origins, some 3000 to 5000 years (for Chinese and ayurvedic medicine, respectively) before the development of "modern medicine." What's old has become new once again. Perhaps the interest in these ancient forms of healing results from the limitations of "modern medicine" and a desire for noninvasive solutions to illness and disease.

CHAPTER 3

The Business of Alternative Medicine

According to the National Health Interview Survey (NHIS), using data from 2002 and reported by Barnes et al. (2004, p. 1), in 1997 American consumers spent $36–$47 billion on alternative and complementary medicine. Of that amount, $12–20 billion was spent on complementary and alternative health practitioners. These out-of-pocket expenses totaled more than out-of-pocket expenses for hospitalizations in the United States and amounted to 50 percent more than out-of-pocket services costs. Spending on herbal products alone represented $5 billion. Clearly, alternative medicine is a growth industry. This chapter explores the impetus behind that growth.

WHAT IS INCLUDED IN ALTERNATIVE AND COMPLEMENTARY MEDICINE?

According to the report *Advance Data from Vital and Health Statistics* (Barnes et al. 2004), 36 percent of U.S. adults age 18 and over use complementary and/or alternative medicine. Otherwise known as CAM, this approach to medicine includes various methods of healing and embraces the following: biologically based practices, defined as "substances found in nature, i.e., herbs, special diets or vitamins"; energy medicine, which involves, according to NCAAM, "the use of energy fields, such as magnetic fields or biofields (energy fields that some believe surround and penetrate the human body)"; manipulative and body-based practices, "based upon manipulation or movement of one of more body parts"; mind–body medicine, which includes "a variety of techniques designed to enhance the mind's ability to affect bodily function and symptoms"; and whole medical systems, which "are built upon complete systems of theory and practice," many of which are derived from other health systems not found in the United States.

The CAM domains most frequently used, according to the report, are mind–body medicine (52.6 percent) and, with prayer excluded, biologically based therapies (21.9 percent). Other therapies, in descending order of usage, include manipulation and body-based therapies (10.9 percent), whole medical systems (2.7 percent), and energy medicine (0.5 percent).

The CAM therapies, as referenced in the NHIS and published in the article by Barnes et al. (2004), include the following: acupuncture; ayurveda; biofeedback; chelation therapy; chiropractic care; deep-breathing exercises; diet-based therapies, including vegetarian diets, macrobiotic diets, the Atkins diet, the Pritikin diet, the Ornish diet, and the Zone diet; meditation; megavitamin therapy; natural products; naturopathy; prayer for health reasons; energy healing therapy; folk medicine; guided imagery; homeopathic treatment; hypnosis; massage; progressive relaxation; qi gong; Reiki (a healing energy therapy based on the use of therapeutic touch); tai chi; and yoga.

I cite these examples as evidence of the broad nature of alternative and complementary medicine, and although it is not the scope of this book to provide an in-depth analysis of each one, it is important for the reader to understand and appreciate the scope of therapies that are included when exploring alternative and complementary medicine.

As the director of the National Center for Health Statistics, Edward Sondick, Ph.D., points out in the Barnes et al. report (2004, p. 5), most of the studies traditionally have focused on conventional medical treatment, but the CAM update illustrates that something new is taking place, that a sizable percentage of the consumer public are taking "their personal health into their own hands" (NCCAM 2004). An interesting finding, although not surprising, is that only 12 percent of the adults using CAM consulted with CAM practitioners, with the majority, 88 percent, being in charge of their own healthcare. Some of the key findings in the Barnes et al. (2004) report, *Complementary and Alternative Medicine Use Among Adults: United States, 2002* (*Advance Data from Vital and Health Statistics,* No. 343, May 27, 2004) with regard to who uses CAM are as follows:

• Fifty-five percent of adults were most likely to use CAM because they believed that it would help them, when combined with conventional treatments.

- Fifty percent thought CAM would be interesting to try.
- Twenty-six percent used CAM at the request of a conventional medical practitioner.
- Thirteen percent used CAM because they felt that conventional medicine was too expensive.

Looking at the demographic profile of who uses CAM in the Barnes et al. (2004) article, the Centers for Disease Control and Prevention (CDC) found the following (NCCAM 2004): More women than men use CAM; those with higher educational levels tend to use CAM more than less educated individuals; individuals who have been hospitalized in the previous year use CAM more frequently than those who have not been hospitalized in the previous year; and former smokers, compared with current smokers or those who have never smoked, tend to use CAM to a greater degree. Racially and ethnically, the breakdown of CAM usage with megavitamins and prayer versus its usage without megavitamins and prayer is as follows: Asians, 61.7 percent versus 43.3 percent; blacks, 71.3 percent versus 26.2 percent; Hispanics, 61.4 percent versus 28.3 percent; and whites, 60.4 percent versus 36.9 percent.

Prayer for one's own health was the most frequently used form of CAM (43 percent), followed by prayer for others (24 percent); natural products, which included herbs, botanicals, and enzymes (19 percent); deep breathing (12 percent); participation in a prayer group for one's own health (10 percent); meditation (8 percent); chiropractic care (8 percent); yoga (5 percent); massage (5 percent); and diet-based therapies, such as Atkins, Pritikin, Ornish, and Zone (4 percent) (Barnes et al. 2004).

The diseases most commonly resulting in the use of CAM therapy, according to Barnes et al. (2004, p. 4), included the following, with musculoskeletal conditions or recurrent pain being the most frequently cited reasons for CAM usage:

- Backache: 16.8 percent
- Headache: 9.5 percent
- Neck pain: 6.6 percent
- Joint aches: 4.9 percent
- Anxiety/sleep disorder: 4.9 percent
- Stomach upset: 3.7 percent
- Neck ache: 3.1 percent
- Recurrent pain: 2.4 percent
- Insomnia: 2.2 percent

The natural products most frequently used with CAM, which include nonvitamin, nonmineral natural products, are the following (Barnes et al. 2004): echinacea (40.3 percent), ginseng (24.1 percent), ginkgo biloba (21.1 percent), garlic supplements (19.9 percent), glucosamine (14.9 percent), St. John's wort (12.0 percent), peppermint (11.8 percent), fish oils and omega fatty acids (11.7 percent), ginger (10.5 percent), and soy (9.4 percent).

Alternative medicine is a business indeed, and as in any business, there will be charlatans who prey on unsuspecting patients in search of the "cure." This is not to say that there are no quality clinicians dedicated to medicine and the care of their patients; there clearly are. However, the purpose of this book is to give an overview of alternative and complementary medicine, and this includes providing a reasonable assessment of conventional medicine as well. If conventional medicine had all the answers, there would be no need to explore alternatives.

If Samuel Nussbaum, M.D. and Chief Medical Officer of Anthem, Inc. (2003), was correct when he stated that "50 percent of medicine is science based," then many of the protocols currently used in modern medicine lack the rigors of good science. In other words, 50 percent of treatment protocols currently in use do not have the scientific justification necessary to establish their efficacy. That being the case, then much of what we consider "modern medicine," in many respects, is a high-cost, high-stakes trial-and-error proposition. That's not a criticism, but a statement of fact, and science is about facts and known quantities.

In support of Dr. Nussbaum's contention that "50 percent of medicine is science based," a study conducted by McGlynn et al. through the RAND Corporation (2003) explored the levels of care received versus levels of care recommended for 7000 patients nationwide. In their research they found that in the 7000 patients studied, irrespective of income, race, or geography, only 55 percent of the patients received the recommended care. This applied to both chronic and acute conditions.

The study by McGlynn et al., titled "The Quality of Health Care Delivered to Adults in the United States," looked at 439 indicators of care for thirty acute and chronic conditions and included preventive care. McGlynn and her colleagues found that 54.9 percent of study participants received the recommended care in prevention, 53.5 percent received the recommended care for acute conditions, and 56.1 percent received the recommended care for chronic conditions. Further, in assessing the level of recommended screenings and protocols for follow-up care, McGlynn et al. (2003) reported that only 52.2 percent received the recommended screenings and 58.5 percent met the criteria for follow-up care. The researchers' conclusion sums up their results quite well: "The deficits we have identified in adherence to recommended processes for basic care pose serious threats to the health of the American public. Strategies to reduce these deficits in care are warranted" (2003, p. 2645).

Since the correct diagnosis is fundamental in determining the proper treatment, it stands to reason that if the diagnosis is not correct, then the treatment protocol that follows is not going to be effective, which may shed light on the high costs and suboptimal outcomes often experienced by patients. Additionally, for serious health conditions that could deteriorate into acute conditions (e.g., high blood pressure and heart attack), the inability to get a correct diagnosis at the onset and establish sound treatment protocols, which can reduce symptoms and decrease the risk of worsening conditions, makes the report of McGlynn et al. all the more important.

Additional research by the Institute of Medicine (2000), Legorreta et al. (2000), McBride et al. (1998), Ni et al. (1998), and Perez-Stable and Fuentes-Afflick (1998) indicates that in excess of 50 percent of patients in their research with the following conditions were "managed inadequately": diabetes, hypertension, tobacco addiction, hyperlipidemia, congestive heart failure, depression, and chronic atrial defibrillation (irregular heartbeat).

Further, if we accept that the time period from point of discovery of a "cure" to its adaptation into medical practice is roughly seventeen years, as stated by Balas (2001), if you're suffering from a debilitating condition, seventeen years may be unacceptable. The wheels of medicine— particularly academic medicine—tend to turn very slowly.

Alternative medicine, obviously, takes in a wide range of options, many that are relatively inexpensive, like megavitamins and especially prayer, which doesn't cost a thing other than attention and time. Other therapies included in alternative medicine involve chiropractic care, yoga, massage, and various diet-based therapies, all of which have price tags attached to them. There are other "alternative therapies" advertised frequently in the news: various weight-loss products, exercise equipment, and other remedies to reduce weight and tighten abdominal muscles. All of those products should be reviewed with caution. When the profit motive is introduced into healthcare and when there is no official oversight of products marketed, exploitation is possible. Not every product, remedy, or piece of equipment will work. Caveat emptor, or "buyer beware," seems a reasonable approach to take. None, or very few, of these products are regulated through traditional means, and they are not approved by the FDA.

However, again, it's important to point out that FDA approval is not necessarily a guarantee that a product will be effective and safe 100 percent of the time. Vioxx, a drug that was approved by the FDA but has been linked to an increased incidence of sudden cardiac death among certain groups of patients, is a case in point. Despite the FDA's approval of Vioxx, reports of negative findings on cardiac involvement were evident in the initial clinical trials. However, given that the data were proprietary, the key researcher on the team was forbidden from releasing them. The incident that led to the recall involved an astute data analyst at a large managed care company on the West Coast. This analyst noticed a spike in sudden cardiac deaths among members in the managed care company's database. Pursuing that finding, the analyst found that the common denominator in those deaths appeared to be the drug Vioxx. The managed care company took that information to the FDA, which in turn brought pressure to bear on Merck, the manufacturer of Vioxx, to withdraw it from the market.

In a news report, one of the chief scientists at the FDA remarked that as a result of the funding relationships researchers have with pharmaceutical firms (i.e., the proprietary nature of the research; pharmaceutical firms own the rights to the research and control any release of that research to the public), the public is "virtually defenseless" with regard to the safety and efficacy of prescription drugs. That is a very strong statement.

What this means to those involved in healthcare research is that the rigors of scientific testing and particularly concerns for both safety and efficacy can be jeopardized when sources of funding have "a stake" in a particular outcome. Clearly, pure science is about seeking the truth. In the case of pharmaceutical products, science is about testing a drug's efficacy in treating particular diseases, in addition to understanding any risks that the drug poses. The ideal pharmaceutical product is the one that provides the maximum benefit (addresses the problem) at the least risk (a sound safety profile) to the patient.

When the science underlying the research is questionable, things play out this way: the public, without any medical knowledge, rely on the advice of doctors, who in turn rely on the data from the pharmaceutical firm. If the safety and efficacy data on a product are incomplete or inaccurate, doctors will unwittingly prescribe the drug and patients will unwittingly take it, as prescribed, putting their health at risk. A remedy is only as good as the science that supports it. If the science is not sound, the outcomes are going to be problematic.

Similar cautions should be applied to the use of alternative therapies, particularly those that can have a compounding effect when used in combination with prescription medications (i.e., herbal remedies). Formal scientific evaluations have not been conducted on most alternative therapies, and caution is recommended when one is combining alternative therapies with conventional medicine, as pointed out by David M. Eisenberg, M.D., in his article "Advising Patients Who Seek Alternative Medical Therapies" (1997). Eisenberg reports that he and his colleagues determined that 60 million Americans used alternative therapies, at a cost of $13.7 million, with 425 million office visits to some 338 million practitioners. Eisenberg's report also claimed that 70 percent of patients never acknowledged their use of alternative therapies to their standard practitioners.

There is a growing national trend in which third-party payers provide coverage for "expanded benefits," which include alternative therapies. The concern Eisenberg (1993) raises, which is a valid one, is how the conventional practitioner can be expected to advise patients who use alternative therapies without complete knowledge about such therapies or their effectiveness. Concerns of litigation were also identified in the co-management of patients who jointly use alternative and traditional therapies. These are legitimate concerns, particularly if the alternative therapy has a poor outcome.

Clearly, complementary and alternative medicine is a growth industry, either as a result of conventional medicine's limitations or because of the ineffectiveness of options available through traditional means (e.g., cancer reappearing after regimens of chemotherapy). Where can individuals locate reliable, valid information on alternative therapies? An Internet search for information on alternative therapy led to more than 900,000 entries, many of which were sales-oriented Web sites. A PubMed search for cost and other information on alternative therapies returned 1846 entries, encompassing a wide range of applications. Which are to be believed; which are safe, effective, and reasonable? It is not the intent of this book to evaluate all of those therapies; rather, this book provides critical issues to consider and broad guidelines for those interested in pursuing alternative therapies, with input from skilled and reputable practitioners from both ends of the spectrum, traditional and alternative. Individuals must follow what they deem reasonable for themselves and their circumstances. As a resource for readers, I have included, in Appendix A, the National Center for Complementary and Alternative Medicine's "Get the Facts: 10 Things to Know about Evaluating Medical Resources on the Web," which lists ten questions that can serve as a guide to evaluating the legitimacy of information available on the Internet.

Clearly, it is wise to consider the potential risks and rewards of any therapy. There are certain therapies that are relatively risk free, such as dietary changes, moderate exercise, massage, prayer, relaxation techniques, and cognitive therapies. There are other therapies, however, that could pose a danger (for example, supplements taken in conjunction with conventional prescription drugs). Eisenberg (1997) provides the example of unintended drug interactions of certain chemotherapeutic agents, with known toxicity to the liver, taken in combination with high-dose herbs or supplements for which there is little data on pharmacological impact.

Eisenberg (1997) provides a step-by-step strategy to guide conventional practitioners in working with patients who seek alternative treatments, with the assumption that the medical evaluation has been done and conventional treatments already offered:

1. Ask the patient to identify the principal symptom.
2. Maintain a symptom diary.
3. Discuss the patient's preferences and expectations.
4. Review issues of safety and efficacy.
5. Identify a suitable licensed provider.
6. Provide key questions for the alternative therapy provider during initial consultation.
7. Schedule a follow-up visit (or call) to review the treatment plan.
8. Follow up to review the response to treatment.
9. Provide documentation.

A comparable step-by-step strategy for the patient might be useful, one that parallels Eisenberg's guidelines for the practitioner. The patient's strategy would include the following:

1. Be direct about symptoms and conditions you're seeking treatment for, including all prescription medications and alternative therapies currently being used, as well as the diet and exercise regimen being followed.
2. Maintain your own diary on all of the above factors, to share with the practitioner.
3. Voice your preferences and reasonable expectations.
4. Pay attention to issues of efficacy and safety, and ask for the science underlying both.
5. Listen to advice about licensed providers; not all alternative practitioners are practicing good medicine.
6. Ask questions regarding the scientific justification for invasive therapies, procedures, or medications.
7. Review treatment plans as needed.

8. Follow up with responses to treatment, both positive and negative.
9. Provide some documented evidence of the benefits or drawbacks of the treatment.

Three things should be kept in mind when one is pursuing medical remedies: (1) Practitioners, be they conventional or alternative, get paid whether you get well or not. (2) Your health should be your top priority, as you'll be living in your body for the rest of your life. (3) There is no better medicine you can give yourself than proper nutrition and adequate exercise, regardless of your condition. Additionally, no prescription or "magic bullet" that I'm aware of will substitute for these proactive and preventive behaviors. There is a price to be paid for poor nutrition and lack of exercise, and it typically comes at the expense of health.

A large part of the healing partnership between a patient and a practitioner involves honesty and respect. This holds true whether the practice is conventional or alternative medicine. The healing partnership involves a shift from the traditional parent–child relationship of doctor–patient toward a co-equal, adult–adult partnership. This requires that patients take responsibility for their health, in its entirety, and view the practitioner not as a miracle worker but as someone trained in medicine who has knowledge and expertise in the respective field. In the arena of alternative medicine, the primary responsibility for health maintenance rests on the shoulders of the patient. The "healing partnership" requires an understanding and appreciation of that premise and what it requires of the patient. Not all patients are willing to assume that responsibility.

The flip side of the coin is that practitioners must be aware, particularly if they are practicing conventional medicine, that there is much they did not learn in medical school about nutrition and alternative and complementary medicine and its impact on health. Much remains to be learned about alternative therapies and the potential value of these therapies with respect to a variety of health conditions. Not all practitioners may be willing to participate in this "healing partnership" model.

Mediating these difficulties is perhaps the biggest challenge of all in the evaluation of alternative therapies. Overcoming biases and advancing the course of health is without question the ultimate goal. One prerequisite to this goal is to keep an open mind and listen to both science and reason, with the understanding that a lack of science doesn't necessarily mean a remedy is bad, and that scientific justification doesn't necessarily mean that a therapy will work. There is much left to be learned in medicine.

Andrew Weil, M.D. (1983, p. 47), puts the healing arts in proper perspective when he so eloquently states,

In our society, the commonality of religion, magic and medicine is obscured. Our medical doctors have narrowed their view to pay attention only to the physical body and the material aspects of illness. As a result, they cannot practice the healing magic of Hermes because they do not see or integrate the nonphysical forces that animate and direct the physical body and the material aspects of illness. For the same reason, many doctors cannot come up with a better definition of health than "absence of disease." They do not grasp the concept of wholeness as perfection that is the root meaning of the word, nor realize that health and illness are particular manifestations of good and evil, requiring all the help of religion and philosophy to fully understand and all the techniques of magic to manipulate.

CHAPTER 4

Why Consumers Seek Alternative Treatments

There are a number of reasons people seek alternative treatments for health conditions. The primary reason is that either traditional medicine cannot offer a solution or the options available through traditional medicine, such as surgery, radiation, or chemotherapy, are not desirable. Some people seek alternative remedies to satisfy their curiosity; friends may have responded well to such therapies, and their experience sets the stage for exploration. Some may use alternative therapies due to an inability to afford prescription medication. Finally, many people simply become disenchanted with traditional medicine and become interested in exploring their own personal pathway to health. This chapter explores who these consumers are and what they're hoping to find with alternative treatments.

WHEN THE BEST THAT MEDICINE HAS TO OFFER ISN'T ENOUGH

When someone has been diagnosed with cancer and has had one treatment of chemotherapy, which has not been successful, and a second round of chemotherapy is recommended, the patient may opt to explore other options. Success is not guaranteed with the alternative route, but neither is there a guarantee through the traditional route. This patient may choose to explore alternative means of treating the cancer, either through nutritional supplements or through other available options.

As stated previously in this book, there are numerous pathways to healing that are categorized under the heading "alternative and complementary medicine," namely, according to the NIH's National Center for

Complementary and Alternative Medicine (NCCAM), Chinese medicine, mind–body integration, biologically based therapies, manipulation and body-based methods, and energy therapies.

Prayer, which is an ancient custom, is considered a type of alternative and complementary medicine. Larry Dossey, M.D. and holistic health practitioner, more than any other researcher has addressed the importance of prayer in several of his books: *Be Careful What You Pray For . . . You Just Might Get It: What We Can Do about the Unintentional Effects of Our Thoughts, Prayers, and Wishes; Prayer Is Good Medicine: How to Reap the Healing Benefits of Prayer;* and *Healing Words: The Power of Prayer and the Practice of Medicine.*

Dossey (2001b, p. 227) cites the research on intercessory prayer by Randolph Byrd, M.D., a staff cardiologist at the University of California–San Francisco. Byrd worked with 393 patients in the coronary care unit at San Francisco General Hospital in 1988. The study involved patients assigned to a group receiving intercessory prayer outside the confines of the hospital or to a control group. It was a double-blind study, meaning that none of the groups involved (patients, doctors, or nurses) knew which patients were in the treatment group or the control group. The outcome was that the patients who were prayed for did better than the control group on several counts. Although the statistical tests were not significant in this category, there were fewer deaths among patients who were prayed for.

Dossey (2001b, p. 227) reported the study results as follows:

> They [the prayed-for group] were less likely to require endotracheal intubation and ventilator support; they required fewer potent drugs, including diuretics and antibiotics; they experienced a lower incidence of pulmonary edema; and they required cardiopulmonary resuscitation less often.

Although, from a scientific standpoint, much criticism has been directed at the use of prayer and the study of prayer as an avenue for healing, Dossey (2001b, p. 227) points out that although Byrd's study design was not ideal, it established the principle that distant intercessory prayer "can be studied like a drug in humans, in a controlled fashion in a sophisticated medical environment. . . . [Byrd's study] helped break a taboo against prayer as a subject of medical research."

Prayer, therefore, is one example of a complementary adjunct to traditional medicine that, in many cases, has contributed to the health restoration of patients. Traditional medicine, which historically has scoffed at prayer as nonsensical, is now giving credence to the power of prayer in healing. Prayer is certainly not science, but many clinicians, regardless of specialty, will admit (if they've been in practice for some time) that they've seen cases where there was no scientific reason to explain why a particular patient recovered. Again, in these cases, the choice as to whether prayer was a critical component of the healing rests with the believer.

In a life-threatening medical crisis, it is not a question of opting for either traditional therapy or prayer; standard therapy is essential to save the patient's life. However, prayer for oneself or for someone else seems to be a reasonable adjunct to traditional therapy and one that should be considered. It has often been said that there are no atheists in foxholes. If you're suffering from a serious health condition, prayer might be an option to consider.

Consumers may seek alternative treatments due to limited options available. This was the subject of an article published in *Forbes* magazine titled "Just Say No" (Langreth 2004). The article detailed the cost of prescription drugs and provided a holistic approach to this problem. One of the individuals profiled was a 56-year-old retired dietary supervisor from West Virginia. He was on fifteen different medications and had undergone a coronary bypass procedure. He commented that it was difficult for him to walk to the mailbox without doubling over in pain. He was 40 pounds overweight and had recurrent heart problems, which necessitated another intervention.

Due to his overall health problems, this man was not a good candidate for a second bypass. Fortunately, the Dean Ornish diet for reversing coronary heart disease was an option his insurance company had available, and the man chose to participate. Several months later, the man had lost the weight, eliminated fourteen of the fifteen medications, and felt "like a new man." All that was required to achieve these remarkable results was a willingness to adhere to a nutritious diet and exercise program to reduce weight and improve health.

In *Prayer Is Good Medicine: How to Reap the Healing Benefits of Prayer* (1996, p. 49), Larry Dossey addresses the issue of prayer and its efficacy in the health restoration equation:

> Prayer works. More than 130 controlled laboratory studies show, in general, that prayer or a prayerlike state of compassion, empathy, and love can bring about healthful changes in many types of living things, from humans to bacteria. This does not mean prayer always works, any more than drugs and surgery always work but that, statistically speaking, prayer is effective.
>
> Hope heals. Faith helps mobilize a person's defenses and assists in getting well, and optimism leads generally to better outcomes. Hundreds of case histories and scientific studies affirm this observation. As a single recent

example, psychiatrist Thomas Oxman and his co-workers at Dartmouth Medical
School investigated the role "religious feeling and activity" might play in
232 patients over fifty-five years of age undergoing cardiac surgery. Their
finding: Those who derive at least some strength and comfort—hope!—
from religion are more likely to survive longer after cardiac surgery than
those who do not.

Hopelessness kills. Numerous studies in humans show that we die as a
result of dire beliefs and a sense of overwhelming futility.

OPTIONS AVAILABLE ARE NOT ATTRACTIVE

A pertinent example illustrates an important point in looking at
options available and then exploring other avenues that could resolve
the problem. The case is uterine fibroids, with a hysterectomy and bilateral oophorectomy as the treatment solution. An underlying thyroid
condition goes undetected and worsens, a subsequent thyroid imbalance
is diagnosed several years later, and a thyroidectomy with radiation is
recommended.

Given the poor health outcomes associated with the initial surgical procedure, hysterectomy, the patient decides to conduct her own research
into the causal factors of the malfunctioning thyroid in an attempt to avoid
a second surgical procedure. The underlying culprit contributing to the
malfunctioning thyroid has a dietary component—insulin resistance, or
the inability to metabolize sugars and carbohydrates normally. Again,
research is required to devise a suitable dietary regimen to resolve the
insulin resistance. After following the indicated regimen, the patient
reverses the weight gain and, miraculously, the cholesterol, glucose,
blood pressure, and thyroid levels return to normal.

The patient had consulted with national "experts," and diagnoses
ranged from hypothyroidism to hyperthyroidism to thyroid toxicosis,
unspecified. There was no consensus on the diagnosis and thus no consensus on the treatment. Invasive procedures to remedy an ill-defined health
problem seemed excessive. A simple accurate diagnosis provided the
solution. Maintenance of a proper diet essentially was able to solve the
problem, whereas an invasive procedure likely would have compounded
the issue. In this case, the options offered by traditional medicine were not
attractive and did not seem reasonable; they seemed excessive and offered
no guarantee of success.

Further, the speed with which the diagnosis and surgical recommendations were presented seemed excessive. Second opinions and conflicting
diagnoses suggested that perhaps there was a missing element, something
the doctors themselves did not understand, that could provide the answer.

This proved to be the case. I am the patient described in the previous paragraphs, and I enjoy excellent health today as a result of my willingness to explore alternative options and my belief that perhaps there was a simple solution to this health issue.

In her book *Medicine and Culture* (1988), which is a cross-cultural analysis of practice patterns in the United States, Germany, England, and France, Lynn Payer points out that the United States is frequently referred to as the "God-Sakers," as in "For God's sake, do something!" Practice patterns in the United States are considered very aggressive, and invasive surgical procedures are far more common in the United States than in other industrialized nations. Rather than being used as the last line of defense, surgery is often selected as the first. This is not the case in other countries.

Payer (1988) states that the United States performs six times the number of "cardiac bypass operations as English doctors." Hysterectomies, performed rarely in France, have become the most popular nonobstetric surgical procedure performed on women in the United States. The primary reason for the difference is the way the female anatomy is viewed and the practice patterns that stem from that philosophy within each country. Hysterectomy is seen as a highly invasive procedure in France and one of last resort, typically performed in cases where the woman's life is at stake. Further, the French view is to keep the female anatomy intact unless there is scientific justification to do otherwise.

In direct contrast is the approach in the United States. Hysterectomy, the most invasive procedure for treating uterine fibroids, is also the most widely used procedure, with 37 percent of all women in the United States undergoing hysterectomy by age 65. There are less invasive procedures available, such as myomectomy and uterine artery embolization, but neither of these is used to the same extent as hysterectomy. Further, oophorectomy, the removal of both ovaries at the time of hysterectomy, is a common practice in many regions of the United States. According to the *Hysterectomy Surveillance Report* (CDC 2002) by the Centers for Disease Control and Prevention in Atlanta, 55 percent of the hysterectomies were done in conjunction with bilateral oophorectomies. The traditional thinking is that since childbearing is no longer an issue, "as long as we're in there, we might as well take them out." Additionally, there has been a traditional concern regarding the risk of ovarian cancer, although scientific evidence indicates that only 5 percent of the 55 percent of women who undergo bilateral oophorectomy have clinical indications for cancer. As a consequence, 50 percent of women undergoing this procedure are doing so without the clinical justification to support it or the long-term health outcomes data to substantiate the practice. Oophorectomy is one of a number of invasive procedures that lack solid scientific outcomes data to justify its widespread usage.

It's been widely known for decades and proclaimed by physicians around the world that nutrition and exercise play a major role in one's health. The absence of either or both of these elements inevitably has negative impacts on the body. Although nutrition plays a vital role, there is little taught in the traditional medical school curriculum about its importance. Cheraskin et al. (1974, p. 4) illustrate the lack of knowledge about nutrition by doctors with a statement by Dr. Jean Mayer of Harvard University: "We have just completed a study to find out what the average doctor at Harvard knows about nutrition. . . . What we found is this—the average doctor at Harvard knows a wee bit more about nutrition than his secretary, unless his secretary has a weight problem, in which the average secretary knows a wee bit more about nutrition than the average doctor."

A recent major study by the Women's Health Initiative (Gardner 2006) on diet and its impact on postmenopausal women found that a low-fat diet does not reduce the incidence of breast or colorectal cancer or coronary heart disease in women. Although this is a puzzling finding and is confusing to many, it points out the incomplete state of science underlying nutrition and weight loss. It also may shed light on the necessity for a reduction in refined carbohydrates and an increased intake of protein in the diet. Jacques Rossouw, Women's Health Initiative (WHI) project officer at the National Heart, Lung, and Blood Institute, states, "The issue isn't over." The WHI is a fifteen-year study involving 50,000 postmenopausal women. The findings were published in the February 8, 2006, issue of the *Journal of the American Medical Association.*

If the CDC's (2002) figures are accurate, 55 percent of women undergo bilateral oophorectomies during hysterectomy and 37 percent of the total population of women in the United States undergo hysterectomy by age 65. New data by Parker et al. (2005) indicate that oophorectomies performed without clinical evidence of cancer may in fact increase the risk of heart disease and contribute to premature death. Thus, the new findings on diet, although important, may need to be reviewed against the backdrop of these more recent studies. Perhaps the incidence of coronary heart disease has to do more with complex issues still poorly understood, such as the prevalence of invasive procedures that may contribute to insulin resistance (often a precursor to coronary heart disease), than with diet alone. Perhaps analysis of the causal factors of insulin resistance postoperatively may assist in reducing the incidence of coronary heart disease, which is the leading cause of death in women in the United States.

Jerome Avorn, M.D., chief of pharmacoepidemiology at Brigham & Women's Hospital and author of *Powerful Medicines: The Benefits, Risks and Costs of Prescription Drugs* (2004), claims that the WHI study results (2002) indicating increased risk of heart disease, cancer, and stroke among subjects taking hormone replacement therapy (HRT), provides us with the largest "medically induced health epidemic in U.S. history" (Avorn 2004, p. 43). If that is the case, diet is merely one small component of health and cannot compensate for damage done by ingesting, at the recommendation of experts, a potentially carcinogenic substance (hormones in HRT).

There are those who criticize the stance against HRT in the WHI (2002) study. These individuals state that the sample was skewed toward older women, who may have had existing health problems, and that there are many gynecologists who continue to advocate HRT as a necessary and valuable resource for postmenopausal women. Each woman must be aware of the existing research both for and against HRT and must make her own decision regarding such treatment.

Since the WHI study results were issued, the FDA has modified its recommendations regarding the use of HRT, stating that it should be used "low-dose, short-term," which is a more conservative approach but not one supporting a ban on HRT. However, at the same time, the United Nations Health Advisory Group has placed HRT on its list of "known carcinogens" (Ross 2005). Again, each woman must make an informed choice, in conjunction with her gynecologist, in terms of what is most appropriate for her. The example of HRT points out the inexact science underlying treatment protocols in this and many areas of healthcare, and the controversies that surround traditional "gold standard treatments."

Gary Null, Ph.D., a nationally known syndicated talk show host, consumer advocate, and author, spoke at the American Academy of Anti-Aging Medicine in Chicago in August 2005. He discussed the issue of nutritional supplements as an avenue of healing. He also has published *Women's Health Risks Associated with Orthodox Medicine—Part 2* (2002) with Debra Rasio, M.D., and Martin Feldman, M.D. In that text Null points out that research on women's health, specifically, the treatment of uterine fibroids, appears problematic, and the "cure" may be worse than the condition in some instances. In the United States 46 million women are candidates for developing uterine fibroids, with 1.6 million newly diagnosed cases each year and 625,000 procedures performed annually. These statistics give one a sense of the magnitude of the impact of diagnostic and treatment protocols on the populations served and the critical importance of having good science beneath these protocols, not to mention the need for these protocols to be followed to ensure there is clinical justification for the procedures.

As indicated previously, hysterectomy, the removal of the uterus, is the most common nonobstetric surgical procedure performed on women in the United States, with 37 percent of all U.S. women undergoing a hysterectomy by age 65. Michael Broder, M.D., and colleagues (2000) studied the application of the American College of Obstetricians and Gynecologists (ACOG) criteria sets (diagnostic and treatment protocols that govern these procedures, as defined by ACOG) as well as the RAND/UCLA appropriateness method in evaluating clinical appropriateness of hysterectomies performed at one capitated medical group on the West Coast.

Broder and his fellow researchers found that 70 percent, or 367 of 497 hysterectomies performed, did not meet the level of care recommended by the expert panel (RAND/UCLA appropriateness method) and 76 percent, or 54 of 71 hysterectomies performed using the ACOG criteria sets, did not meet the ACOG criteria for hysterectomy. "The most common reasons for recommendations for hysterectomies considered inappropriate were lack of adequate diagnostic evaluation and failure to try alternative treatments before hysterectomy" (2000, p. 1). What this means to the consumer is that, in many instances, these invasive procedures may not be clinically justified. Further, invasive procedures without clinical merit come with certain risks and quality-of-life outcomes that may not be evident until after the surgery.

There are two additional problems in this area of medicine that should be noted. First, the benchmarks for evaluating success are mortality rates and surgical error (e.g., perforation of the bowel). Although, from a clinical standpoint, these are clearly important, hysterectomies are not considered life-threatening, so mortality is not an appropriate benchmark here. Also, unintentional perforation of organs or other surgical error is an evaluation of the surgeon, not a determination of whether the procedure is appropriate and returns the patient to full functioning. Additionally, there are no long-term outcomes available for these procedures, which is problematic from a scientific standpoint. It is akin to putting one's life savings into an investment that has data for only two years out. If you knew that the investment had only short-term results available and had never been evaluated long-term, would you put your life savings into it?

CONCLUSION

Consumers seek alternative treatments for a variety of reasons. The primary reason appears to be twofold: Either traditional medicine cannot offer a solution, or the options available from traditional medicine are not attractive. In addition, curiosity may lead some to explore alternative therapies given friends who have used them with positive results. Or perhaps disenchantment with one's state of health serves as a compelling reason to explore alternative treatments. With 1997 statistics indicating that between $36 and $47 billion was spent on complementary and alternative medicine, clearly there is an active interest among consumers to explore healing pathways beyond the confines of conventional medicine.

SECTION TWO

Controversies

CHAPTER 5

Do Alternative Therapies Work?

This chapter explores the usefulness of alternative therapies as well as ways to protect yourself if you pursue alternative therapies. Not all supplements are safe, and not all are proven to be effective. However, the same can be said regarding branded pharmaceutical products that have been approved by the FDA, as the case of Vioxx points out. Vioxx, a pain relief product, was recalled by the FDA but returned to the market within several weeks as a result of the manufacturer's effective lobbying efforts.

Dr. Sam Nussbaum, the Chief Medical Officer of Anthem, Inc., one of the largest managed care companies in the United States, reported in a presentation to the Disease Management Congress in 2003 that less than 50 percent of medicine is science based (Nussbaum 2003). In short, we are uncertain about many interventions currently utilized in traditional health-care as well. We have much to learn about health and healing in general, whether we're talking about traditional or alternative medicine.

As we explore the efficacy of alternative therapies, we must first look at the efficacy of conventional practices, namely the costs and outcomes of prescription drug usage. What are we spending and what are we getting in return for that investment? Jerry Avorn, in his book *Powerful Medicines: The Benefits, Risks and Costs of Prescription Drugs,* states it plainly:

> We currently spend more than $200 billion a year on medications in the United States. . . . Spending on prescription drugs has become the fastest-growing component of all American health care costs, rising 13–19 percent per year and doubling between 1995 [and] 2002. . . . Our outspending the rest of the world on drugs and other medical care might be worth doing if it produced better health outcomes for Americans but it doesn't. . . . The

OECD [developed world] data show that the United States ranks nineteenth
out of thirty countries in life expectancy at birth, fourteenth of twenty-nine
in life expectancy at birth, fourteenth of twenty-nine in life expectancy at
age sixty-five, and twenty-fourth out of thirty in infant mortality. (Avorn
2004, p. 217)

If the amount of spending resulted in an equally large increase in good
health, the United States would be enjoying much better outcomes than
we currently are experiencing. We're clearly spending more on healthcare, but the returns in health outcomes do not equal the financial outlay.

One possible glimpse into why the costs are so high, and some of the
results of those expenditures, can be found in a report by the Institute of
Medicine. *To Err Is Human* (1999) reported that "medication-related
errors for hospitalized patients cost roughly $2 billion annually." A
detailed analysis of some of those costs is provided by Bates et al. (1997).
Their research assessed healthcare utilization associated with adverse
drug events and included 4108 admissions of eleven medical and surgical
units in two tertiary-care hospitals over a six-month time period. Their
conclusion, published in the article "The Costs of Adverse Drug Events in
Hospitalized Patients," was that the estimated post-event costs for an
adverse drug event (ADE) were $2595 for all ADEs and $4685 for preventable ADEs. Bates et al. projected total estimated costs for a 700-bed
teaching hospital at $5.6 million (for all ADEs) and $2.8 million (for preventable ADEs).

In some of the research published (Institute of Medicine 1999, 2000),
prescription drugs are given as the fourth leading cause of death in the
United States. Some of the underlying issues include side-effect profile,
contraindications, combination drug involvement, lack of safety of the
drugs themselves, and errors in delivery of the drugs.

A balanced approach to looking at both prescription drugs and alternative therapies involves first answering the million-dollar question, do they
work? A second, equally important question is, what risk do they entail to
the patient? The third question is, what is the cost to the patient?

If we consider the National Health Interview Survey, specifically
Advance Data from Vital and Health Statistics No. 343 (Barnes et al.
2004), which utilized interviews conducted with 31,044 adults age 18 and
older, the results indicate that 62 percent of adults used complementary
and alternative medicine (CAM) (including prayer for health reasons) in
the twelve months prior to the date of interview. When prayer was eliminated from the forms of CAM, the use of alternative therapies was reduced
to 36 percent. There were ten common forms of CAM used: prayer for one's
own health (43 percent), prayer by others for one's health (24.4 percent),

natural products (18.9 percent), deep breathing exercises (11.6 percent), participation in a prayer group for one's own health (9.6 percent), meditation therapies (3.5 percent), chiropractic care (7.5 percent), yoga (5.1 percent), massage (5 percent), and diet-based therapies (3.5 percent).

CAM was most widely used to treat the following conditions: "back pain or back problems, head or chest colds, neck pain and neck problems, joint pain and stiffness, and anxiety or depression" (Barnes et al. 2004, p. 4). The demographics on those who used CAM included individuals who thought that CAM, coupled with conventional medical treatments, would help (54.9 percent) and those who thought it would be interesting to try (50.1 percent).

Further, the demographics on CAM therapy, including megavitamins and prayer, are interesting. More women (69.3 percent) were likely to use CAM than men (54.1 percent). Individuals age 85 and older (70.3 percent) were more likely to use CAM than those between 18 and 29 years of age (53.5 percent). The intermediate age groups had the following levels of CAM usage: 30–39 (60.7 percent), 40–49 (64.1 percent), 50–59 (66.1 percent), and 70–84 (68.6 percent) (Barnes et al. 2004). Racially, there were some differences as well. Blacks (71.3 percent) had the highest rate of CAM usage, followed by Asians (61.7 percent), Hispanics (61.4 percent), and whites (60.4 percent).

In addition, people with more education used CAM therapy, including megavitamins and prayer, to a greater degree than did those with less education. Those with a bachelor of arts (B.A.) degree (66.7 percent) tended to use CAM to the greatest extent; people with a master of arts (M.A.), Ph.D., or professional degree (65.5 percent) used CAM second most frequently. Those with some college (64.7 percent) were followed by people with associate of arts (A.A.) degrees (64.1 percent). The lowest rates of usage of CAM including prayer were high-school graduates or their equivalent (58.3 percent), followed by those with less than a high-school education (57.4 percent).

Do alternative therapies work? If we look at megavitamins alone, there is much in the research that points to their effectiveness. The clinicians listed in the 2005 Orthomolecular Medicine Hall of Fame all built their reputations on innovative approaches to health, on detoxification, and on "varying the concentrations in the human body of substances that are normally present," as Linus Pauling, Ph.D., the two-time Nobel Prize winner, so aptly stated (Pauling 1968).

Dr. Max Gerson's therapy involved the finding that cancer was a result of both toxicities and deficiencies. By administering vegetable juices, which are rich in nutrients and fluids, to empty the kidneys, Gerson found that the body was often able to heal itself (Orthomolecular Medicine Hall of Fame 2005). Albert Szent-Gyorgyi, Ph.D., a Nobel Prize winner in 1933 for the discovery of vitamin C, not only found that ascorbic acid could prevent scurvy but predicted that it would inevitably be used in the treatment of cancer (Orthomolecular Medicine Hall of Fame 2005). Fredrick Klenner, M.D., worked with high doses of vitamin C and found it to have therapeutic effects in the treatment of polio. He also found consistent cures for a wide range of both bacterial and viral infections following treatment with vitamin C (Orthomolecular Medicine Hall of Fame 2005).

Stephen Sinatra, M.D., metabolic cardiologist, makes the following comment in his book *The Sinatra Solution: Metabolic Cardiology*: "Although hundreds of scientific papers have been published in noteworthy scientific and medical journals describing the individual roles of these naturally occurring compounds in preserving the energy health of your heart, skeletal muscle, and other tissues, you've probably never heard or read about the exciting combination of D-ribose, L-carnitine, and Coenzyme Q10" (2005, p. 22).

Sinatra goes on to say that ignorance and deep-rooted reliance on pharmaceuticals by clinical cardiologists will prevent many patients who do not benefit from conventional treatments alone from reaping the benefits of these three nutrients, although they are utilized by many board-certified cardiologists in the United States, Europe, and Japan.

Sinatra attributes the lack of use of these nutrients and the reluctance to grant them credibility to "political bias, insufficient marketing, economics, and ignorance regarding the results of real science" (2005, p. 23). The fact that the PubMed Web site features 1254 articles published in scientific and medical journals attesting to the effectiveness of Coenzyme Q10 and 5769 entries for the equivalent term "ubiquinone" is a fitting conclusion to Sinatra's point. The volume of articles available tends to nullify the "no science available, not enough data on which to base an argument" objection.

Abram Hoffer, M.D., is another clinician who provides an answer to the question, do alternative therapies work? Hoffer believed that vitamin C was effective in the treatment of cancer. Andrew Saul, Ph.D., in a review of the book by Hoffer and Linus Pauling, *Vitamin C and Cancer: Discovery, Recovery and Controversy* (1999), refutes the three primary criticisms of vitamin C for treatment of cancer: that it is ineffective against cancer; that it interferes with conventional therapies; and that it is, in itself, harmful to the patient (Saul 2000).

The facts, according to Saul, are as follows: "There are many controlled studies demonstrating vitamin C's efficacy in the treatment of cancer; vitamin C reduces the side-effects of chemotherapy, surgery and radiation therapy[;] some of the benefits include reduced nausea, little or no hair loss, [and] reduced swelling after radiation [and] improved and shortened recovery time from surgery; and vitamin C appears to be unusually safe, with substantive scientific data to support that conclusion." Saul "considers it essential as an adjunct to traditional therapy for cancer, given that there is no known cure for cancer" (Saul 2000).

How effective are other alternative therapies, such as megavitamins, in other clinical areas, including heart disease and mental illness (e.g., schizophrenia and manic depression)? There are a number of scientists, award winners from the 2004 Orthomolecular Medicine Hall of Fame, who have done significant work in these areas. Dr. Linus Pauling described "orthomolecular medicine" as the utilization of the "right molecules in the right concentration" (1968).

Decades before the work of Pauling, William McCormick, M.D., a Canadian, was interested in exploring the benefits of vitamin C in the treatment of cancer. McCormick found in his laboratory research indicating that smoking one cigarette resulted in the reduction of 25 mg of ascorbic acid in the body. That observation, coupled with McCormick's earlier finding that "poor collagen formation was due to vitamin C deficiency," led McCormick to conclude that these deficiencies were the culprit in everything from "stretch marks to cardiovascular disease and cancer." His findings served as the basis for Pauling and Ewan Cameron in their advocacy of large doses of vitamin C to combat cancer (Orthomolecular Medicine Hall of Fame 2004).

Roger J. Williams, Ph.D., another recipient of the Orthomolecular Medicine Hall of Fame (2004) award, was an advocate for vitamin B_5, otherwise known as pantothenic acid, and is touted as having made more vitamin-related discoveries at the University of Texas Clayton Biochemistry Institute than any researcher at any other laboratory in the world. The following quote is attributed to him: "The nutritional microenvironment of our body cells is crucially important to health, and deficiencies in this environment constitute a major cause of disease" (Orthomolecular Medicine Hall of Fame 2004).

Three researchers in orthomolecular medicine who focused on nutritionals and their use in the treatment of mental illness were Carl C. Pfeiffer, M.D., Ph.D.; Alan Cott, M.D.; and Humphrey Osmond, M.D. Pfeiffer found that schizophrenia was a result of chemically induced metabolic disorders and that eliminating those deficiencies through nutritionals was the remedy. His quote regarding the use of nutritionals is as follows: "For every drug that benefits a patient, there is a natural substance that can achieve the same effect" (Orthomolecular Medicine Hall of Fame 2004).

Cott applied fasting to the treatment of manic-depressive illness, following the example set by a Russian clinician, Dr. Yuri Nicholay, in his treatment of 10,000 patients suffering from mental illness (i.e., manic depression). Cott placed his patients on a regimen that included exercising and drinking two quarts of water daily. As a result, at the end of week 1 many patients no longer needed their prescription medications (Orthomolecular Medicine Hall of Fame 2004). Cott is the author of *Help for the Learning Disabled Child: The Orthomolecular Treatment.*

Finally, Osmond focused his work on high doses of niacin in the treatment of schizophrenia patients. He found that amounts in excess of 17,000 mg daily, 1000 times the FDA's recommended daily allowance (RDA), was surprisingly not toxic and had therapeutic effects in the treatment of schizophrenia (Orthomolecular Medicine Hall of Fame 2004).

All of the aforementioned researchers have shown through their work that there is another pathway to health—that of orthomolecular medicine.

Other evaluations of alternative therapies and their effectiveness include the work of Laura Patton, M.D. At a 1997 conference of the Washington Health Policy Forum with the Group Health Cooperative of Puget Sound, Patton presented an article titled "The Role of the Consumer in Coverage Decisions." The article discussed a survey that had been conducted with 492 members who had used various forms of alternative or complementary medicine offered by the cooperative in May 1997, including acupuncture, naturopathy, and massage. Seventy-six percent of the members had had the condition requiring alternative therapy for longer than one year.

Forty-six percent of the members rated the care received from their conventional physician as very helpful (16.5 percent) or moderately helpful (29.9 percent) (Patton 1997). In contrast, care received from the CAM provider was rated as extremely helpful by 51.9 percent and as moderately helpful by 12.4 percent. The respondents perceived a slight (25 percent) or substantial (24 percent) decrease in their use of "the conventional team," for a total of 49 percent. They also perceived a slight (26 percent) or substantial (56 percent) decrease in their use of prescription medications. Finally, the respondents stated that they would definitely (70 percent) or probably (15 percent) return to the same CAM provider if they "had to do it all over again," for a total favorable response of 85 percent (Patton 1997).

In answering the question of the efficacy of alternative therapies, how do we evaluate the alternative therapy most widely used—prayer? Many in the scientific community would answer that prayer alone is not an effective remedy when one is dealing with a life-threatening condition. Others, like Larry Dossey, M.D., are staunch advocates of prayer in conjunction with conventional medicine. What is the value of prayer and its place in modern medicine? Andrew Weil, M.D., probably stated it best in his book *Health and Healing: Understanding Conventional and Alternative Medicine*:

> Restoring that which is broken is the function of religion, the word means "to bind again." . . . In our society, the commonality of religion, magic and medicine is obscured. Our medical doctors have narrowed their view to pay attention only to the physical body and the material aspects of illness. They do not grasp the concept of wholeness as perfection that is the root meaning of the word, nor realize that health and illness are particular manifestations of good and evil, requiring all the help of religion and philosophy to understand and all the techniques of magic to manipulate. (Weil 1983, p. 47)

The importance of prayer and its value in maintaining health is a certainty, but how does one go about quantifying the benefits of prayer? According to the National Health Information Survey (Barnes et al. 2004), prayer is one of the most widely used of all alternative therapies Does it work? How does it work? When does it work? How do you put God (whatever your version of God may be) to the test?

Sociologists refer to the difference between the sacred and the profane. The profane is everything that stems from our daily, ordinary lives, whereas the sacred refers to an entirely different realm, one that inspires awe and wonder. You can catch the profane world on the 11:00 news— with its killings, war, and destruction—and be left with considerable fear and anxiety. The sacred realm is the unseen world, that which is ever constant and powerful and holds the capacity for miracles.

In the days immediately following September 11, 2001, Americans witnessed a transformation of the profane into the sacred. There was unity instead of division, not just in the United States but abroad as well. People came together; strangers helped strangers. There was a groundswell of the best of humanity, which was witnessed on the news. I believe that that groundswell we were witnessing was a spiritual experience. In the tragedy of 9/11, we humans tapped into our divinity to help ourselves and each other deal with what we were experiencing. Since then we've returned to divisiveness, but in the days immediately after 9/11 something remarkable occurred. I believe that it was the sacred spirit working through us all, and we put forth our best because we felt compelled to help others who were suffering.

Weil's reference to religion, philosophy, and magic as being necessary to the healing process makes health as much about spirituality as it is about surgery. If, as Weil says, the function of religion is to heal what is broken, and if dis-ease occurs as a result of the body breaking down in some respect, then exploration of the spiritual must be considered as a component of healing.

The body's ability to renew itself is a remarkable thing. Deepak Chopra, physician and New Age guru, writes,

> We've learned that the lining of your stomach is replaced about every five days. It takes about a month for your skin to be retread. In about six weeks your liver has turned over, and within just a few months, most of the calcium and phosphorus crystals that make up your skeleton have come and gone. Every year 98 percent of all the atoms in the human body have been exchanged. After a course of three years, you would be hard pressed to find an atom that was a part of you then, which could still be considered yours now. (Chopra 2001, p. 32)

Our physical renewal and transformation is taking place, without any effort on our part, in divine order. Chopra encourages his readers to see the body "not as a static machine but rather as a field of energy and intelligence, constantly renewing itself" (Chopra 2001, p. 32).

By shifting our view of healing and recognizing that the body has an enormous capacity for regeneration, we can change our perception of health and healing. Frequently, when we change our perception, our reality begins to change as well.

Prayer, then, is a request for a remedy that the individual has not been able to summon of his or her own accord. The data from the National Health Information Survey (Barnes et al. 2004) document that prayer is not bound by gender, as men and women alike use it. It is not bound by racial or ethnic divisions, as all racial and ethnic groups use it to some degree. Nor is it bound by age, as both young and old use it. Annual income also does not influence its usage; the low-income as well as the high-income groups use it to varying degrees. Healing miracles occur across all divisions, with no single group having a lock on the miraculous, which would seem to be in accordance with all that is representative of the spiritual realm.

Quantifying prayer is a difficult task. PubMed has 1156 entries on "Prayer for Healing." Some of those articles document significant results when prayer was tested scientifically in controlled settings (e.g., hospitalized patients with coronary heart disease). There are also articles that do not show significant results but suggest that prayer be encouraged or suggested as a useful adjunct to traditional therapy. Although various statistical analyses may not show hard evidence of prayer's usefulness, personally, I would be reluctant to conclude that it doesn't work. I may need to use prayer someday in a health crisis of my own or for the benefit of a loved one, and I would not want to be on record as stating that prayer is of no value in the healing process.

Joseph Campbell—former theologian, professor of theology at Sarah Lawrence College for decades, and author of the book *The Power of Myth* (1991)—gives a convincing argument in that book about the power of the sacred. He states that all of the world's religions have strikingly similar themes throughout. He also makes the point that these religions were conceived in different parts of the world, by very different peoples and cultures, prior to communication, and yet they bear striking similarities. This realization convinced Campbell that some type of inexplicable power resides in the universe, which is called by different names and approached under different belief systems. We often refer to that power as "the sacred," "divinity," or "the supernatural" because it is outside the realm of everyday understanding.

The concept of faith is a vital part of religious belief systems, as well as healing. Faith is the belief in something that we cannot see, and the word *faith* comes from the Latin root word *fidere*, meaning "to trust." That is part of the paradox of faith: how does one believe in something one cannot see? Another aspect of faith and spirituality is the ability to surrender what we think we know and to let into our lives the shaft of light (God, whatever you conceive God to be).

Critics of prayer point out the difficulties in determining its effectiveness due to the problem of testing it scientifically. These issues were noted in a March 26, 2006, article by Rob Stein, a syndicated columnist from the *Washington Post*. Stein confirms that prayer is the most widely used "complement to mainstream medicine, outpacing acupuncture, herbs, vitamins and other alternative remedies" (2006, p. A9). In the study that prompted Stein's article, a team of researchers put prayer to the test, using the tools of science. The results of the research were "mixed and highly controversial" (Stein 2006, p. A9). Skeptics claimed that the work had significant flaws and described it as "a misguided waste of money that irresponsibly attempts to validate the supernatural with science" (Stein 2006, p. A9).

The result of intercessory prayer, or prayer on behalf of others, as reported by cardiologist Randolph Byrd (Stein 2006, p. A9), was that the prayed-for groups in the study required fewer drugs and less assistance in breathing. The criticisms of this and similar studies were that the positive health outcomes reported were difficult to "trace directly to prayer itself and could possibly have been the result of a chance event" (Stein 2006, p. A9). Richard Sloan, a behavioral scientist quoted in the article, referred to the positive conclusions as "the sharp-shooter effect" (Stein 2006, p. A9), where a round of ammunition is emptied into the side of a barn and then, after the shots are fired, a bulls-eye is drawn. Scientific studies, according to Sloan, "have to predict in advance what effect you may have" (Stein 2006, p. A9).

An article by Malcolm Ritter, published in the March 31, 2006, *Lexington Herald-Leader* and titled "Strangers' Prayers Don't Help Patients Recover, Study Finds," points out that, according to Dr. Charles Bethea, cardiologist at the Integris Baptist Medical Center in Oklahoma City, "intercessory prayer under our restricted format had a neutral effect" (Ritter 2006, p. A4). The $2.4 million study, touted as the "largest and best designed" study to test the medical benefits on intercessory prayer (Ritter 2006, p. A4), included 1800 patients at six different medical centers. The results were as follows: 59 percent of patients who knew they were being prayed for developed complications, whereas 52 percent of those who were told that intercessory prayer was a possibility developed complications. Dr. Harold G. Koenig, director of the Center for Spirituality, Theology and Health at Duke University Medical Center, commented, "Science is not designed to study the supernatural," and the results did not surprise him. "There is no god in either the Christian, Jewish or Muslim scriptures that can be constrained to the point that they can be predicted" (Ritter 2006, p. A4).

Allopathic medical authorities' skepticism about prayer extends to other types of complementary and alternative medicine as well. Marcia Angell, M.D., and Joseph Kassirer, M.D., editors of the *New England Journal of Medicine*, one of the most respected journals in medicine, state in their article "The Risks of Untested and Unregulated Remedies" that "it is time for the scientific community to stop giving alternative medicine a free ride" (1998, p. 839).

The editors of the *Journal of the American Medical Association*, Phil Fontanarosa, M.D., and George Lundberg, M.D., state that "there is no alternative medicine. There is only scientifically proven, evidence-based medicine . . . or unproven medicine, for which scientific evidence is lacking" (Fontanarosa and Lundberg 1998, p. 1618).

Barry Beyerstein attributes the use of CAM to "common errors in reasoning" stemming from social and cultural factors such as anti-scientific attitudes; psychological phenomena such as wishful thinking and the will to believe; and the illusion that an ineffective therapy works when the outcome actually may be due to placebo effect or spontaneous remission (Beyerstein 2001).

Wallace Sampson describes CAM therapies as "anomalous practices for which claims of efficacy are either unproved or disproved" (2001). Sampson goes on to point out that CAM therapies in most medical schools are not presented in a way that allows for rigorous critique or analysis of their claims. Of the fifty-six CAM courses taught in U.S. medical schools from 1995 to 1997, only four were taught with the curricular method oriented to criticism. Sampson concludes the article by encouraging this critical approach for CAM course offerings in the medical school curriculum.

In conclusion, it is not the purpose of this chapter to provide an exhaustive overview of alternative therapies and their irrefutable value. You will find as many articles that deny the effectiveness of alternative and complementary forms of healthcare as you will articles that support it. The intent of this chapter is to provide you with a sampling of alternative and complementary forms of healthcare, such as prayer and orthomolecular medicine (megavitamins), and encourage you to explore whether such treatments have value. As Chopra so aptly states, "Reality is the result of perception, which is a selective act of attention and interpretation" (2001, p. 23).

CHAPTER 6

Should Alternative Medicine Be Regulated by the Government?

This chapter addresses the benefits and the drawbacks of government regulation of alternative treatments. The National Center for Complementary and Alternative Medicine, an arm of the National Institutes of Health, is charged with evaluating various forms of complementary and alternative therapies, including herbal supplements. Given that Americans spent $5 billion on herbal supplements in 1997, clearly there is an interest in supplements among the American public as well as a need to evaluate the benefits and risks of alternative therapies.

The issues behind government regulation of alternative therapies should involve the safety and efficacy of the products for the consumers taking them. It is not entirely accurate to state that FDA approval and regulation guarantee the safety and efficacy of conventional medical procedures and prescription drugs. To provide an accurate analysis, this chapter begins with findings by the Institute of Medicine (IOM) (2000) regarding the U.S. healthcare system and some of the flaws one is likely to find within it. This report provides a means by which to conduct an accurate analysis of government regulation of traditional medicines and treatments and to put the regulation of alternative and complementary forms of healthcare in proper perspective.

The IOM report (1999) *To Err Is Human: Building a Safer Health System* considers the increasing problem of medical errors and related concerns for patient safety. The report states that between 44,000 and 98,000 individuals die each year in the United States as a result of medical errors.

Medical errors claim more lives annually in the United States than motor vehicle accidents (43,458), breast cancer (42,297), or AIDS (16,516). The report also indicates that 7000 additional lives are lost each year in the United States as a result of medication-related mistakes, 16 percent more than the rate of deaths from work-related injuries. A fact sheet produced by the Agency for Healthcare Research and Quality (AHRQ) titled *Medical Errors: The Scope of the Problem* (2000) points out that medical errors cost $37.6 billion annually, with $17 billion of these costs being preventable. The errors do not occur solely in hospitals; the IOM report states that according to the Massachusetts State Pharmacy Board, 2.4 million prescriptions are improperly filled in that state each year.

The IOM defines a medical error as "the failure to complete a planned action as intended or the use of a wrong plan to achieve an aim." Adverse events are defined as "injury caused by medical management rather than by the underlying disease or condition associated with treatment, such as a life-threatening allergic reaction to a drug when the patient has known allergies" (IOM 1999, p. 1).

The AHRQ report (2000) points out a number of areas in which errors occur:

> Diagnostic error, such as misdiagnosis leading to an incorrect choice of therapy, failure to use an indicated diagnostic test, misinterpretation of test results, and failure to act on normal results; equipment failure, such as defibrillators with dead batteries or intravenous pumps whose valves are easily dislodged or bumped, causing increased doses of medication over too short a period; infections, such as nosocomial and post-surgical wound infections; blood transfusion–related injuries, such as giving a patient the blood of the incorrect type; [and] misinterpretation of other medical orders, such as failing to give a patient a salt-free meal, as ordered by a physician. (AHRQ 2000, p. 1)

Statistics on adverse events include a study in which the IOM (1999) reviewed 1133 medical records and found that 70 percent of the adverse events that occurred were preventable, 6 percent potentially preventable, and 24 percent not preventable. The AHRQ report (2000) indicates that according to a 1999 study based on a chart review of medical records in Colorado and Utah, 54 percent of surgical errors could have been prevented. Clearly, these reports suggest that navigating the healthcare system, as well as taking prescription drugs as recommended by your doctor, can be a dangerous undertaking. These statistics underscore the need to be an informed consumer.

The issues of safety and efficacy play a central role in the debate over regulation of alternative and complementary therapies. From a clinical standpoint, however, the concern focuses on issues of liability resulting from the use of unregulated therapies and recommendations of untested therapies or co-managing patients who utilize those therapies. There are as many opinions on these issues as there are publications.

David Eisenberg's article "Advising Patients Who Seek Alternative Medical Therapies" (1997) outlines the more critical issues surrounding the regulation of alternative therapies, namely the challenges imposed by the co-management of patients who are accessing both traditional and alternative medicine. Eisenberg states that a review of the current medical literature fails to provide "unequivocal documentation of the safety or efficacy of the overwhelming majority of alternative therapies." He provides several exceptions to that statement, namely spinal manipulation for acute back pain, acupuncture for the treatment of nausea, and relaxation and certain behavioral therapies for the treatment of chronic pain and insomnia. He also comments that there are risks involved with alternative therapies and cautions against relying on these therapies when conventional treatments may resolve the problem.

Peter Curtis, M.D., and Susan Gaylord, Ph.D., (2005) in their article "Safety Issues in the Interaction of Conventional, Complementary and Alternative Health Care," point out some of the safety issues regarding the combined use of alternative and traditional forms of healthcare, such as errors in treatment and medical management, adverse effects of pharmaceuticals, risk for the patient, as well as "quality control issues, licensing, regulation and misrepresentation with dietary supplements." Other concerns with alternative and complementary forms of healthcare include "drug/herb interactions, laboratory diagnosis and lack of communication between clinicians and patients" (2005, p. 6).

To counter those concerns, authors in alternative medicine provide different views. One of these authors, is Richard Walters, whose book *Options: Alternative Cancer Therapy Book* (1993) points out that two of three people diagnosed with cancer succumb to the disease. In addition, he reports that "the war on cancer has been a colossal failure despite hundreds of billions of dollars spent on research and treatment" (1993, p. 1).

Walters points out that over 50 percent of cancer patients "routinely receive chemotherapy drugs, which can cripple a person's chance of survival." He outlines and refutes four myths that surround alternative cancer therapies: "All alternative therapies are worthless; alternative cancer therapists are quacks—unscrupulous, unlicensed, untrained in medicine, out for a fast buck; patients who seek alternative therapies are driven by desperation [and are] . . . ignorant, gullible or both; and alternative cancer therapies are 'unproven,' therefore untested and unscientific" (1993, pp. 4–14).

Walters refutes the first myth, that "all alternative cancer therapies are worthless," by stating that success rates with alternative therapies vary widely. He cites Gary Null's (1987, p. 10) research on the efficacy of alternative therapies as ranging from "2 to 20" percent in cases of terminal cancer. He cites Ralph Moss, author of *The Cancer Industry*, who reports a baseline five-year remission rate of 4 to 5 percent with alternative therapies for cancer treatment (1989, p. 98).

Walters refutes the second myth, that "alternative cancer therapists are quacks—unscrupulous, unlicensed, untrained in medicine, out for a fast buck," by stating that in Cassileth's research published in the *Annals of Internal Medicine* (1984), 60 percent of the 138 alternative cancer practitioners reviewed were medical doctors, with the remainder having advanced degrees in biology, chemistry, or other sciences. Each practitioner must be evaluated on his or her own merits. As mentioned previously, Linus Pauling, Ph.D., the founder of orthomolecular medicine and a Nobel Prize winner, was a staunch advocate of the benefits of megadoses of vitamin C in the treatment of cancer. There is significant scientific research that supports Pauling's claims. Moreover, whether a Nobel Prize winner and molecular biologist should be considered a quack is best left up to the reader to decide.

Walters refutes the third myth, that "patients who seek alternative therapies are driven by desperation [and are] . . . ignorant, gullible or both," by stating that alternative cancer therapies tend to be sought by well-educated, affluent patients and that conventional practitioners tend to be supportive of them. He cites Cassileth's (1984) research showing that alternative therapies tended to be approved by primary physicians "30 percent of the time," and demonstrating that highly educated persons were drawn to alternative therapies by the desire to take more control over their health and the realization that conventional medicine has its limitations.

Walters dispels the fourth myth, that "alternative cancer therapies are 'unproven,' therefore untested and unscientific," by citing research indicating the presence of seventy-two alternative cancer therapies designated as unproven methods on the American Cancer Society (ACS) blacklist, of which 44 percent had not been investigated, 11 percent had yielded positive results, and 16 percent resulted in inconclusive findings.

Cancer is a complicated and frequently fatal disease. There is as of yet no cure. There are many patients for whom conventional therapies seem to eliminate the cancer; however, there are just as many patients who die from the disease after receiving conventional treatment. Ruling out all alternative therapies as useless is just as extreme as ruling out all conventional therapies as useless. There is much that we don't understand about the disease process of cancer, and thus it is rash to make such generalized pronouncements about alternative therapies. Rather, judgment as to the efficacy or futility of various forms of alternative treatment should be rendered only after thorough testing and collection of evidence.

A recent article by Lauran Neergaard (2006) points out that a study on chemotherapy side effects sheds new light on health outcomes. The study, which assessed the risks of chemotherapy in 35,000 patients under age 64 with breast cancer, found the following results: "Roughly one in six wind up in the emergency room or hospitalized because of side effects like infection, low blood counts, dehydration or nausea." The incidence of side effects in this study was three to four times higher than in previous studies. Dr. Michael Hassett, from the Dana-Farber Cancer Institute in Boston, led the research. Researchers extracted data from insurance claims on women who had breast cancer and ended up in the hospital after treatment, attempting to discern if the outcomes were chemotherapy related. They found that 61 percent of the breast cancer patients with chemo either visited the emergency room or were hospitalized, compared with 42 percent who did not have chemotherapy. Dr. Joseph Kay of the Tufts–New England Medical Center writes, "Better understanding of the risks is especially important for those patients who choose chemo despite a good prognosis, when it could increase their chances of survival by less than 5 percent." Neergaard concludes her article by saying, "Of course the extra care meant extra medical bills. Hassett estimated that serious chemo side effects could cost health plans up to $45 million a year."

A recent article on current cancer treatments by John Carey (2006) profiles Dr. David Eddy, heart surgeon turned economist, who is touted as "the father of evidence-based medicine." Evidence-based medicine is a healthcare reform movement that focuses on science-based protocols, and the need for data that support the efficacy of protocols used in medicine. Dr. Eddy's experience in dealing with the lack of evidence-based medicine and the "consumer mindset" that seeks new treatments, even in the absence of evidence establishing their efficacy, is enlightening. Carey writes,

> As a consultant on Blue Cross insurance coverage decisions, Eddy testified on the insurers' behalf in high profile court cases, such as bone marrow transplants for breast cancer. Women and doctors demanded the treatment, even though there was no evidence it saved lives. Insurers who refused coverage usually lost in court. "I was the bad guy," Eddy recalls. When clinical trials were actually done, they showed the treatment costing . . . $50,000–$150,000 didn't work. The doctors, who pushed the painful, risky procedure on women "owe this country an apology," Eddy says. (Carey 2006, p. 177)

One of the more interesting studies cited by Walters is the research of Harold Foster, Ph.D., reported in "Lifestyle Changes and the 'Spontaneous' Regression of Cancer: An Initial Computer Analysis" (1988). Foster's research reviewed 200 cases of spontaneous remission in cancer and concluded that "88 percent of the persons had made major dietary changes, switching to a strict vegetarian diet and avoiding white flour, sugar and canned or frozen foods—before their dramatic tumor regression or complete remission occurred." Many also used vitamins, minerals, and detoxification procedures in conjunction with dietary changes. Foster's research illustrates the impact of diet and nutrients on the healing process, neither of which is given major emphasis in conventional medicine.

As stated previously, some of the issues surrounding the regulation of alternative and complementary forms of healthcare involve safety and efficacy. Other legitimate concerns involve politics and control of medicine. At a meeting of the American Academy of Anti-Aging Medicine, holistic practitioners expressed concern that government regulation of many of the forms of therapy they currently use with success could force them out of business. Other issues focus on liability in the co-management of patients who are using conventional medicine as well as alternative and complementary forms of healthcare. How do conventional practitioners address their concerns, and how legitimate are liability concerns?

On the issues of safety and efficacy, you can find data to support both conventional medicine as well as alternative and complementary forms of healthcare. Whom do you believe? Whom do you trust? What works and what doesn't? The one absolute regarding alternative and complementary forms of healthcare is the importance of taking a more active approach to one's healthcare—in a sense becoming one's own health maintenance organization. Not all people are willing to do that. Further, the proper and effective use of alternative medicine involves mobilizing various healing forces, which include diet, exercise, prayer—whatever one must do to restore one's health. It is tempting to look for a simpler route, preferably through medication or a "magic bullet" approach, rather than taking a more active role in addressing health problems.

Keep in mind that change comes to medicine slowly. According to the IOM, innovations in medicine take roughly 17 years from the point of conception to integration into the mainstream. Further, in response to the introduction of a new treatment form, even with substantial public interest, the conventional medical community characteristically exhibits considerable reluctance, if not outright defiance. This was the case with the genesis of the NCCAM, as medical historian James C. Whorton points out in his book *Natural Cures: The History of Alternative Medicine* (2002). The initial government funding for evaluating the effectiveness of "the most promising alternative therapies" was a mere $2 million. However, administrators at the NIH apparently were displeased that the NCCAM received *any* funding and felt that political pressure rather than scientific consensus was granting legitimacy to alternative medicine. In the midst of pressure to begin research on alternative medicine, there were detractors: "The Berlin Wall [of medicine] was coming down," and some thought the Office of Alternative Medicine (the precursor to NCCAM) was "one step removed from the 'Office of Astrology'" (2002, p. 294).

CHAPTER 7

Should Managed Care Provide Coverage for Alternative Therapies?

The U.S. healthcare system is based on the disease model, the most costly of all models. People access the healthcare system when they've developed a health problem or when they become symptomatic. In most cases, managed care provides coverage for treatment of a disease but not for precautionary measures that could prevent or limit the disease. For example, managed care plans cover treatment of cancer, but many do not provide coverage for smoking cessation aids. Managed care bears the cost of treatment for obesity-related diseases such as hypertension and diabetes, as well as coverage for bariatric surgical procedures for the morbidly obese, but many plans do not provide coverage for health club memberships or incentive programs that focus on prevention, such as through weight loss. Many argue that the disease model needs to shift toward preventive care, which entails some additional costs in the short run but substantial cost savings over the long term.

David Eisenberg, M.D., points out in his article "Advising Patients Who Seek Alternative Medical Therapies" that some things are beginning to change. There has been a trend among third-party payers to provide alternative therapies as "expanded-benefits." "Oxford Health Plan began a program whereby chiropractic, acupuncture and naturopathy became available to the Plan's 1.5 million subscribers as paid benefits" (1997). Eisenberg's concerns focus on issues of responsibility on the part of the conventional practitioner who co-manages patients with alternative practitioners using therapies that have limited scientific data to support them.

Safety issues that govern alternative and complementary medicine, according to Peter Curtis, M.D., and Susan Gaylord, Ph.D., (2005) include "errors in treatment and medical management, adverse effects of pharmaceuticals and defining risk for patients." With respect to dietary supplements, issues of "quality control, licensing, regulation and misrepresentation" are cited. Other issues pointed out in Curtis and Gaylord's research are drug interactions between prescription medication and herbal remedies, and fragmented communications or lack thereof between clinicians. These are all legitimate concerns.

Concerns over the co-management of patients by alternative practitioners and conventional practitioners, both from a health and from a liability standpoint, appear to dominate the literature. The efficacy of alternative therapies, side effects of combining prescription drugs with alternative supplements, and uncertainty over which therapy is addressing the problem and which is impeding progress are frequently discussed.

Statistics that provide insight into the magnitude of attitudinal shifts regarding treatment modalities and interest in the exploration of alternative forms of healing can be found in an article by Eisenberg et al. (1998). In a randomized phone survey of 2055 adults in 1997, investigators found that the use of alternative therapies increased from 34 to 42 percent and office visits to alternative practitioners increased from 427 million to 629 million, a 47 percent increase, "exceeding total visits to all U.S. primary care physicians." Conservative estimates indicate that nearly $27 billion is spent annually for alternative and complementary forms of healthcare.

Additional concerns from the standpoint of managed care, beyond liability issues of co-management of patients, is the reported lack of scientific evidence supporting the efficacy of various forms of alternative and complementary forms of healthcare.

In research by Studdert et al. (1998) the focus was on malpractice issues with regard to practitioners who deliver alternative therapies and legal guidelines governing a regulated form of therapy, conventional medicine, versus an unregulated form of therapy, alternative and complementary medicine. Malpractice claims against chiropractors, massage therapists, and acupuncturists for the years 1990–1996 were found to be fewer than claims against traditional practitioners in the same time frame.

A pertinent issue surrounding the use of conventional medicine with alternative and complementary medicine is, what guidelines are used to govern their joint use? Are there standards for this governance in academic medical centers, tertiary care hospitals, and community-based hospitals? If so, what are they?

Research by Cohen et al. (2005) sheds light on some of these important issues. In an article titled "Emerging Credentialing Practices, Malpractice Liability Policies, and Guidelines Governing Complementary and Alternative Medical Practices and Dietary Supplement Recommendations," Cohen and colleagues looked at nineteen hospitals and their policies governing the integration of traditional and complementary/alternative medical therapies and providers. Their survey included twenty-one academic health centers and thirteen non–academically affiliated hospitals. The nineteen institutions that responded included eleven tertiary care hospitals, six community hospitals, one free-standing center, and one university-based rehabilitation hospital.

Their conclusion was that none of the institutions had a consistent approach to "provider mix and authority within the integrated team, with minimum requirements for professional liability coverage, informed consent and hiring status." Less than 33 percent had formal policies regarding dietary supplements, and the supplements in the pharmacy "lacked consistent, evidenced-based rationales regarding brands to include or exclude."

Cohen et al. (2005) provided the following formal conclusions:

> Hospitals are using heterogeneous approaches to address licensure, credentialing, malpractice liability and dietary supplement use in developing models of integrative care. The environment creates significant impediments to the delivery of consistent clinical care and multiple evaluations of the safety, efficacy and cost-effectiveness (or lack thereof) of CAM therapies (or models) as applied to management of common medical conditions. Consensus policies need to be developed.

Are their ethical issues for clinicians to consider when either co-managing patients with joint allegiance to conventional and alternative practitioners, or referring patients to a complementary or alternative practitioner? If so, what are they? Karen Adams et al. (2002) touch on these issues in their article "Ethical Considerations of Complementary and Alternative Medical Therapies in Conventional Medical Settings." They suggest the application of a risk-benefit model as one method for determining the appropriateness of complementary and alternative medical therapy. Their model includes

> severity and acuteness of condition; the curability of the illness by conventional forms of treatment; the degree of invasiveness, associated toxicities and side effects of the conventional treatment; the availability and quality of evidence of utility and safety of the desired CAM treatment combined with the patient's knowing and voluntary acceptance of those risks; and the patient's persistence of intention to use CAM therapies.

As a result of the lack of current regulatory oversight of CAM thera-pies and concerns over their efficacy, the risk-benefit model appears to be a reasonable approach on the part of clinicians to the co-management of patients or their referral to complementary practitioners. This risk-benefit model should have as its underlying purpose to provide, as Adams et al. (2002) so aptly conclude, recommendations that are "clinically sound, ethically appropriate and targeted to the unique circumstances of individual patients."

Understanding the quality-of-life issues the patient must deal with as well as the beliefs and value system that prompt the patient to seek a rem-edy for the particular health problem should be at the forefront of the practitioner's mind in consulting with the patient and recommending treatment options. Eisenberg et al. (1998) noted that $27 billion was spent on alternative and complementary forms of healthcare in 1997, the bulk of which was not covered by insurance. This level of out-of-pocket expenses speaks volumes concerning the degree of dissatisfaction among con-sumers with the limitations of conventional medicine and their willing-ness to explore other pathways to health, even at their own expense.

Kenneth Pelletier, M.D., notes in his book *The Best Alternative Medi-cine* (2000) that, to date, there is no centralized database reporting type of CAM coverage by insurance carrier, nationwide. The more progressive states appear to have taken the lead in providing CAM coverage, but little is available in the way of comparisons to draw from.

In a review of the educational Web sites of the major managed care companies in the Bluegrass region of Kentucky (United Healthcare, Anthem, and Humana), it is reported that most are focused on customiz-ing health plans to suit the needs of the consumer, not unlike the automo-bile insurance companies, with various types of coverage and deductible ranges. Their approach appears to be based on the insurance models used in the automobile industry. If you're a safe driver and are the only house-hold member licensed to drive, you would purchase a policy with the highest deductible with collision, as the probabilities are that you will not have an accident or need to file a claim. The benefit to you as a consumer is that you pay less in premiums.

Continuing with the model of insurance in the automobile industry, if you live in a household with two teenagers who have just received their driver's licenses and tend to be careless drivers, you clearly require a dif-ferent type of policy. To determine the type of coverage needed, you would have to factor in their ages, their levels of responsibility, and the probabili-ties of their becoming involved in accidents and getting speeding tickets. As a result, the type of coverage required would tend to be more expensive, based on the law of averages, their teenage status, and the probabilities of speeding tickets and accidents. This cumulative "risk factor" would place them in a high-risk, high-cost category. The result is that you'll pay more for coverage, as they represent a likelihood of higher costs to the insurer.

Health Savings Accounts, in principle, seem to apply a comparable approach in customizing health care coverage to the consumer. If you're in excellent health, have no preexisting conditions, and are within the normal weight range for your height, then your health plan will be one with high deductibles and minimal coverage, as the probability is high that you will not need extensive healthcare services. On the other hand, if you or your family members have significant health conditions, requiring numerous prescriptions and frequent office visits, your coverage will be more costly.

Consumer Web sites for the managed care companies surveyed include generic information on Health Savings Accounts. Some programs are geared toward patient education, for example, preparing patients for weight loss surgery. There are wellness programs focused on mailings to patients reminding them of various screenings and support programs for those with chronic conditions, such as diabetes, to enhance health outcomes. Various types of care coordination programs are available, such as a 24-hour, on-call RN program to answer questions from members, as well as sources of information on patient safety listing reports and publications from the Institute of Medicine, as well as patient alerts from the Agency for Health Research Quality.

Some of the more progressive managed care companies had sites allowing consumers to access the quality rating of the hospital where they are scheduled to have surgery, as well as the clinician's date of graduation and the educational facility providing the clinician's medical training. Some managed care companies had sites called "Condition Centers," where consumers with asthma or diabetes can access information and education about managing their conditions more successfully. There were sites that provided access to medical libraries, clinical drug libraries, and audio libraries offering information on health topics, and there were also sites that provided information and support on first pregnancies, coronary vascular disease and ongoing heart health, and rare neurological diseases, including lupus, multiple sclerosis, and cystic fibrosis.

With respect to CAM coverage by insurance companies, Pelletier (2000, p. 281) conducted research on eighteen insurance companies in 1997 and found that the majority provided some coverage for "nutrition counseling, biofeedback, psychotherapy, acupuncture, preventive medicine, chiropractic, osteopathy, and/or physical therapy." Very few offered total coverage of CAM therapy, "with 22 percent offering sixteen to twenty therapies, 39 percent offering eleven to fifteen therapies, and 39 percent offering six to ten therapies. Smaller companies offered a greater number of CAM therapies than did larger ones."

Pelletier's research into CAM coverage, which is probably one of the most comprehensive in the literature, outlines the types of policies available, from the most to the least comprehensive. The most comprehensive plans covered visits to CAM practitioners including "chiropractors, naturopaths and acupuncturists." The second tier of CAM coverage offered discounted rates for CAM practitioners of 10 to 30 percent. The third tier of coverage consisted of companies that offer a CAM rider policy, in which additional are costs incurred by the member either monthly or through a co-payment, and include benefits for "chiropractic services, acupuncture, naturopathy and massage." The fourth tier of CAM coverage included "other limited benefit forms." Covered benefits included Dr. Dean Ornish's diet for reversing coronary heart disease.

Pelletier found that regions of the country that appeared to have the most widespread use of CAM therapies included the Pacific Northwest, California, New England, and the upper Midwest, typically the areas most active in embracing cultural change.

Research conducted by Cleary-Guida et al. (2001) on insurance coverage for CAM therapies, reported under the title "A Regional Survey of Health Insurance Coverage for Complementary and Alternative Medicine: Current Status and Future Ramifications," assessed three states in the Northeast, namely New York, New Jersey, and Connecticut. The researchers found that "almost all insurers surveyed covered chiropractic services, less than half covered acupuncture, usually for chronic pain management . . . coverage of massage therapy was minimal and usually associated with either physical therapy or chiropractic treatment. Other CAM services received negligible coverage." They also commented that the wide variation in policies, practitioner licensing requirements, and health plans themselves made the analysis of CAM coverage quite confusing.

The impact of state legislation on the use of CAM therapies was demonstrated in the research conducted by Sturm and Unutzer (2000–2001) and reported under the title "State Legislation and the Use of Complementary and Alternative Medicine." They used data from a survey of 10,000 individuals to assess CAM usage, insurance coverage, and the effect of state regulations. Their findings were that "insurance mandates to cover CAM providers were significantly associated with increased coverage of CAM, but not with increased use of CAM providers. Liberalization of physician licensure to practice CAM is associated with significantly increased CAM use, as are practice laws authorizing nonphysician CAM providers." Additionally, in states with multiple CAM laws, insurance coverage for CAM visits was found to be significantly lower than for states without the practice laws.

Tindle et al. (2005), in their article "Trends in Use of Complementary and Alternative Medicine by U.S. Adults: 1997–2002," determined which types of CAM therapies had been used to the largest extent and a provided a description of those who utilized CAM therapies. They compared two national surveys of CAM use: the Alternative Health/Complementary and Alternative Medicine supplement to the 2002 National Health Interview Survey (NHIS), consisting of 31,044 subjects; and a 1997 national survey of 2055 subjects. Their conclusions: "Herbal therapy was the most widely used (18.6 percent), with 38 million U.S. adults, followed by relaxation therapy (14.2 percent), representing 29 million U.S. adults, followed by chiropractic (7.4 percent), representing 15 million U.S. adults." Those who used CAM tended to be age 40 to 64, female, and non-black/non-Hispanic, with annual incomes of $65,000 and above. The greatest increase in CAM usage between 1997 and 2002 was seen in herbal medicine (12.1–18.6 percent) and yoga (3.7–5.1 percent).

A comprehensive review of the issues surrounding insurance coverage of CAM therapies as well as efficacy arguments can be found in Bruce Barrett's article "Alternative, Complementary and Conventional Medicine: Is Integration upon Us?" Barrett noted that in 2003, the date of the article's publication, four in ten Americans could be expected to use complementary and alternative medicine. In the state of Washington, coverage of CAM therapy has been given a legislative mandate, as a result of which "integrated" delivery systems coupling conventional and alternative/complementary systems have begun to emerge.

The initial resistance and antagonism toward alternative and complementary forms of healthcare are beginning to be replaced with a degree of acceptance by conventional medicine. Barrett attributes that shift partly to the more than 5000 randomized controlled trials under way to evaluate various complementary and alternative forms of therapy. Additionally, the provision of CAM therapies involves issues of consumer demand and economics; payments totaling roughly $27 billion annually cannot be excluded as a factor contributing to its acceptance into the mainstream.

Signs of the shift toward acceptance by the mainstream include the following:

> The majority of medical schools now offer courses in CAM; widespread agreement that medical schools should include education regarding CAM; experience at . . . the University of Wisconsin, where an evening, elective CAM course, for two years running, had the highest enrollment rate in the medical school's history; residencies offering and requiring rotations in

CAM; and a post-residency fellowship in integrated medicine through the University of Health Sciences Center in Tucson, graduating the first generation of physician-CAM-specialists in the country. (Barrett 2003, p. 420)

Barrett (2003, p. 423) points out the critical factors that will determine CAM's integration into the mainstream: "While political and economic forces are clearly involved, it is the underlying belief system, world view, or philosophical orientation of individuals—replete with values, preferences, prejudices and desires—that will control the direction and scope of this social process."

The problems (barriers) and the opportunities (facilitators) of integration, as outlined by Barrett, provide a comprehensive overview of the issues at stake and include

belief in the effectiveness of CAM, among patients, healthcare providers and health care system decision-makers; competition for patients (facilitators) versus cost containment (barriers); consumer demand (facilitators) versus fear of liability (barriers); evidence of efficacy (facilitators) versus momentum, i.e., habits and ingrained behaviors (barriers); lack of effectiveness of conventional medicine (facilitators) versus lack of availability (barriers); evidence of cost effectiveness (facilitators) versus lack of efficacy evidence (barriers); low overall costs (facilitators) versus lack of insurance coverage (barriers); and lower risks of CAM therapies (facilitators) versus lack of standards, credentialing and regulation (barriers). (Barrett 2003, p. 422)

Margaret A. Colgate's (1995) research into the integration of CAM with twelve managed care companies and two trade unions provides insight into the factors that contributed to the successful integration of chiropractic, acupuncture, and biofeedback: "gaining accreditation for its educational system; licensing its practitioners; developing standards of practice guidelines; and conducting research to establish efficacy and safety." She points out that the success experienced in obtaining third-party reimbursement is the result of the companies and unions implementing strategies of their own, as well as meeting standards set by the biomedical community and by the insurance systems.

The potential barriers and facilitators to the integration of CAM into mainstream medicine that Barrett identifies constitute a case of "good news/bad news," as most of the factors he points to are both facilitators and barriers. I'm reminded of the Chinese translation of "crisis" as "opportunity riding on dangerous winds." If CAM therapies are here to stay, then forward-thinking individuals will need to begin the process of translating perceived "problems" into opportunities. That change in thinking will, in large part, determine the success or failure of the integration process itself.

CHAPTER 8

Pharmaceuticals versus Alternative Therapies

This chapter will focus on the choice of pharmaceuticals over alternative therapies in the treatment of disease and will outline some of the controversies in this arena. The Institute of Medicine reports that errors in prescription medication cost roughly $2 billion dollars annually (Institute of Medicine 1999). A second report published by the Institute of Medicine (IOM) claims that "medical errors kill more people per year than breast cancer, AIDS or motor vehicle accidents" (Institute of Medicine 2000).

What this means to the average consumer is that there are risks and benefits in taking any prescription medication. Further, if consumers are taking multiple medications, the side-effect profile of multiple prescriptions could qualify as a medical condition of its own. Jerry Avorn (2004, p. 217) points out that $200 billion annually is currently spent for prescription medication in the United States, making prescription medication the most rapidly escalating area of healthcare, with a growth rate of 13 to 19 percent annually. Although the United States spends more than any other industrialized nation on prescription drugs, we do not have the most favorable health outcomes in exchange for those expenditures. We're spending more but getting less.

According to the Agency for Health Research Quality report *Medical Errors: The Scope of the Problem* (2000), medical errors account for roughly $37.6 billion annually in wasted expenditures and poor health outcomes, even deaths in many instances, and $17 billion of those expenditures are thought to be due to preventable errors. The

National Patient Safety Foundation statistics (AHRQ 2000) indicate the following:

- "Forty-two percent of respondents had been affected by a medical error, either personally or through a friend."
- "Thirty-two percent of the respondents indicated that the error had a permanent negative effect on the patient's health."

If consumers are concerned about safety issues, they certainly have a right to be, based on the responses in this survey. When 42 percent of respondents either have been adversely affected by a medical error or know someone who has, that is justification for concern. Further, when 32 percent have suffered a permanent negative effect on their health, it makes one pause to question the process they've gone through and to identify what can be done to avoid further problems in the future.

A second survey, by the American Society of Health-System Pharmacists, indicated that Americans have great concern over the following: "Being given the wrong medication (61 percent); being given two or more medicines that interact in a negative way (58 percent); and complications from a medical procedure (56 percent)" (AHRQ 2000).

Ivan Illich, in his book *Medical Nemesis* (1976), uses the term *iatrogenic*, meaning "caused by the physician," to refer to medical conditions that are caused or exacerbated by prescription drugs, invasive procedures, radiation, and other interventions used in conventional medicine. When one recalls that in 2000 the United States spent more on healthcare than any other industrialized nation—$1.4 trillion—and ranked thirty-seventh in health system effectiveness, one is forced to question where the dollars went. Other nations that spent far less than the United States had better outcomes in two specific areas where healthcare expenditures count: life expectancy and disability-adjusted life expectancy. These figures should raise questions among those who look to the healthcare system as a panacea for resolving complicated health conditions and who fail to take greater responsibility for their own healthcare through diet and exercise.

A PILL FOR SHYNESS?

One significant issue within the pharmaceutical industry is the medicalization of various conditions. A recent commercial on television for a "block-buster antidepressant" indicated that it could be used to treat shyness. The spot showed a young professional man unable to present his material before a corporate board meeting. After taking the new product, he not only was able to give the presentation but won the account.

I would question the authenticity of a drug that claims to "cure" shyness. Shyness, after all, may be a personality characteristic, one that is sometimes referred to as introversion, not a medical condition to be "cured."

A concern of many with respect to the use of prescription drugs is the quality of the science underlying their effectiveness and the challenges posed by potential "conflicts of interest" of the scientists charged with evaluating their efficacy. A recent news article (Vergano 2006) illustrates the point. The article highlights a recent study (forthcoming in the journal *Psychotherapy and Psychosomatics*) investigating the financial ties of the medical experts who created the *Diagnostic and Statistical Manual for Mental Disorders* (*DSM*), the manual used "as the basis for insurance payments for psychiatric treatments, including drugs." The study evaluated 170 medical experts who participated in writing the two most recent editions of this manual to assess whether they had financial ties to companies whose products are represented in the manual. Of the 170 experts, 56 percent had "one or more ties" to the pharmaceutical industry. In the area of schizophrenia and mood disorders, more than 80 percent of the panel for "anxiety disorders, 'medication-induced-movement disorders,' and premenstrual dysphonic disorder had financial ties" (Vergano 2006, p. 6A).

The journal *PLOS Medicine* is quoted as accusing the pharmaceutical industry of "disease mongering," or manufacturing diseases such as "restless leg syndrome" and of "widening definitions to sweep up more patients" (Vergano 2006, p. 6A). As Lisa Cosgrove of the University of Massachusetts–Boston, the lead author of the study, points out, "No blood tests exist for the disorders in the *DSM*. It relies on judgments from practitioners who rely on the manual." Ken Johnson, a pharmaceutical industry spokesman, responded that the "health care professionals on these panels have 'impeccable integrity and base their decisions on independent judgments and research'" (Vergano 2006, p. 6A).

Financial conflicts of interest do not necessarily mean that the science is compromised, but they certainly bring up an issue of concern with respect to objectivity. Ideally, the science and recommendations of efficacy stemming from that science should be straightforward. When undisclosed financial conflicts of interest become part of the equation, a red flag of caution is raised.

Another area of concern with respect to prescription drugs was illustrated in a study (Radley et al. 2006), published in the *Archives of Internal Medicine*, of off-label prescribing—that is, prescribing a medication for indications other than the condition or disease for which it was officially approved. Such medications may lack the scientific evidence to support the off-label usage. Drs. David Radley, Stan Finkelstein, and Randall

Stafford evaluated 160 commonly used drugs and their prescription patterns from the *2001 IMS Health National Disease and Therapeutic Index*, a nationally representative sample. The researchers' intent was to evaluate the frequency of off-label drug use as well as the degree of scientific evidence supporting the off-label prescribing. They found that in the year 2001, "there was an estimated 150 million off-label mentions (21 percent of overall use) among the sampled medications." Off-label use was most common with cardiac medications (46 percent), with the exception of antihyperlipidemic and antihypertensive agents. Anticonvulsants (46 percent) were highly represented in off-label prescribing, with gabapentin (83 percent) and amitriptyline hydrochloride (81 percent) having the highest percentage of off-label usage. The authors note that most off-label usage had "little or no scientific support." They concluded, "Off-label medication use is common in outpatient care, and most occurs without support. Efforts should be made to scrutinize underevaluated off-label prescribing that compromises patient safety or represents wasteful medication use."

A Cox News Service article (2006) with the headline "Medicine 'More Guesswork than Science'" begins with the question "Are Americans taking too much medicine that doesn't really do much good?" It went on to say, "Even today, with a high-tech health care system that costs the nation $2 trillion a year, there is little or no evidence that many widely used treatments and procedures actually work better than various cheaper alternatives."

GOT SCIENCE?

A feature story in *BusinessWeek* magazine (Carey 2006) highlights the work of Dr. David Eddy, a cardiac surgeon turned health economist, who coined the term *evidence-based medicine* in the early 1980s. Evidence-based medicine demands underlying scientific justification for the medication or treatment approach—in other words, the evidence and the data establishing that the treatment options used actually work to correct the problem.

Eddy's interest in evidence-based medicine stems from his experience as a cardiac surgeon at Stanford Medical Center in the 1970s. When he asked whether there was evidence to support many of the protocols utilized to treat patients, the response from colleagues was no. In fact, the protocols used were developed primarily as a result of "rules and traditions handed down over the years, as opposed to real scientific proof" (Carey 2006, p. 75).

As a result of that conversation, Eddy concluded that computer models could be designed to mimic clinical trials and could be used to evaluate the efficacy of treatment options. He first looked at diabetes and compared the conventional approach with an alternative treatment of aspirin and generic drugs to lower cholesterol and blood pressure. When put to the test, the alternative option proved superior to the conventional approach in reducing the incidence of heart attack and stroke, which are common with diabetes.

Kaiser Permanente's Care Management Institute, the group to which Eddy first presented his model, has since implemented his alternative treatment approach with roughly one million subjects in their care. The good news is that Eddy's model is, in fact, improving the care of those individuals as well as reducing costs. It was the first managed care company in the United States to implement Dr. Eddy's novel approach. The company was also instrumental in having the drug Vioxx removed from the market as a result of a spike in sudden cardiac deaths among members in its database.

To illustrate the pervasiveness of the lack of evidence-based medicine in many areas of medicine, Eddy frequently conducted his version of the litmus test at medical specialty meetings. He would ask the group to identify a typical patient and a standard treatment and conclude with the treatment result. Eddy would then ask the society's president to read the results of the group exercise. The result was that the predictions of success for various procedures had no consensus and ranged from 0 to 100 percent. The participants, in an attempt to quantify the results, came up with different answers. Eddy's comment on that: "I've spent 25 years proving that what we lovingly call clinical judgment is woefully outmatched by the complexities of medicine. . . . Go to one doctor, get one answer. . . . Go to another, and you get another one" (Carey 2006, p. 76).

Rather than waste precious lives and resources, Eddy's computer model, dubbed "Archimedes," is designed to mimic through technology the biology of the body and to evaluate the efficacy and cost of treatment options. The computer model, designed by Eddy and particle physicist Len Schlessinger, compares treatment approaches through a program that simulates a thirty-year clinical trial in thirty minutes, with initial results modeling Eddy's prediction. Dr. Richard Kahn, chief scientific officer of the American Diabetes Association, comments, "It is at least 10 times better than the model we use now, which is called thinking" (Carey 2006, p. 75).

Gerard Anderson, director of the Center for Hospital Finance and Management at Johns Hopkins University's Bloomberg School of Public Health, states in the article, "The investment in health care in the U.S. is just not paying off" (Carey 2006, p. 78). An executive of healthcare at one of the largest corporations in the United States comments, "There is a massive amount of spending on things that really don't help patients, and even put them at greater risk. Everyone that's informed on the topic knows it, but it is such a scary thing to discuss that people are not willing to talk about it openly" (Carey 2006, p. 78).

Dr. Paul Wallace, senior advisor at Kaiser Permanente's Care Management Institute, points out that "the popular version of evidence-based medicine is about proving things, but it is really about transparency, being clear about what we know and don't know" (Carey 2006, p. 78). One obvious implication is that when medicine doesn't have the evidence to support the protocols being used, the consumer needs to be informed that the outcomes are simply not there, that medicine simply doesn't know what works or does not work. Studies reflect that when patients are presented with the science (or lack of it) underlying treatment options, they tend to select less invasive, more conservative options. The critical issue is for the patient to fully understand the options available (informed consent).

BARIATRICS AND BYPASSES

Another example of the medicalization of certain conditions, on a par with the use of pharmaceuticals to treat shyness, is bariatric surgery used in the treatment of the morbidly obese. The condition of morbid obesity, which in the past was simply known as being overweight, is now a high-growth area of healthcare, primarily because morbid obesity has recently been classified as a medical condition and covered by insurance. There are substantial risks with this procedure, particularly if the patient has comorbidities—other conditions that go hand in hand with obesity. These comorbidities include high blood pressure and diabetes.

Not only is bariatric surgery risky in itself, but research has shown that if the patient does not make necessary changes in diet and exercise after the weight loss, then once the surgical procedure has been reversed, the weight returns and health conditions are compounded. The patient seeking a "magic bullet"—a procedure or pill that will eliminate all health problems, with no risk and preferably in short order—is simply living in a fool's paradise. There are no magic bullets. It's often stated in the literature by scholars, clinicians, and holistic health practitioners alike that the majority of health problems can be mediated through diet and exercise alone. If so, then the individual holds the power to make changes. This is the true, unheralded "magic bullet."

A *Forbes* magazine cover story (Langreth 2004), discussed in Chapter 1, illustrates this point. The article provides a comprehensive overview of the most common health conditions experienced by Americans, the costs involved with prescription drug coverage, and the costs involved with alternative therapies. Further, it describes the case of Wesley Miller, which is useful to keep in mind, as it illustrates the risks and benefits on both sides of the aisle: conventional medicine versus alternative therapies.

Miller, a retired food service worker from West Virginia, underwent a coronary triple-bypass procedure in 1994. In 2001 he was taking sixteen different prescription drugs, among them Lipitor for cholesterol, Glucotrol for diabetes, and three diuretics to lower blood pressure. The blockages had returned, but Miller was a high-risk patient and surgery was not advisable. Fortunately, he discovered Dr. Dean Ornish's "low-tech" regimen of low fat, daily exercise, stress reduction, and group support. The outcome: his angina lessened, he lost 49 pounds in eight months, his cholesterol level decreased from 243 to 110, and his blood sugar fell into normal range. Miller felt that his life had been given back to him.

It was fortunate for Miller that he was not a candidate for a second bypass procedure, because the alternative approach that included diet, exercise, and noninvasive methods to address stress reduction proved to be the solution. This is one of thousands of examples that illustrate the long-term benefits of alternative therapies and the use of simple, commonsense measures to address serious health problems in preference to prescription drugs and invasive procedures that can have significant long-term health outcomes that are less than ideal.

CONVENTIONAL MEDICAL WISDOM: HORMONE REPLACEMENT THERAPY

Another example that illustrates the iatrogenic effects of traditional healthcare, with its use of prescription drugs, is hormone replacement therapy (HRT), which has been widely used for decades in the United States to treat menopausal and postmenopausal women. Considered the "gold standard" treatment, HRT, which constitutes an attempt to replace the estrogen no longer produced by an aging woman's ovaries with estrogen extracted from other sources (such as pregnant mares' urine—hence the brand name Premarin), was touted as the "fountain of youth" for women and was thought to prevent heart disease as well as slow the aging process and maintain mental acuity. The Women's Health Initiative (2002) study results provided a very different conclusion. Avorn (2004, p. 23) observed, "Many years later modern scientific studies revealed that the long-term ingestion of the horse-urine extract was useless for most of its intended purposes, and that it caused tumors, blood clots, heart disease and perhaps brain damage." Avorn described the debacle as the largest "medically induced health epidemic in U.S. history" (2004, p. 23).

In short, the "gold standard" was doing more harm than good and had been doing so for forty-plus years. When I heard the results of the Women's Health Initiative study, my first reaction was to wonder how many other protocols currently touted as the "gold standard" are in fact creating or compounding health conditions instead of resolving them.

SALES TRUMPING SCIENCE

One last issue with respect to prescription drugs involves the focus on sales to the detriment of science in the drug industry, as recently pointed out in another *Forbes* article (Langreth and Herper 2006). Jurgen Drews, a former Roche research chief, points out, "The dominance of marketing over research has done real damage to company pipelines" (2006, p. 96). He was referring to the fact that actual research in innovative, life-saving drugs has lapsed, with a greater emphasis and more dollars being directed toward sales, as evidenced by the fact that eighty-seven major drugs have lost their patent protection since 2002, with only twenty new drugs recently approved by the FDA for their replacement.

Direct-to-consumer pharmaceutical advertising, which had been prohibited before the 1990s, has contributed to the increased spending on sales by the drug industry. "Ad spending in the U.S. has soared eight-fold in nine years to $4.8 billion," according to Nielsen Monitor-Plus (Langreth and Herper 2006, p. 97). "TV spots ply supposed low-risk, quick fixes to millions of people: Try Zoloft to get happy; gobble a state-of-the-art pain pill when aspirin would work fine. Drugs designed for a narrow set of patients end up in the hands of a far broader audience" (Langreth and Herper 2006, p. 97). Dr. Robert Centor, a University of Alabama internist, comments that the advertising "creates demand where there's not even disease" (Langreth and Herper 2006, p. 97).

For the pharmaceutical industry, making a market, or creating consumer demand, requires the medicalization of a problem, whose resolution takes the form of a prescription medication. The problem of sleeplessness (insomnia) is a case in point. Langreth and Herper (2006, p. 98) report that there has been a 48 percent increase in the use of sleeping pills in the last five years, with 43 million prescriptions written each year. With respect to the efficacy of these new drugs—what they offer that's "bigger and better" compared with existing products—John Abramson from

Harvard points out that "the newer drugs are no better than older ones costing about one-tenth as much. . . . Has insomnia become an epidemic in the past five years? Or are the makers skillfully leading Americans to an expensive drug?" (Langreth and Herper 2006, p. 102).

The entire issue with prescription drugs boils down to concerns of safety and efficacy—does the drug correct the problem, and at what risk to the patient? Some of the clinical trials evaluating these issues may be skewed in favor of the drug manufacturer. A recent study published in the *American Journal of Psychiatry* found that in twenty-one studies evaluating the efficacy of drugs manufactured by Lilly and Johnson & Johnson to treat schizophrenia, "90 percent of the time conclusions favor the sponsor's drugs" (Langreth and Herper 2006, p. 100). A second study, published in the *Archives of Internal Medicine*, reviewed fifty-six studies of painkillers and found that none of the studies indicated the sponsor's drug to be inferior (Langreth and Herper 2006, p. 100).

Jack E. Rosenblatt, a psychiatrist, comments, "The comparative studies are a joke. They are comical. A lot of the scientific literature these days is worthless. The whole process has been corrupted" (Langreth and Herper 2006, p. 102).

A QUESTION OF TRUST

So, the issues come down to the question of trust. Whom do you believe? What choices do you make? Do you opt for conventional medicine or alternative therapies? Those are decisions only you can make. However, others can provide guidance for those choices. Listen to what they say, weigh the risks and benefits, and make your own decision. Andrew Weil (1983, p. 24), an integrative practitioner, provides a risk-benefit model to evaluate conventional versus alternative therapies that certainly provides food for thought.

"Regular medicine is the most effective for dealing with many common and serious problems, namely acute trauma, acute infections associated with bacteria, protozoa, some fungi, parasites and a few other organisms; acute medical emergencies and acute surgical emergencies," says Weil (1983, p. 24). In other words, these are the strengths of conventional medicine—what, in his opinion, it can do and what, in his experience, works.

Weil goes on to discuss the weaknesses of conventional medicine:

> I would look elsewhere for help if I contracted a severe viral disease, like hepatitis or polio, or a metabolic disease like diabetes. I would not seek allopathic treatment for cancer, except for a few varieties, or for such chronic ailments as arthritis, asthma, hypertension, multiple sclerosis or

many other chronic diseases of the digestive, circulatory, musculoskeletal and nervous systems. Although allopaths give lip service to the concept of preventive medicine, for practical purposes they are unable to prevent most diseases that disable and kill people today. (Weil 1983, p. 24)

Clearly, there are prescription drugs that are beneficial and life-saving for millions. However, this chapter is dedicated to looking at both sides of the equation, which includes analyzing the benefits and risks of both alternative therapies and prescription drugs.

The downsides of alternative therapies have been pointed out by many researchers and include questions of safety and efficacy. Curtis and Gaylord (2005) identify some of the safety concerns as "errors in treatment and medical management; adverse effects of pharmaceuticals; and defining risks for patients." Their cautionary tale involves complementary and alternative therapies related to dietary supplements: issues of quality control, licensing, regulation, and misrepresentation. Other issues involve drug interactions with prescription drugs and herbal remedies, and difficulties in communication between conventional and alternative practitioners.

Barry Beyerstein, a staunch critic of the void of science underlying alternative therapies, begins his article (2001) with the following question: "Why do so many otherwise intelligent patients and therapists pay considerable sums for products and therapies of alternative medicine, even though most of these either are known to be useless or dangerous or have not been subjected to rigorous scientific testing?" He goes on to point out that patients who subscribe to alternative therapies are making errors in reasoning, such as wishful thinking and believing that an alternative therapy has worked when, in fact, the disease may have just run its course.

Wallace Sampson, another critic of alternative therapies, states that "CAM therapies are anomalous practices for which claims of efficacy are either unproved or disproved" (2000). He criticizes the advocacy approach to introducing and teaching CAM therapies in medical schools, in place of a critical assessment approach, as being a critical contributing factor to the problem. Of the fifty-six courses in CAM therapy taught in medical school curricula from 1995 through 1997, only four encouraged critique or analyses. He also claims that one of the reasons behind CAM's "unwarranted acceptance" is the alteration of standards for evaluation, which he claims is highly problematic.

One commonly practiced alternative therapy is prayer. Much has been written about the use of prayer, and according to the National Center for Complementary and Alternative Medicine at NIH, it is the most widely used alternative therapy, cutting across boundaries of race, class, gender, and geography. A recent $2.4 million study, the "largest scientific test of its kind" (Ritter 2006, p. A4), concluded that the patients in the study showed no benefit from intercessory prayer (i.e., being prayed for by others).

In this study, surgical patients were divided into three groups of 600 each, with one group knowing that they were being prayed for, the second group knowing intercessory prayer was a possibility, and the third group not prayed for. Complications from the surgical procedures were reviewed 30 days following the procedure. The results were that 59 percent of prayed-for patients developed complications, versus 52 percent of those who knew that prayer was a possibility.

In this study, contrary to the claims of Larry Dossey, Weil, and numerous other authors in alternative medicine, intercessory prayer appeared to have a negligible effect on the patients involved in the study. Dr. Harold Koenig, director of the Center for Spirituality, Theology and Health at Duke University, did not find the results of the study surprising and pointed out that there are inherent challenges in applying the tools of science to study the supernatural. He concludes the article with the following statement: "There is no god in either the Christian, Jewish or Muslim scriptures that can be constrained to the point that they can be predicted" (Ritter 2006, p. A4).

CHAPTER 9

Culture and Health: Who Bears Responsibility for Health and Healthcare?

In July 2000, the World Health Organization (WHO) published *World Health Report 2000,* based on the WHO Global Programme on Evidence for Health Policy in conjunction with the regional offices of the WHO. The report evaluated 191 countries worldwide on five indicators of health system effectiveness, using a composite score. The WHO was interested in what each country spent on healthcare and what it received for those expenditures. The United States spent $1.4 trillion at that time, more than any other country in the study, yet ranked thirty-seventh in overall system effectiveness (WHO 2000).

In terms of morbidity and mortality rates, the United States fared no better than the other industrialized nations, most of which spent a fraction of the dollar amount that Americans spent (WHO 2000). Further, citizens of many European countries such as France, Italy, and Spain outlived U.S. men and women by several years in terms of both life expectancy and disability-adjusted life expectancy (WHO 2000). The obvious question is, if the dollars we're spending are not reducing the incidence of disease, death, or disability, than what is the value of the expenditures?

Doing what works means assessing the return on investment of healthcare expenditures. Are we investing wisely? A recent news article points out that the United States leads the pack in rates of diabetes, heart disease, stroke, lung disease, and cancer, regardless of educational level or socioeconomic status (Johnson and Stobbe 2006). Spending more apparently does not equate to better health. Dr. Michael Marmot, epidemiologist and coauthor of the study, says that the primary question that should be up for discussion is, "Why isn't the richest country in the world the healthiest country in the world?" The article reports that the United States spent roughly $5200 per capita, in contrast to England, which spent roughly half of that amount; yet the Americans fared worse than the British, not better. Gerard Anderson, a chronic disease specialist in international health at Johns Hopkins University, comments, "I knew we were less healthy, but I didn't know the magnitude of the disparities." Explanations for the differences ranged from lack of money to excessive stress in the lives of Americans. In an analysis of the obesity problem in the United States, with computer models generating hypothetical parallels with lifestyle-related risk factors common among Americans superimposed on the British, Americans remained more disease-prone than the British.

The actual statistics comparing rates of disease were reported as follows: "Americans reported twice the rate of diabetes compared to the English (12.5 percent to 6 percent); for high blood pressure (42 percent for Americans versus 34 percent for the English); cancer showed up in 9.5 percent of Americans versus 5.5 percent of the English" (Johnson and Stobbe 2006, p. A3). The study was published in the *Journal of the American Medical Association* and was based on the 2002 Health and Retirement Survey in the United States and the 2002 English Longitudinal Survey of Aging.

A news article released about a month later stated that Canadians can now be added to the list of "foreigners who are healthier than Americans" (Stobbe 2006, p. B10). The article reports on a recent study by Dr. Steffie Woolhandler, soon to be published in the *American Journal of Public Health*, that found "Americans are 42 percent more likely than Canadians to have diabetes, 32 percent more likely to have high blood pressure, and 12 percent more likely to have arthritis" (Stobbe 2006, p. B10).

The article further reports that "about 21 percent of Americans said they were obese, compared with 15 percent of Canadians. And about 13.5 percent of the Americans admitted to a sedentary lifestyle, versus 6.5 percent of Canadians" (Stobbe 2006, p. B10). An interesting finding was that although more Canadians (19 percent) than Americans (17 percent) smoked, and more Americans (92 percent) than Canadians (83 percent) had had Pap smears in the last five years, Canadians had fewer deaths from cervical cancer than Americans (Stobbe 2006, p. B10). Less than 1 percent of Americans reported having to wait to see a physician, versus 3.5 percent of Canadians, and 9.9 percent of Americans reported being unable to afford prescription drug coverage, versus 5.1 percent of Canadians.

The study was based on a survey of 5200 Americans and 3500 Canadians age 18 and older (Stobbe 2006, p. B10).

THE WORLD HEALTH ORGANIZATION LOOKS AT HEALTH SYSTEM EFFECTIVENESS

The message from the WHO director general in the *World Health Report 2000* (WHO 2000, p. vii) focuses on three questions: "What makes for a good health system?" "What makes a health system fair?" "How do we know whether a health system is performing as it should?" The report looked at the following indicators: overall level of health and distribution of health; overall level of health system responsiveness (combination of patient satisfaction and responsiveness of the healthcare system) and distribution of responsiveness within the healthcare system (quality of healthcare among various socioeconomic groups); fairness in financial contribution (who pays the costs); overall goal attainment; health expenditure per capita; and performance on level of health and overall health system performance. A composite score was used to rank overall health system performance.

As mentioned earlier, in 2000 the United States spent $1.4 trillion on healthcare, but its composite score on health system performance put it merely in thirty-seventh place.

Taking each of the criteria used to evaluate the 191 countries, the United States had the following results: in health level of the population, as indicated by the disability-adjusted life expectancy levels, the United States ranked twenty-fourth. According to the report, the average level of population health is "most easily understood as the expectation of life lived in equivalent full health, without chronic, disabling disease" (WHO 2000, p. 146). The second component of that particular criterion, distribution of health, assesses health inequality within the population, using child survival rates as a leading indicator. In that instance, the United States ranked thirty-second (WHO 2000, p. 155).

For the second indicator applied by WHO, the level of health system responsiveness, the assessment was based on responses from 2000 informants in key countries and included the following elements of responsiveness: "dignity; autonomy and confidentiality; prompt attention; quality of basic amenities; access to social support networks during care; and choice of care provider" (WHO 2000, p. 147). These elements were each given a score from 1 to 10. Scores were then tabulated and included in a composite score. The United States ranked first in the level of system responsiveness. The second part of the component was the distribution of responsiveness within each country. The same informants who responded to the first part of the health system responsiveness question were also asked to develop the information for the second part by identifying disadvantaged groups or by including absolute poverty levels and access to healthcare. In this section of the report the United States' rank ranged between third and thirty-eighth, indicating a wide range of scores on the level of health system responsiveness (WHO 2000, p. 155).

In the third component of the assessment, health system effectiveness, the WHO looked at fairness in financial contribution—that is, what contribution the household made to the financing of the health system. The equation was determined based on "the ratio of total household spending on health to its permanent income above subsistence" (WHO 2000, p. 148). On this particular component, fairness in financial contribution, the United States ranked fifty-fourth to fifty-fifth out of the 191 countries.

The fourth component, overall goal attainment, consisted of a composite measure including "the level of health, the distribution of health, the level of responsiveness, the distribution of responsiveness and fairness of financial contribution" (WHO 2000, p. 149), which was based on the WHO survey of more than 1000 public health practitioners in 100 select countries. The United States' score on overall goal attainment put it in fifteenth place (WHO 2000, p. 155).

Although health expenditure per capita in international dollars was not one of the elements of the composite score, it clearly is significant. In assessing dollars spent per capita on healthcare, the United States exceeded all other nations in the study in dollars spent. In the year 2000, total healthcare expenditures were $1.4 trillion, as mentioned earlier.

As for the fifth component, overall performance on level of health, and the composite ranking on health system effectiveness, we find the following conclusions. The index of performance on the level of health focused on how well health systems "translated expenditure into health on the disability-adjusted life expectancy" (WHO 2000, p. 155). The second part of that equation, overall health system performance, matched achievement to expenditures: "maximum attainable composite goal achievement was estimated using a frontier production model relating overall health system achievement to health expenditure and other non–health system determinants represented by educational attainment" (WHO 2000, p. 150). In this area, performance on level of health, the United States ranked seventy-second. To give you a sense of the other countries receiving comparable scores, Bosnia/Herzegovina was ranked at seventieth, Nicaragua at seventy-fourth, Argentina at seventy-first, and Yugoslavia at sixty-ninth (WHO 2000). Further, on the composite index ranking each country on overall health system performance, the United States ranked thirty-seventh out of 191 countries globally. Countries in this category with superior rankings include Australia (thirty-second), Chile (thirty-third), and Dominica (thirty-fifth) (WHO 2000, pp. 152–55).

Jerry Avorn points out that the Organization for Economic Cooperation and Development (OECD) compared the United States and nineteen industrialized nations in 2000, including "most of western Europe, Japan, Australia and Canada. In those nations the total average per capita price tag for all medical care, converted to U.S. dollars, was just $1696 per year. In the United States, it was $4165—about two and a half times the average, with the per capita for 2004 over $6000" (Avorn 2004, p. 220). Avorn also notes that although expenditures were twice as high in the United States, "OECD data show that the U.S. ranks nineteenth out of thirty countries in life expectancy at birth, fourteenth of twenty-nine in life-expectancy at age sixty-five, and twenty-fourth out of thirty in infant mortality. . . . [O]f all the nations tracked by OECD, only South Korea, Slovakia, Hungary, Poland, Mexico and Turkey recorded worse numbers than we did" (Avorn 2004, p. 220).

In terms of satisfaction with the healthcare system, Avorn reports, "in the five-country survey, 44 percent of American patients reported being dissatisfied with the nation's health care system, with 48 percent identifying its high cost as a major problem—over twice the rate observed in any of the other countries studied. A larger study of nationally representative samples of over seven thousand people across the same five countries found that 79 percent of U.S. respondents thought the health care system needed to undergo fundamental change or be rebuilt completely" (Avorn 2004, p. 221).

Donald Barlett and James Steele conclude, with reference to the WHO *World Health Report* data, that "many countries around the world take far better care of their people, achieve better results from their health care systems and do it all with fewer dollars" (Barlett and Steele 2004, p. 13). They go on to draw comparisons:

> In 2001, per capita healthcare spending in the United States amounted to $4,887. That was 75 percent more than the $2,792 that Canada spent. Yet, Canadians expect to live two and a half years longer than Americans. The Canadian life-span at birth: 79.8 years. The American: 77.1 years. U.S. spending was 205 percent greater than Spain's, yet the Spanish can expect to live 2.1 years longer. As for the Japanese, with a life span of 80.9 years, the world's longest, they can expect to live nearly four years longer than Americans. This even though Japan's per capita spending on health care is only 41 percent of U.S. outlays. (Barlett and Steele 2004, p. 19)

In sum, "Americans pay for a Hummer but get a Ford Escort" (Barlett and Steele 2004, p. 13).

So who bears responsibility for health and healthcare? Clearly, in the United States we have a fee-for-service system and a free-market economy. If you're a large pharmaceutical company, that is clearly to your benefit, as there are no caps on what you can charge. However, employers are paying through the nose as a result of that free-enterprise "no caps" system, as are consumers with the escalation of premium hikes. When you hear on the news that upstate New York is shuttling busloads of senior citizens across the border into Canada so that they can purchase their blood pressure medications, it gives you pause.

Additionally, countries included in the WHO report had various payment systems; some were publicly financed, which was the case for many of the Eastern European countries, and some were privately financed, such as the United States. Many of the countries used a combination of the two, such as Medicare and Medicaid, two publicly financed programs that operate in conjunction with the primary fee-for-service, free-market approach in the United States. Whichever payment system was used, the countries that appeared to have healthier populations, as evidenced by longevity as well as low infant mortality rates, incorporated healthier diets and more exercise into the cultural pattern, which set them apart from industrialized nations that didn't fare as well—such as the United States.

Kenneth R. Pelletier, M.D., in looking at countries that have healthy populations, discussed the health of Swedish nationals, who attracted his attention because Sweden has enjoyed the world's longest life expectancy since the early 1960s. Pelletier cited Dr. Richard F. Tomasson's research from the University of Mexico to explain those longevity rates. The main factors believed to contribute to this longevity were compulsory national health insurance; the relatively high status of even the lowest socioeconomic groups; a structured and relatively tight social order; low infant mortality rates; a relatively low rate of cigarette and alcohol use; and a relatively low consumption of meat and sugar, with a high consumption of fish (Pelletier 2000, p. 307). The cultural components of lifestyle and diet certainly play a critical role in the health of Sweden's citizens.

ONE'S PERSPECTIVE DEPENDS ON WHERE ONE SITS AT THE HEALTHCARE TABLE

In looking at issues of culture and health, the reality of where one sits at the table of healthcare makes a definite difference in how one perceives the issues surrounding healthcare. A recent article by Charles Lauer in

Modern Healthcare underscores the point. Lauer points out that the opportunities are endless to expand the industry and "contribute to the nation's economy." According to Lauer, the state of healthcare is good—at least from a business point of view. There are abundant career opportunities in administration as well as for doctors, nurses, and volunteers. For entrepreneurs looking for ways to reduce expenditures or get a better return on investments, healthcare provides significant opportunities. Profits increased in the hospital industry from $17 billion to $22.6 billion in 2003, and both operations and reimbursement were strong in 2004. As a result of the growth in the healthcare industry, a 14 percent gain in healthcare portfolios was reported by Commonfund for the year 2003. Information technology is reported to be a growth area in the healthcare industry as hospitals invest in this technology to reduce errors and streamline the accessing and storage of medical records. Data analytics companies are applying information technology to cost reduction models in high-cost, high-volume arenas. Hospitals are in a building boom, with new construction to the tune of $32 billion in 2005 and an estimated $35 billion for 2006. There were 652 mergers and acquisitions within the industry in the first nine months of 2004, representing $140 billion (Lauer 2005). From a business standpoint, the healthcare field is booming and the future is bright.

From the standpoint of health of the population, the picture is different. In a recent article, Danica Kirka points out that 50 percent of children in North and South America will be overweight by 2010, with scientists expecting "profound impacts on everything from public health care to economies" (Kirka 2006). The researchers cited by Kirka concluded that obesity rates of school-age populations increased in "almost all of the countries for which data was available." These trends tend to be fueled by sedentary lifestyles and the accessibility of junk food. Researchers predict that as obesity seems to be carried into adulthood, these children will tend to retain these health patterns as they age, with an increased likelihood of heart disease, stroke, and other comorbidities of the extra weight.

Another unique perspective providing a cultural snapshot of U.S. healthcare is offered by a group of Amish exercising their lobbying power (Millman 2006). When a regional hospital opened in Pennsylvania Dutch country in 2004, the "Plain People" lobbied for discounted rates from the hospital on the grounds that they paid, in cash, roughly $5 million annually for health services. As part of their separation from the secular world, the Amish opt not to use insurance or Medicare. They also tend not to file malpractice claims, because of their belief that the outcome is in God's hands.

The Amish group successfully negotiated discounted rates of upwards of 40 percent through their willingness to mobilize forces. Their negotiating strategy was "No deal, no patients." Health Management Associates and the Heart of Lancaster Regional Medical Center agreed to the discounted rates. Heart of Lancaster "wasn't worried about risking steep losses if elaborate surgeries went awry: [Amish] patients generally don't want such procedures. 'If you're paying out of pocket, you'll hunt for bargains,' says Lee Christenson, chief executive of Heart of Lancaster, who bargained with the [Amish] elders. 'Basically, the Amish won't pay for healthcare they don't need'" (Millman 2006).

The Amish point of view certainly is a new way of looking at healthcare. The fact that they don't accept Medicare and they pay for healthcare services in cash makes them a unique group to deal with, and a powerful one. Because they pay in cash they are not interested in paying for services that they do not need—a concept that is too remote for most consumers to comprehend. As a result of third-party payer groups underwriting services, most consumers simply don't care what procedures or medications they get, as long as they don't involve a co-pay. For most consumers, premiums and co-pay amounts are the extent of their concern. The fact that the Amish pay out of pocket for everything makes them a true consumer group, in every sense of the word. The fact that they successfully negotiated a 40 percent reduction in their healthcare rates speaks to the power of the $5 million annually that they represent, as well as their "pay as you go" philosophy.

In reviewing the various initiatives under way by managed care companies, it appears that some provide incentives for members to take more control of their health. However, many do not. The need to have an incentive to get healthy, rather than doing so as a personal choice, says a great deal about the American consumer. Apparently, many are not interested enough to make changes if it does not benefit them directly, such as through Health Savings Accounts. Health does not become an issue until one has a problem with it, and then it becomes very important. This concept is related to the "disease model" that currently is central to healthcare, and it suggests that a shift toward a model focused on prevention is needed.

Other issues surrounding culture and health involve the safety and efficacy in clinical trials of new products released onto the market, as discussed in an article (Burton 2006b) focusing on criticism by Senator Charles Grassley (R-Iowa) aimed at Northfield Laboratories and the clinical trials under way at thirty-one hospitals in eighteen states of Northfield's blood substitute product, PolyHeme. Critics such as Grassley consider the research design unethical because of the lack of informed consent on the part of the patients. Grassley wrote to the U.S. Food and Drug Administration (FDA), "I am personally troubled that for all intents and purposes, the FDA allowed a clinical trial to proceed which makes the inhabitants of these communities "potential guinea pigs," without their consent and, absent consent, without full awareness of the risks and benefits of the blood substitute" (Burton 2006b, p. D5).

Grassley's letter came on the heels of a *Wall Street Journal* article the month before (Burton 2006a) reporting that ten out of eighty-one surgical patients in a previous PolyHeme study who received the substitute blood had suffered heart attacks, compared "with 0 of 71 who got blood." Two of the hospitals in the study had halted the study since the February 22 article was published, but other hospitals remained in the study.

Northfield Laboratories argued, "We believe the protocol is appropriate to evaluate a new therapy with potential lifesaving capability addressing a critical unmet clinical need." Referring to a federal rule that allows non-consent studies in certain circumstances, the company said, "We have adhered scrupulously to the rule, and are committed to conducting the study with the utmost concern for patient safety" (Burton 2006b, p. D5). The challenge, it appears, involves informed consent in a clinical trial. The Human Subjects Protection Act mandates that any subject involved in a clinical trial be informed of the risks and benefits of the trial, including any side effects that may be evident from earlier clinical trials.

The same month, the same publication reported on a lawsuit against Merck & Co. in response to a heart attack the plaintiff claimed was a result of his taking the analgesic Vioxx, and which left him disabled. The article mentions that "Merck withdrew Vioxx from the market in September of 2004, following a study that linked the drug to an increased risk of heart attacks and strokes in patients taking the drug for 18 months or longer. The company now faces 10,000 lawsuits" (Won Tesoriero 2006, p. D5). Vioxx had shown cardiac side effects in the early clinical trials, but it was FDA-approved nonetheless and released onto the market. A large managed care company on the West Coast noticed that the product was correlated to the sudden cardiac deaths of a number of individuals in the company's database, and the drug was later pulled from the market. The case of John Darby in Atlantic City, New Jersey, is one of thousands that are now being heard in courts across the country.

Compelled to address these health problems, consumers are seeking alternative remedies. As a result of this consumer demand, there is a growing interest among conventional practitioners in the area of alternative and complementary medicine, as referenced by James C. Whorton in his book *Natural Cures: The History of Alternative Medicine* (2006). He points out that in December 1997 the editorial board of the *Journal of the American Medical Association* made the announcement that "unconventional medicine" ranked third out of eighty-six subjects of interest and importance to their readers (Whorton 2002, p. x). A special issue of the journal, focusing on the topic of "unconventional medicine," was published in November 1998. In that issue the editors reviewed clinical trials of seven alternative therapies, including chiropractic, acupuncture, yoga, and herbs, with four of the seven trials indicating positive results. As Whorton (2002, p. x) points out, it appears that even conventional practitioners are now "fooling around" with alternative medicine.

Whether the issue is life expectancy, the health of the population, health system effectiveness, the escalating costs of prescription drug coverage, uninformed consent of subjects in a clinical trial, or a negotiated discount in healthcare prices, culture plays a critical role in health. All of the issues discussed in this chapter point to pressing problems within the healthcare industry and, in the case of the Amish, innovative solutions to those problems. Who bears responsibility for healthcare? Clearly, the most effective solution puts responsibility on the shoulders of the individual, as there are few doctors who can force people to eat properly, exercise, and refrain from activities that jeopardize health. Beyond that, however, the answer to the question of who is responsible—the individual, the employer, the government, or managed care—in large part will be determined by where one sits at the healthcare table.

CHAPTER 10

The Future of Health and Healthcare

The United States has one of the best acute care healthcare systems in the world. If you are a motor vehicle accident or burn victim, the U.S. healthcare system offers a level of technology and quality of care surpassing all other industrialized nations. Demographics, however, point to the fact that the bulk of our high-cost, high-volume patient populations fall in the chronic disease category.

Some of the most difficult challenges to be addressed are the escalating costs of healthcare, particularly in light of the aging baby boom generation; the high costs of errors in the diagnosis and treatment protocols of various medical problems; the need to improve the underlying science in diagnostic and treatment protocols (i.e., evidenced-based medicine); the urgency of providing healthcare coverage to the 45 million uninsured Americans (Gross 1998, p. 1971); the extensive use and costs of prescription drugs; and the importance of enlisting the participation of all Americans in taking greater responsibility for their health and healthcare through improved diet and increased exercise.

A recent news report (Berliner 2005) on the cost of healthcare for General Motors (GM) reported that $1500 of the cost of every vehicle manufactured goes to pay for the healthcare costs of GM employees and retirees. GM spends more on healthcare than it does for its most basic raw material—steel. At one time in the United States, GM was a powerhouse among automobile manufacturers. As a result of GM's decline in sales and the high costs of healthcare, its future seems uncertain. This chapter explores the future of health and healthcare in the United States and focuses on escalating healthcare costs and the impact of those costs on various sectors of the economy. In addition, the chapter discusses the managed care industry's various approaches to cost containment.

The article "Americans Pay More, Get Less for Health Care: Survey Looks at U.S. and Other Western Nations," written by Rob Stein of the *Washington Post* and published in the *Lexington Herald-Leader,* reported that "Americans pay more when they get sick than people in other Western nations and receive more confused, error-prone treatment" (p. A5). The article, based on results from a Harris Interactive survey that looked at 7000 sick adults in the United States, Australia, Canada, New Zealand, Britain, and Germany, concluded that "Americans were most likely to pay at least $1,000 in out-of-pocket expenses. More than half went without needed care because of cost and more than a third endured mistakes and disorganized care when they did get treated" (Stein 2005, p. A5).

Donald L. Barlett and James B. Steele state the following about healthcare:

> Everywhere there is uneasiness. Almost everyone knows somebody who has experienced the reality of what healthcare has become—a friend or relative who has no coverage, a young person who can't pay the premiums, a parent whose child needs expensive specialized treatment, or an elderly person who can't afford prescription drugs. "Why should people have to worry about their healthcare, something this basic?" asked a retired Colorado executive who has lived in Europe and Asia and who has seen the national healthcare systems of other nations. "No other country permits this. It's a crime." (2004, p. 24)

The United States reportedly spends more on healthcare than any other industrialized nation, roughly 15.3 percent of the gross domestic product (GDP) in 2003 and a much higher percentage than Germany, France, Japan, Italy, and Canada (Avorn 2004).

THE HIGH COST OF ERRORS IN THE DIAGNOSIS AND TREATMENT OF MEDICAL PROBLEMS

The Institute of Medicine (IOM), a widely respected independent organization based in Washington, D.C., and composed of leaders in medicine from throughout the United States, published two reports outlining healthcare in the United States. Those reports, *Crossing the Quality Chasm* and *To Err Is Human*, point out the flaws in the U.S. healthcare system and areas that require correction. Some of the findings were highlighted in the report *The Chasm in Quality: Select Indicators from Recent Reports*:

- Each year between 44,000 and 98,000 Americans die as a result of medical errors. In a random sample of adults, only 55 percent of patients received recommended treatment, with little difference found in the care recommended for prevention, for addressing acute episodes, and for treating chronic conditions.
- The annual cost of medication-related errors for hospitalized patients is roughly $2 billion.
- The 41 million Americans who are uninsured have consistently worse medical outcomes than those who are insured, and they face a greater risk of dying prematurely.
- The average time from the discovery of improved forms of treatment to their use in routine patient care is 17 years.
- Eighteen thousand Americans die annually from heart attacks because they did not receive preventive medications, although they were eligible for them.
- Each year more people die from medical errors than from breast cancer, AIDS, and automobile accidents combined.
- More than 50 percent of patients who have diabetes, hypertension, tobacco addiction, hyperlipidemia, congestive heart failure, asthma, depression, or chronic atrial defibrillation are being managed inadequately.

A recent issue of *Time* magazine featured the headline "What Doctors Hate About Hospitals: An Insider's View of What Can Go Wrong and How You Can Improve Your Odds of Getting the Right Treatment." One of the articles asks the question "What scares doctors most?" The answer is "Being the patient."

The article features a number of stories on healthcare strategies to address a health condition, but with a twist—the patients are the doctors themselves or family members of doctors. Their experience as doctors, while providing them with knowledge of the pitfalls and glitches inherent in the healthcare system, did not provide them with the ability to avoid such problems. The case of Donald Berwick, M.D., was of particular interest. His wife's hospitalization for a spinal cord problem was his "baptism by fire" into the healthcare system. His comments about the experience are as follows: "No day passed—not one—without a medication related error. Tests were repeated, data misread, information lost. And this was at a top hospital. The errors were not rare: they were the norm" (Gibbs and Bower 2006, p. 47).

Other doctors whose experiences were highlighted include Sherwin Nuland, a surgeon. Dr. Nuland's daughter required a brain shunt to correct a medical problem. As a result of complications, four surgeries were required before the problem was corrected. Dr. Nuland's response to this situation was: "I had to be restrained [with respect to his dealings with the doctors]. . . . I knew how badly it was affecting them emotionally" (Gibbs and Bower 2006, p. 45).

Internist Lisa Freedman, who was also part owner of her health maintenance organization (HMO), had to take the HMO to task to get a mammogram performed to evaluate a lump in her breast. The guidelines specified coverage of mammograms every 24 months, and Lisa wanted one at 18 months. According to Freedman, "They didn't even do a biopsy . . . one look and the radiologist said: 'you've got breast cancer'" (Gibbs and Bower 2006, p. 43).

The final profile in the Gibbs and Bower article was that of Dr. Robert Johnson, a surgeon. After breaking a bone in his wrist, he contacted his friend, a top-flight hand surgeon. After recovering from anesthesia, Johnson learned that a "slip of a [surgical] tool had damaged the vital bone" (Gibbs and Bower 2006, p. 48). Johnson sued both the hospital and his friend, and a settlement was reached prior to trial. The article points out that Johnson remained friends with the hand surgeon but lost his own career as a surgeon.

A recent episode illustrates the escalating costs of healthcare in the United States and the problematic, substandard outcomes often experienced despite the high cost. The Dartmouth Atlas Project, operated by the Center for Evaluative Clinical Sciences at Dartmouth Medical School, evaluates health resource allocation and utilization nationwide. Their goal is to improve both healthcare and health systems. One of the project's most important reports is *The Care of Patients with Severe Chronic Illness: A Report on the Medicare Program by the Dartmouth Atlas Project* (2006), which evaluated Medicare beneficiaries who have at least one of the twelve chronic illnesses that together account for more than 75 percent of all U.S. healthcare spending. The results indicate that getting more in the way of medical services does not result in better outcomes.

In fact, more care can be harmful in some cases, as documented in the article by Fisher and Welch (1999) "Avoiding the Unintended Consequences of Growth in Medical Care: How Might More Be Worse?" The research findings indicate that more frequent medical care does not result in better care, improvement in survival, or enhanced quality of life. As Pulitzer Prize–winning journalists Barlett and Steele have pointed out, "Americans pay for a Hummer but get a Ford Escort" (2004, p. 13).

The concept of "paying more but getting less" is also the backdrop for an article by Reed Abelson titled "Hospitals Fight for Heart Patients Paid For by Medicare." The article begins by noting that "hospitals across the United States covet patients such as Robert E. Wilson," a 79-year-old Indiana man with coronary vascular disease. He is a Medicare patient, and Abelson points out, "Medicare pays generously for cardiac care—so generously that hospitals and doctors scramble after that business" (2003, p. A1).

The article notes that "cranes have been raised over construction sites in places like Milwaukee, Phoenix and Houston. . . . The General Accounting Office, the investigative arm of Congress, counted at least 26 specialty hospitals under construction across the country" (Abelson 2006, p. A1). Roughly $100 billion is spent each year on inpatient hospital care that is paid for by Medicare, which makes it a lucrative niche in healthcare.

Robert Wilson, the 79-year-old patient profiled in the article, has undergone "two open-heart operations, five angioplasties, three cardiac catheterizations and an implanted defibrillator." In addition, "he checked into the Heart Center of Indiana to get his first stent, a tiny bit of wire scaffolding that helps keep arteries open" (Abelson 2006, p. A1). He will receive, the article notes, "room service," with meals provided by an executive chef.

According to the article, Congress is "turning its attention to the growth of specialty hospitals. The Senate version of the Medicare bill would make it harder for doctors to invest in and refer patients to such hospitals, and full-service hospitals are lobbying hard for the provision" (Abelson 2006, p. A1). Abelson notes that hospitals don't disclose their profit margins for specific procedures, such as a coronary bypass. However, Becky Nelson, the president of Sioux Valley Hospital in South Dakota, indicates that "cardiac procedures are 'absolutely our highest-margin business'" (Abelson 2006, p. A1).

A report from the Center for Studying Health System Change, a nonprofit research group, notes, "Improving clinical quality did not appear to be a driving force for new facilities or services. Given these market conditions, provider competition could, alternatively, result in high use rates and costs" (Abelson 2003, p. A1). Dr. John Birkmeyer, a surgeon from Dartmouth Medical School, indicates that a typical coronary bypass could generate $20,000 per procedure.

Dr. Samuel R. Nussbaum, the chief medical officer of Anthem, Inc., one of the largest managed care companies in the United States, comments: "The incentives are terribly misaligned" (Abelson 2006, p. A1). The question that should be asked is, are the clinical characteristics of the patient driving the procedures, or are there other forces at work that have little relevance to medical needs? Mr. Wilson, the 79-year-old patient in the article, is probably not aware of any of these issues surrounding his care, but he certainly needs to be.

REVISITING THE USE, COSTS, AND RISKS OF PRESCRIPTION DRUG COVERAGE

In Barlett and Steele's book *Critical Condition: How Health Care Became Big Business and Bad Medicine*, an example of the side effects of prescription drug use is given. The example provides a cautionary tale for consumers. The drug is Rezulin, a Parke-Davis drug that was released in 1997. The news media was positive in its coverage of the drug, and an endocrinologist "hailed Rezulin as a unique drug, the first in its class" (Barlett and Steele 2004, p. 252) and offered patients the opportunity to reduce their use of other drugs and consolidate with one—Rezulin. Also included was information that the endocrinologist was "beginning a study at New York's Albert Einstein College of Medicine where he's looking into whether Rezulin may even stop diabetes before it occurs in high-risk patients" (Barlett and Steele 2004, p. 252).

USA Today and *The New York Times* both touted the benefits of Rezulin, with *USA Today* stating that Rezulin "may reduce or eliminate the need for insulin shots for nearly 1 million diabetics. Of the patients who take Rezulin, 15 percent might be able to stop insulin shots, officials said." *The New York Times* quoted an FDA official as saying that adverse effects "appeared to be rare and relatively mild, including infection, pain and headache." Barlett and Steele point out that "the only cautionary note was that 'animal studies suggest that the drug should be prescribed with caution for patients with advanced heart failure or liver disease'" (2004, p. 253). Unfortunately (or fortunately, as the case may be), three years after those news releases, Rezulin had to be pulled from the market due to deaths and required liver transplants among patients who had taken the drug.

A second example (Avorn 2004) of the concern with new prescription drugs and the unwitting doctors who prescribe them is the case of Prosicor, an antihypertensive product designated for patients who were "starting a lifetime of therapy." A representative from the manufacturer provided samples to a doctor, and the doctor placed his next patient, a woman in her sixties, on the drug (the woman was also on a number of other antihypertensive agents). The doctor did not know that the drug had the potential for fatal interactions when combined with other agents. The woman developed acute kidney failure and subsequently suffered a stroke. After being comatose for three weeks, her family authorized the removal of artificial life support, and she died.

Avorn (2004, p.15) points out that in the ensuing months, more information became available regarding Prosicor's propensity to drop a patient's pulse to dangerously low levels, as well as its tendency to inhibit metabolization of cardiovascular drugs taken concurrently with Prosicor, which could result in acute renal failure. Avorn ends the case description by stating that after one year on the market Prosicor was removed, and the manufacturer cited pharmacokinetic interactions for its removal. "Some time later Paul [the sales representative] left the company. A number of suits are pending against the drug maker."

These clearly are exceptional cases, and many of the prescription drugs that millions of Americans take are beneficial, some even lifesaving. I cite these cases for the following reason: in most instances the FDA does not approve alternative treatments as safe and effective, but it is equally important to keep in mind that drugs that have been touted as safe and effective *and* approved by the FDA come with no guarantee that they will be helpful and no warranty against harm. In both of the cases mentioned here, the doctors prescribed the drugs innocently enough, based on the knowledge that FDA approval and indications for specific conditions justify their usage; however, FDA approval was not sufficient to ensure their safety and efficacy in these instances.

Estrogen, which has been used for decades in the United States to treat menopausal women, provides a cautionary tale with respect to two areas—the use of prescription drugs and how conventional medical wisdom sometimes is simply wrong. Jerry Avorn's book *Powerful Medicines: The Benefits, Risks and Costs of Prescription Drugs* provides a synopsis of what led to the hormone replacement therapy debacle in "The Pregnant Mare's Lesson":

> In a former British colony, most healers believed the conventional wisdom that a distillation of fluids extracted from the urine of horses, if dried to a powder and fed to aging women, could act as a general tonic, preserve youth, and ward off a variety of diseases. The preparation became enormously popular throughout the culture, and was used widely by older women in all strata of society. Many years later modern scientific studies revealed that long-term ingestion of the horse-urine extract was useless for most of its intended purposes, and that it caused tumors, blood clots, heart disease, and perhaps brain damage. (Avorn 2004, p. 15)

As stated in Chapter 4, for decades hormone replacement therapy (HRT) was used as the "gold standard" treatment for menopausal and postmenopausal women. It was indicated as having "cardio-protective" effects and was reported in respected scientific journals as being effective in treating depression and incontinence as well. The first study to cast a new light on its usage was the HERS (Heart and Estrogen-Progestin Replacement Study) report, published in 1998 and discussed in an article in the *Journal of the American Medical Association* titled "Randomized Trial of Estrogen Plus Progestin for Secondary Prevention of Coronary Heart Disease in Postmenopausal Women" (Hulley et al. 1998).

The intent of HERS was to test women who had a preexisting heart condition to assess HRT's "heart-protective" effect. The results of the trial were that those given estrogen not only did *not* enjoy a heart-protective effect, but in fact experienced significantly more heart attacks than those taking the placebo. Further, higher rates of both blood clots and gallbladder disease were reported among the subjects taking estrogen.

Additionally, while HERS test results were being published, the National Institutes of Health (NIH), at the behest of the Women's Health Initiative (WHI), had undertaken a major study exploring the long-term health outcomes of 16,000 women randomly assigned to estrogen or placebo. When the 1998 HERS study was published, the NIH questioned whether it was ethical to continue its long-term study in light of estrogen's potential to cause harm to patients.

In July 2002, officials at WHI decided to halt the study for ethical concerns. Some of the results of the study were confirmed (WHI 2002): estrogen did not prevent senility; in fact, the study found that cognitive function seemed to worsen in patients taking estrogen. The conclusion, according to Avorn (2004, p. 15), was that a drug "taken by millions of women to preserve their health and youth turned out to be worthless for that purpose and instead caused heart disease, cancer, stroke, blood clots and perhaps even brain damage."

OTHER HEALTHCARE ISSUES

As mentioned previously, there are numerous issues facing healthcare, including escalating costs, particularly in light of the aging baby boom generation; the high costs of errors in medicine; the need to improve the science underlying diagnostic and treatment protocols; the urgency of insuring the uninsured; and the importance of enlisting the participation of all Americans in taking greater responsibility for their health.

Underlying all of these issues, however, is the way healthcare is perceived and delivered and the need to approach healthcare from an entirely new perspective. Eleanor W. Davidson highlights some of these changes in her article "A Whole New Way of Thinking about Healthcare" (2004). In that article, Davidson discusses critical points from Donald M. Berwick's book *Escape Fire*. Berwick is a pediatrician and founder of the Institute for Healthcare Improvement, a nonprofit organization that focuses on addressing errors in medicine and other pressing issues facing the healthcare system. The "escape fire" metaphor stems from a case study in organizational change among the Mann Gulch firefighters in 1949, originally written about by Karl Weick in his book *Sensemaking in Organizations* (1995). The Mann Gulch firefighters were faced with tremendous winds, a difficult terrain, and a fire that was rapidly approaching. The foreman of the firefighters ordered his men to build an "escape fire" (burn the grass around them, leaving them with an oasis that would allow them to escape the fire, since the grass couldn't burn twice) to enable them to survive (he realized they couldn't outrun the main fire). His recommendation was counterintuitive to everything the men knew about firefighting. Very few listened to his recommendation to build the escape fire, and they died as a result. Berwick claims that changes in healthcare must come from counterintuitive measures, rather than from more of the same, which is not sufficient to solve the problem. The "escape fire" that he advocates for healthcare includes three major changes: access, science, and relationships.

Open access is defined as "access to health and healing," which Berwick points out "does not necessarily mean face to face meetings between practitioner and patient. . . . Half or more encounters . . . maybe 80 percent of them—are neither wanted by patients nor deeply believed in by professionals."

With respect to science, the help that is offered ideally should be based on knowledge—specifically, good science, or what has come to be known as "evidence-based medicine." According to Berwick, the model of healthcare should be initiated with a commitment to excellence and must incorporate a commitment to safety for patients and staff alike.

The third element, relationships, is embodied in the statement that "interaction is not the price of care, it is the care itself." This involves a paradigm shift in the way that interactions with patients are viewed. According to Berwick, "Our current system acts as if interactions with patients were the burden it must bear so it can deliver the care . . . [but in fact] interaction is care."

Escape Fire challenges us to view change within healthcare from a new perspective. In her discussion of Berwick's book, Davidson asks, "Why do people hold on to their heavy tools, lose agility and endanger co-workers and patients? Does this happen in medicine? Does our identity become fused with our tools?"

Why do practitioners continue to advocate highly invasive mastectomies when breast-conserving treatments for cancer have been available for the past twenty years? Monica Morrow, M.D., in an October 17, 2002, article in the *New England Journal of Medicine*, "Rational Local Therapy for Breast Cancer," points out that according to one study, among 29 percent of college-educated patients mastectomy was the only treatment option offered during the consultation. Are oncologists "wed" to their invasive tools, even in the face of science that offers less invasive options? What about thoracic surgeons and coronary bypass procedures, psychiatrists and medications, gynecologists and hysterectomies? Why are hysterectomies, the most invasive procedure, utilized most frequently in the treatment of uterine fibroids when less invasive procedures, such as uterine artery embolization, are available?

Being "wed" to the traditional tools of medicine in practice protocols and being unable or unwilling to entertain less invasive options results in less-than-optimal solutions. Getting different results in healthcare requires a different way of thinking, "dropping the old tools," and doing things differently.

Whose responsibility is healthcare? If most conditions are "self-limiting," meaning that they are self-created, then whose responsibility is it to address those issues? Obesity is one area that illustrates this problem of accountability. Carla L. Plaza, in an article titled "State Focuses on Health Issues to Minimize Future Healthcare Costs" and published in the journal *Healthcare Financial Management*, looks at the obesity rate among children in the United States, which has been increasing since 1960 and, if not checked, is expected to further contribute to escalating costs for providers.

In 2004 legislation was enacted to promote healthy practices among school-age children. This legislation established nutrition standards for food and beverages sold through school vending machines. Lawmakers in thirty-seven states encouraged and educated children on healthy diets and addressed the issue of sedentary lifestyles. As a result of the legislation, thirty-one states expanded physical and health education programs.

Lawmakers in several states have also limited liability claims against food and beverage manufacturers regarding their products' contribution to weight gain, obesity, or health conditions related to obesity. The first state to enact the Commonsense Consumption Act was Louisiana, in 2003; twenty-six states introduced the Act in 2004, and governors of eleven of the twenty-six states approved the legislation. Governor Jim Doyle of the state of Wisconsin vetoed the legislation.

Another critical issue in healthcare is cost and financing. As healthcare costs continue to escalate, employers will pass these costs on to employees and retirees, and fewer benefits will be financed by major employers. As a result, the methods for payment of healthcare continue to change. The magazine *Health and Medicine Week* published an article titled "Study Outlines Three Scenarios for the Future of Healthcare Financing."

In that article, a VHA, Inc. study titled "Dollars and Sense: Strategies for Emerging Payment Scenarios" illustrates how healthcare will be financed and paid for as economic and political factors change over time.

The VHA study looked at three healthcare financing scenarios: "1) cost management driven healthcare—purchasers (employers and government) maintain their role as decision makers and financiers of healthcare coverage, but seek ways to control exposure to escalating costs; 2) consumer-driven healthcare—purchasers take efforts to obtain improved outcomes from their healthcare investments; and 3) purchaser-driven healthcare—purchasers take efforts to obtain improved outcomes from their healthcare investments." ("Study Outlines Three Scenarios" 2003, p. 510)

In the first scenario, the reduction of payments to providers will result in efforts to increase payments from patients directly. In the second scenario, consumers will assume more responsibility in allocating dollars for healthcare services. In the third scenario, as healthcare costs escalate, purchasers will have a greater stake in reducing healthcare expenditures as a result of performance improvement measures for higher quality and improved outcomes (i.e., purchasers will get a better return on their investment).

David Gross, in his article "How Will America Stay Healthy? The Future U.S. Healthcare System: Who Will Care for the Poor and Uninsured?"(1998), addresses the issue of the uninsured as a critical problem caused by the market-based pricing of healthcare, which has reduced the resources typically used to fund indigent care. There are roughly 45 million uninsured Americans. Without healthcare coverage, most do not get the care they need at the early stages of disease and instead access the healthcare system when their conditions reach the acute stage; at the acute stage, treatment is more costly and more problematic.

CONCLUSION

Whether we're focusing on the IOM reports and errors in medicine, the escalating costs of prescription drug coverage, the millions of uninsured Americans, the outmoded and untested clinical protocols being used in medicine, or the need to enlist the engagement of Americans in taking greater responsibility for their health, clearly there are significant problems in healthcare. How and when we begin to address these issues will, in large part, shape the future of this country. Doing more of what we've done in the past will not address the critical issues we face. How we begin to formulate solutions will depend on our ability to assess the effectiveness of current approaches and a willingness to do things differently.

SECTION THREE

References and Resources

Annotated Primary Source Documents

Throughout this book, I have referenced the "state of the healthcare system" through research conducted by the Institute of Medicine, an arm of the National Academy of Sciences of the USA. Their research has been instrumental in educating the scientific community on issues of concern in healthcare. Typically, the consumer public is not aware of these reports, although their contents are clearly of importance to them. My goal is to familiarize the consumer public with their existence and encourage them to become familiar with their content. The two publications that have been referenced numerous times throughout this book were *To Err Is Human* (1999) and *Crossing the Quality Chasm* (2000).

To illustrate the relevance of these reports to the consumer public, a recent *Time* cover story by Nancy Gibbs and Amanda Bower titled "Q: What Scares Doctors Most? A: Being the Patient," (2006) profiles several doctors and their own or their loved ones' experiences as patient. The jacket synopsis states, "Doctors end up at the hospital just like the rest of us. The experience gives them new insight into the problems and risks faced by today's patients: the breakdown of communication between shifts; the clock-punching mentality of residents; the dangers of the latest technology." The insight provided by experiencing the healthcare system first-hand heightens many of the concerns that patients have experienced for quite some time.

Donald Berwick, M.D. (Gibbs and Bower 2006, p. 47), president of the Institute for Healthcare Improvement, experienced the healthcare system first-hand when his wife became ill with a spinal-cord problem. He comments about that experience: "No day passed—not one—without a medication error. . . . tests were repeated, data misread. . . . the errors were not rare, they were the norm."

Experience is a powerful teacher. Until you experience the problem, you only have a distanced view of the situation. When your health or the health of a loved one rests in the balance, it allows you to see the problems from an entirely different perspective and one that may provide a more realistic view of current challenges faced within the healthcare system.

APPENDIX ITEM I: *TO ERR IS HUMAN: BUILDING A SAFER HEALTH SYSTEM*

Health care in the United States is not as safe as it should be—and can be. At least 44,000 people, and perhaps as many as 98,000 people, die in hospitals as a result of medical errors that could have been prevented, according to estimates from two major studies. Even using the lower estimate, preventable medical errors in hospitals exceed attributable deaths to such feared threats as motor vehicle wrecks, breast cancer and AIDS.

Medical errors can be defined as the failure of a planned action to be completed as intended or the use of a wrong plan to achieve an aim. Among the problems that commonly occur during the course of providing health care are adverse drug events and improper transfusions, surgical injuries and wrong-site surgery, suicides, restraint-related injuries or death, falls, burns, pressure ulcers and mistaken patient identities. High error rates with serious consequences are most likely to occur in intensive care units, operating rooms and emergency departments.

Beyond their cost in human lives, preventable medical errors exact other significant tools. They have been estimated to result in total costs (including the expense of additional care necessitated by the errors, lost income and household productivity and disability) of between $17 billion and $29 billion per year in hospitals nationwide. Errors also are costly in terms of loss of trust in the healthcare system by patients and diminished satisfaction by both patients and health professionals. Patients who experience a long hospital stay or disability as a result of errors pay with physicial and psychological discomfort. Health professionals pay with loss of morale and frustration at not being able to provide the best care possible. Society bears the cost of errors, as well, in terms of lost worker productivity, reduced school attendance by children, and lower levels of population health status.

A variety of factors have contributed to the nation's epidemic of medical errors. One oft-cited problem arises from the decentralized and fragmented nature of the health care delivery system or "nonsystem," to some observers. When patients see multiple providers in different settings, none of whom has access to complete information, it becomes easier for things to go wrong. In addition, the processes by which health professionals are licensed and accredited have focused only limited attention on the prevention of medical errors and even these minimal efforts confronted resistance from some health care organizations and providers. Many providers also perceive the medical liability system as a serious impediment to systemic efforts to uncover and learn from errors. Exacerbating these problems, most third-party purchasers of health care provide little financial incentive for health care organizations and providers to improve safety and quality.

Health Care System at Odds with Itself

The Quality of Health Care in America Committee of the Institute of Medicine (IOM) concluded that it is not acceptable for patients to be harmed by the health care system that is supposed to offer healing and comfort—a system that promises, "First, do no harm." Helping to remedy this problem is the goal of *To Err Is Human: Building a Safer Health System*, the IOM Committe's first report.

In this report, issued in September 1999, the committee lays out a comprehensive strategy by which government, health care providers, industry and consumers can reduce preventable medical errors. Concluding that the know-how already exists to prevent many of these mistakes, the report sets as a minimum goal a 50 percent reduction in errors over the next five years. In its recommendations for reaching this goal, the committee strikes a balance between regulatory and market-based initiatives, and between the roles of professionals and organizations.

One of the report's main conclusions is that the majority of medical errors do not result from individual recklessness or the actions of a particular group—this is not a "bad apple" problem. More commonly, errors are caused by faulty systems, processes, and conditions that lead people to make mistakes or fail to prevent them. For example, stocking patient-care units in hospitals with certain full-strength drugs, even though they are toxic unless diluted, has resulted in deadly mistakes.

Thus, mistakes can best be prevented by designing the health system at all levels to make it safer—to make it harder for people to do something wrong and easier for them to do it right. Of course, this does not mean that individuals can be careless. People still must be vigilant and held responsible for their actions. But when an error occurs, blaming an individual does little to make the system safer and prevent someone else from committing the same error.

Strategy for Improvement

To achieve a better safety record, the report recommends a four-tiered approach.

- Establishing a national focus to create leadership, research, tools and protocols to enhance the knowledge base about safety.

Health care is a decade or more behind many other high-risk industries in its attention to ensure basic safety. This is due, in part, to the lack of a single designated government agency devoted to improving and monitoring safety throughout the health care delivery system. Therefore, Congress should create a Center for Patient Safety that would set national safety goals and track progress in meeting them; develop a research agenda; define prototype safety systems; develop, disseminate and evaluate tools for identifying and analyzing errors; develop methods for educating consumers about patient safety; and recommend additional improvements as needed.

- Identifying and learning from errors by developing a nationwide public mandatory reporting system and by encouraging health care organizations and practitioners to develop and participate in voluntary reporting systems.

Under the mandatory reporting system, state governments will be required to collect standardized information about adverse medical events that result in death and serious harm. Hospitals should be required to begin reporting first, and eventually reporting should be required by all health care organizations. This system will ensure a response to specific reports of serious injury, hold health care organizations and providers acountable for maintaining safety, provide incentives to organizations to implement internal safety systems that reduce the liklelihood of erors occuring, and respond to the public's right to know about patient safety. Currently, about a third of the states have mandatory reporting requirements.

Voluntary reporting systems will provide an important complement to the mandatory system. Such systems can focus on a much broader set of errors, mainly those that do no or minimal harm, and help detect system weaknesses that can be fixed before the occurences of serious harm and help detect system weaknesses that can be fixed before the occurrence of serious harm, thereby providing rich information to health care organizations in support of their quality improvement efforts. To foster participation in voluntary systems, Congress should enact laws to protect the confidentiality of certain information collected. Without such legislation, health care organizations and providers may be discouraged from participating in voluntary reporting systems out of worry that the information they provide might ultimately be subpoenaed and used in lawsuits.

- Raising performance standards and expectations for improvements in safety through the actions of oversight organizations, professional groups and group purchasers of health care.

Setting and enforcing explicit performance standards for patient safety through regulatory and related mechanisms, such as licensing, certification and accreditation, can define minimum performance levels for health professionals, the organizations in which they work, and the tools (drugs and devices) they use to care for patients. The process of developing and adopting standards also helps to form expectations for safety among providers and consumers.

Standards and expectations are not only set through regulations, however. The values and norms set by the health professions influence the practice, training and education of providers. Thus, professional societies should become leaders in encouraging and demanding improvements in patient safety, by such actions as setting their own performance standards, convening and communicating with members about safety, incorporating attention to patient safety in training programs, and colaborating across disciplines.

The actions of large purchasers of health care and health care insurance, as well as actions by individual consumers, also can affect the behaviors of health care organizations. Public and private purchasers, such as businesses buying insurance for their employees, must make safety a prime concern in their contracting decisions. Doing so will create financial incentives for health care organizations and providers to make needed changes to ensure patient safety.

- Implementing safety systems in health care organizations to ensure safe practices at the delivery level.

Health care organizations must develop a "culture of safety" such that their workforce and processes are focused on improving the reliability and safety of care for patients. Safety should be an explicit organizational goal that is demonstrated by strong leadership on the part of clinicians, executives and governing bodies. This will mean incorporating a variety of well-understood safety principles, such as designing jobs and working conditions for safety; standardizing and simplifying equipment, supplies and processes; and enabling care providers to avoid reliance on memory. Systems for continuously monitoring patient safety also must be created and adequately funded.

The medication process provides an example where implementing better systems will yield better human performance. Medication errors now occur frequently in hospitals, yet many hospitals are not making use of known systems for improving safety, such as automated medication order entry systems, nor are they actively exploring new safety systems. Patients themselves also could provide a major safety check in most hospitals, clinics and practice. They should know which medications they are taking, their appearance, and their side effects, and they should notify their doctors of medication discrepancies and the occurence of side effects.

Progress Under Way

The response to the IOM report was swift and positive, within both government and the private sector.

Almost immediately, the Clinton administration issued an executive order instructing government agencies that conduct or oversee health-care programs to implement proven techniques for reducing medical errors, and creating a task force to find new strategies for reducing errors. Congress soon launched a series of hearings on patient safety, and in December 2000 it appropriated $50 million to the Agency for Healthcare Research Quality to support a variety of efforts targeted at reducing medical errors.

The AHRQ already has made major progress in developing and implementing an action plan. Efforts under way include:

- Developing and testing new technologies to reduce medical errors.
- Conducting large-scale demonstration projects to test safety interventions and error-reporting strategies.
- Supporting new and established multidisciplinary teams of researchers and health-care facilities and organizations, located in geographically diverse locations, that will further determine the causes of medical errors and develop new knowledge that will aid the work of the demonstration projects.
- Supporting projects aimed at achieving a better understanding of how the environment in which care is provided affects the ability of providers to improve safety.

• Funding researchers and organizations to develop, demonstrate and evaluate new approaches to improving provider education in order to reduce errors.

Casting its net even more broadly, the AHRQ has produced a booklet of practical tips on what individual consumers can do to improve the quality of health-care services they receive. The booklet focuses on key choices that individuals and their families face, such as choosing doctors, hospitals and treatments, and it stresses the importance of individuals taking an active role in selecting and evaluating their care. (This booklet is available on the organization's website at www.ahrq.gov.).

In efforts focused at the state level, during the past year the National Academy for State Health Policy (NASHP) convened leaders from both the executive and legislative branches of the states to discuss approaches to improving patient safety. The NASHP also helped lead an initiative to better understand how states with mandatory hospital error-reporting requirements administer and enforce their programs. (A report on this initiative is available on the organization's website at www.nashp.org). In addition, the Agency for Healthcare Research and Quality has contracted with the National Quality Forum to produce a list of so called "never events" that states might use as the basis of a mandatory reporting system.

Among activities in the private sector, the Leapfrog Group, an association of private and public sector group purchasers, unveiled a market-based strategy to improve safety and quality, including encouraging the use of computerized physician-order entry, evidence-based hospital referrals, and the use of ICUs staffed by physicians credentialed in critical care medicine.

Professional groups within the health-care community also have been active. As but one example, the Council on Graduate Medical Education (COGME) and the National Advisory Council on Nurse Education and Practice (NACNEP) held a joint meeting on "Collaborative Education Models to Ensure Patient Safety." Participants addressed such issues as the effect of the relationships between physicians and nurses on patient safety, the impact of physician-nurse collaboration on systems designed to protect patient safety, and educational programs to ensure interdisciplinary collaboration to further patient safety. (A report on the meeting is available on the COGME's web site at www.cogme.org.)

Pulling Together

Although no single activity can offer a total solution for dealing with medical errors, the combination of activities proposed in *To Err Is Human*, offers a roadmap toward a safer health system. With adequate leadership, attention and resources, improvements can be made. It may be part of human nature to err, but is also part of human nature to create solutions, find better alternatives and to meet the challenges ahead.

For More Information

Copies of *To Err Is Human: Building A Safer Health System* are available for sale from the National Academy Press; or visit the NAP home page at www.nap.edu. The full text of this report is available at: http:// www.nap.edu/books/0309068371/html/.

Support for this project was provided by The National Research Council and The Commonwealth Fund. The views presented in this report are those of the Institute of Medicine Committee on the Quality of Health Care in America and are not necessarily those of the funding agencies.

The Institute of Medicine is a private, nonprofit organization that provides health policy advice under a congressional charter granted to the National Academy of Sciences. For more information about the Institute of Medicine, visit the IOM home page at www.iom.edu.

Committee on Quality of Healthcare in America

William C. Richardson, (Chair), President and CEO, W.K. Kellogg Foundation, Battle Creek, MI

Donald M. Berwick, President and CEO, Institute for Healthcare Improvement, Boston, MA

J. Cris Bisgard, Director, Health Services, Delta Air lines, Inc., Atlanta, GA

Lonnie R. Bristow, Former President, American Medical Association, Walnut Creek, CA

Charles R. Buck, Program Leader, Health Care Quality and Strategy Initiatives, General Electric Company, Fairfield, CT

Christine K. Cassel, Professor and Chairman, Department of Geriatrics and Adult Development, The Mount Sinai School of Medicine, New York, NY

Mark R. Chassin, Professor and Chairman, Department of Health Policy, The Mount Sinai School of Medicine, New York, NY

Molley Joel Coye, Senior Fellow, Institute for the Future, and President, Health Technology Center, San Francisco, CA

Don E. Detmer, Dennis Gillings Professor of Health Management, University of Cambridge, UK

Jerome H. Grossman, Chairman and CEO, Lion Gate Corporation, Boston, MA

Brent James, Executive Director, Intermountain Health Care Institute for Health Care Delivery Research, Salt Lake City, UT

David McK. Lawrence, Chairman and CEO, Kaiser Foundation Health Plan, Inc. Oakland, CA

Lucian L. Leape, Adjunct Professor, Harvard School of Public Health, Boston, MA

Arthur Levin, Director, Center for Medical Consumers, New York, NY

Rhonda Robinson-Beale, Executive Medical Director, Managed Care management and Clinical Programs, Blue Cross Blue Shield of Michigan, Southfield

Joseph E. Scherger, Associate Dean for Primary Care, University of California, Irvine College of Medicine

Arthur Southam, President and CEO, Health Systems Design, Oakland, CA

Mary Wakefield, Director, Center for Health Policy, Research and Ethics, George Mason University, Fairfax, VA

Gail L Warden, President and CEO, Henry Ford Health System, Detroit, MI

Study Staff

Janet Corrigan, Director, Quality of Health Care in America Project; Director, Board of Health Care Services

Molla S. Donaldson, Project Coordinator

Linda T. Kohn, Project Coordinator

Tracy McKay, Research Assistant

Kelly C. Pike, Senior Project Assistant

Auxiliary Staff

Mike Edington, Managing Editor

Kay Harris, Financial Advisor

Suzanne Miller, Senior Project Assistant

Copy Editor

Florence Poillon

APPENDIX ITEM II: *CROSSING THE QUALITY CHASM: A NEW HEALTH SYSTEM FOR THE 21ST CENTURY*

The U.S. health care delivery system does not provide consistent, high quality medical care to all people. Americans should be able to count on receiving care that meets their needs and is based on the best scientific knowledge—yet there is strong evidence that this frequently is not the case. Health care harms patients too frequently and routinely fails to deliver its potential benefits. Indeed, between the health care that we now have and the health care that we could have lies not just a gap but a chasm.

A number of factors have combined to create this chasm. Medical science and technology have advanced at an unprecedented rate during this past half-century. In tandem has come growing complexity of health care, which today is characterized by more to know, more to do, more to manage, more to watch, and more people involved than ever before. Faced with such rapid changes, the nation's health care delivery system has fallen far short in its ability to translate knowledge into practice and to apply new technology safely and appropriately. And if the system cannot consistently deliver today's science and technology, it is even less prepared to respond to the extraordinary advances that surely will emerge during the coming decades.

The public's health care needs have changed as well. Americans are living longer, due at least in part to advances in medical science and technology, and with this aging population comes an increase in the incidence and prevalence of chronic conditions. Such conditions, including heart disease, diabetes and asthma, are now the leading cause of illness, disability and death. But today's health system remains overly devoted to dealing with acute, episodic care needs. There is a dearth of clinical programs with the multidisciplinary infrastructure required to provide the full complement of services needed by people with common chronic conditions.

The health care delivery system also is poorly organized to meet the challenges at hand. The delivery of care often is overly complex and uncoordinated, requiring steps and patient "handoffs" that slow down care and decrease rather than improve safety. These cumbersome processes waste resources; leave accountable voids in coverage; lead to loss of information; and fail to build on the strengths of all health professionals involved to ensure that care is appropriate, timely and safe. Organizational problems are particularly apparent regarding chronic conditions. The fact that more than 40 percent of people with chronic conditions have more than one such condition argues strongly for more sophisticated mechanisms to coordinate care. Yet health care organizations, hospitals and physician groups typically operate as separate "silos," acting without the benefit of complete information about the patient's condition, medical history, services provided in other settings, or medications provided by other clinicians.

Strategy for Reinventing the System

Bringing state-of-the-art care to all Americans in every community will require a fundamental, sweeping redesign of the entire health system, according to a report by the Institute of Medicine (IOM), an arm of the National Academy of Sciences. *Crossing the Quality Chasm: A New Health System for the 21st Century*, prepared by the IOM's Committee on the Quality of Health Care in America and released in March 2001, concludes that merely making incremental improvements in current systems of care will not suffice.

The committee already has spoken to one urgent problem—patient safety— in a 1999 report titled, *To Err Is Human: Building a Safer Health System*. Concluding that tens of thousands of Americans die each year as a result of preventable mistakes in their care, the report lays out a comprehensive strategy by which government, health care providers, industry and consumers can reduce medical errors.

Crossing the Quality Chasm focuses more broadly on how the health system can be reinvented to foster innovation and improve the delivery of care. Toward this goal, the committee presents a comprehensive strategy and action plan for the coming decade.

Six Aims for Improvement

Advances must begin with all health care constituencies—health professionals, federal and state policy makers, public and private purchasers of care, regulators, organization managers and governing boards, and consumers—committing to a national statement of purpose for the health care system as a whole. In making this committment, the parties would accept as their explicit purpose "to continually reduce the burden of illness, injury and disability and to improve the health and functioning of the people of the United States." The parties would also adopt shared vision of six specific aims for improvement. These aims are built around the core need for health care to be:

- Safe: avoiding injuries to patients from the care that is intended to help them
- Effective: providing services based on scientific knowledge to all who could benefit, and refraining from providing services to those not likely to benefit
- Patient-centered: providing care that is respectful of and responsive to individual patient preferences, needs and values and ensuring that patient values guide all clinical decisions
- Timely: reducing waits and sometimes harmful delays for both those who receive and those who give care
- Efficient: avoiding waste, including waste of equipment, supplies, ideas and energy
- Equitable: providing care that does not vary in quality because of personal characteristics such as gender, ethnicity, geographic location and socioeconomic status

A health care system that achieves major gains in these six areas would be far better at meeting patient needs. Patients would experience care that is safer, more reliable, more responsive to their needs, more integrated and more available services that are likely to prove beneficial. Clinicians and other health workers also would benefit through their increased satisfaction at being better able to do their jobs and thereby bring improved health, greater longevity, less pain and suffering, and increased personal productivity to those who receive their care.

Ten Rules for Redesign

To help in achieving these improvement aims, the committee deemed that it would be neither useful nor possible to specify a blueprint for 21st-century health care delivery systems. Imagination abounds at all levels, and all promising routes for innovation should be encouraged. At the same time, the committee formulated a set of ten simple rules, or general principles, to inform efforts to redesign the health system. These rules are:

1. "Care is based on continuous healing relationships." Patients should receive care whenever they need it and in many forms, not just face-to-face visits. This implies that the health care system must be responsive at all

times, and access to care should be provided over the Internet, by telephone and by other means in addition to in-person visits.

2. "Care is customized according to patient needs and values." The system should be designed to meet the most common types of needs, but should have the capability to respond to individual patient choices and preferences.

3. "The patient is the source of control." Patients should be given the necessary information and opportunity to exercise the degree of control they chose over health care decisions that affect them. The system should be able to accommodate differences in patient preferences and encourage shared decision making.

4. "Knowledge is shared and information flows freely." Patients should have unfettered access to their own medical information and to clinical knowledge. Clinicians and patients should communicate effectively and share information.

5. "Decision making is evidence-based." Patients should receive care based on the best available scientific knowledge. Care should not vary illogically from clinician to clinician or from place to place.

6. "Safety is a systems property." Patients should be safe from injury caused by the care system. Reducing risk and ensuring safety require greater attention to systems that help prevent and mitigate errors.

7. "Transparency is necessary." The system should make available to patients and their families information that enables them to make informed decisions when selecting a health plan, hospital, or clinical practice, or when choosing among alternative treatments. This should include information describing the system's performance on safety, evidence-based practice and patient satisfaction.

8. "Needs are anticipated." The system should anticipate patient needs rather than simply react to events.

9. "Waste is continuously decreased." The system should not waste resources or patient time.

10. "Cooperation among clinicians is a priority." Clinicians and institutions should actively colaborate and communicate to ensure an appropriate exchange of information and coordination of care.

Taking the First Steps

To initiate the process of change, Congress should establish a Health Care Quality Innovation Fund—roughly $1 billion for use over three to five years to help produce a public-domain portfolio of programs, tools and technologies of wide-spread applicability, and to help communicate the need for rapid and significant change hroughout the healthcare system. Some of the projects funded should be targeted at achieving the six aims for improvement.

The committee also calls for immediate attention on developing care processes for the common health conditions, most of them chronic, that afflict great numbers of people. The federal Agency for Healthcare Research and Quality (AHRQ) should identify 15 or more common priority conditions. (The agency has requested guidance from the IOM on selection of these conditions, and the Institute expects to issue its report in September of 2002.) The AHRQ then should work with various stakeholders in the health community to develop strategies and action plans to improve care for each of these priority conditions over a five-year period.

Changing the Environment

Redesigning the health care delivery system also will require changing the structures and processes of the environment in which health professionals and organizations function. Such changes need to occur in four main areas:

- "Applying evidence to health care delivery." Scientific knowledge about best care is not applied systematically or expeditiously to clinical practice. It now takes an average of 17 years for new knowledge generated by randomized controlled trials to be incorporated into practice, and even then application is highly uneven. The committee therefore recommends that the Department of Health and Human Services establish a comprehensive program aimed at making scientific evidence more useful and accessible to clinicians and patients.

It is critical that leadership from the private sector, both professional and other health care leaders and consumer representatives, be involved in all aspects of this effort to ensure its applicability and acceptability to clinicians and patients. The infrastructure developed through this public-private partnership should focus initially on priority conditions. Efforts should include analysis and synthesis of the medical evidence, delineation of specific practice guidelines, identification of best practices in the design of care processes, dissemination of the evidence and guidelines to the professional communities and the general public, development of support tools to help clinicians and patients in applying evidence and making decisions, establishment of goals for improvement of care processes and outcomes and development of measures for assessing quality of care.

- "Using information technology." Information technology, including the Internet, holds enormous potential for transforming the health care delivery system, which today remains relatively untouched by the revolution that has swept nearly every other aspect of society. Central to many information technology applications is the automation of patient-specific clinical information. Such information typically is dispersed in a collection of paper records, which often are poorly organized, illegible, and not easy to retrieve, making it nearly impossible to manage various illnesses, especially chronic conditions, that require frequent monitoring and ongoing patient support. Many patients also could also have their needs met more quickly and at a lower cost if they could communicate with health professionals through e-mail. In addition, the use of automated systems for ordering medications can reduce errors in prescribing and dosing drugs, and computerized reminders can help both patients and clinicians identify needed services.

The challenges of applying information technology should not be underestimated, however. Health care is undoubtedly one of the most, if not the most complex sectors of the economy. Sizable capital investments and multiyear commitments to building systems will be needed. Widespread adoption of many information technology applications will also require behavioral adaptations on the part of large numbers of clinicians, organizations and patients. Thus, the committee calls for a nationwide commitment of all stakeholders to building an information infrastructure to support health care delivery, consumer health, quality measurement and improvement, public accountability, clinical and health services research, and clinical education. This commitment should lead to the elimination of most handwritten clinical data by the end of the decade.

- "Aligning payment policies with quality improvement." Although payment is not the only factor that influences provider and patient behavior, it is an important one. The committee calls for all purchasers, both public and private, to carefully reexamine their payment policies to remove barriers that impede quality improvement and build in stronger incentives for quality enhancement. Clinicians should be adequately compensated for taking good care of all types of patients, neither gaining or losing financially for caring for sicker patients or those with more complicated conditions. Payment methods also should provide an opportunity for providers to share in the benefits of quality improvement, provide an opportunity for consumers and purchasers to recognize quality differences in health care and direct their decisions accordingly, align financial incentives with the implementation of care processes based on best practices and the achievement of better patient outcomes, and enable providers to coordinate care for patients across settings and over time.

To assist purchasers in their redesign of payment policies, the federal government, with input from the private sector, should develop a program to identify, pilot test, and evaluate various options for better aligning payment methods with quality improvement goals. Examples of possible means of achieving this end included blended methods of payment designed to counter the disadvantages of one payment method with the advantages of another, multiyear contracts, payment modifications to encourage use of electronic interaction among clinicians and between clinicians and patients, and bundled payments for priority conditions.

- "Preparing the workforce." Health care is not just another service industry. Its fundamental nature is characterized by people taking care of other people in times of need and stress. Stable, trusting relationships between a patient and the people providing care can be critical to healing or managing an illness. Therefore, the importance of adequately preparing the workforce to make a smooth transition into a thoroughly revamped health care system cannot be underestimated.

Three approaches can be taken to support the workforce in this transition. One approach is to redesign the way health professionals are trained to emphasize the six aims for improvement, which will mean placing more stress on teaching evidence-based practice and providing more opportunities for interdisciplinary training. Second is to modify the ways in which health professionals are regulated and accredited to facilitate needed changes in care delivery. Third is to use the liability system to support changes in care delivery while preserving its role in ensuring accountability among health professionals and organizations. All of these approaches likely will prove to valuable, but key questions remain about each. The federal government and professional associations need to study these approaches to better ascertain how they can best contribute to ensuring the strong workforce that will be at the center of the health care system of the 21st century.

- "No better time." Now is the right time to begin work on reinventing the nation's health care delivery system. Technological advances are making it possible to accomplish things today that were impossible only a few years ago. Health professionals and organizations, policy makers and patients are becoming all too painfully aware of the shortcomings of the nation's current system and of the importance of finding radically new and better approaches to meeting the health care needs of all Americans. Although *Crossing the Quality Chasm* does not offer a simple prescription—there is none—it does provide a vision of what is possible and the path that can be taken. It will not be an easy road, but it will be most worthwhile.

The full text of this report is available at: http://www.nap.edu/books/0309072808/html

Support for this project was provided by: The Institute of Medicine; the National Research Council; The Robert Wood Johnson Foundation; the California Health Care Foundation; the Commonwealth Fund; and the Department of Health and Human Services' Health Care Finance Administration; Public Health Service; and Agency for Health Research Quality. The views in this report are those of the Institute of Medicine on the Quality of Health Care in America and are not necessarily those of the funding agencies.

The Institute of Medicine is a private, nonprofit organization that provides health policy advice under a congressional charter granted to the National Academy of Sciences. For more information about the Institute of Medicine, visit the IOM home page at www.iom.edu.

Committee on Quality of Healthcare in America

William C. Richardson, (Chair), President and CEO, W.K. Kellogg Foundation, Battle Creek, MI

Donald M. Berwick, President and CEO, Institute for Healthcare Improvement, Boston, MA

J. Cris Bisgard, Director, Health Services, Delta Air lines, Inc., Atlanta, GA

Lonnie R. Bristow, Former President, American Medical Association, Walnut Creek, CA

Charles R. Buck, Program Leader, Health Care Quality and Strategy Initiatives, General Electric Company, Fairfield, CT

Christine K. Cassel, Professor and Chairman, Department of Geriatrics and Adult Development, The Mount Sinai School of Medicine, New York, NY

Mark R. Chassin, Professor and Chairman, Department of Health Policy, The Mount Sinai School of Medicine, New York, NY

Molley Joel Coye, Senior Fellow, Institute for the Future, and President, Health Technology Center, San Francisco, CA

Don E. Detmer, Dennis Gillings Professor of Health Management, University of Cambridge, UK

Jerome H. Grossman, Chairman and CEO, Lion Gate Corporation, Boston, MA

Brent James, Executive Director, Intermountain Health Care Institute for Health Care Delivery Research, Salt Lake City, UT

David McK. Lawrence, Chairman and CEO, Kaiser Foundation Health Plan, Inc. Oakland, CA

Lucian L. Leape, Adjunct Professor, Harvard School of Public Health, Boston, MA

Arthur Levin, Director, Center for Medical Consumers, New York, NY

Rhonda Robinson-Beale, Executive Medical Director, Managed Care Management and Clinical Programs, Blue Cross Blue Shield of Michigan, Southfield.

Joseph E. Scherger, Associate Dean for Primary Care, University of California, Irvine College of Medicine

Arthur Southam, President and CEO, Health Systems Design, Oakland, CA

Mary Wakefield, Director, Center for Health Policy, Research and Ethics, George Mason University, Fairfax, VA

Gail L Warden, President and CEO, Henry Ford Health System, Detroit, MI

Study Staff

Janet Corrigan, Director, Quality of Health Care in America Project; Director, Board of Health Care Services

Molla S. Donaldson, Project Coordinator

Linda T. Kohn, Project Coordinator

Shari K. Maguire, Research Assistant

Kelly C. Pike, Senior Project Assistant

Auxiliary Staff

Mike Edington, Managing Editor

Jennifer Cangco, Financial Advisor

Consultant
Rona Brier, Brier Associates

APPENDIX ITEM III: *COMPLEMENTARY AND ALTERNATIVE MEDICINE USE AMONG ADULTS: UNITED STATES, 2002 (ADVANCE DATA FROM VITAL AND HEALTH STATISTICS, NUMBER 343, MAY 27, 2004)*

Patricia M. Barnes, M.A., and Eve Powell-Griner, Ph.D., Division of Health Interview Statistics; and Kim McFann, Ph.D., and Richard L. Nahin, Ph.D., National Center for Complementary and Alternative Medicine, National Institute of Health

Abstract

Objective—This report presents selected estimates of complementary and alternative medicine (CAM) use among U.S. adults, using data from the 2002 National Health Interview Study (NHIS), conducted by the Centers for Disease Control and Prevention's (CDC) National Center for Health Statistics (NCHS).

Methods—Data for the U.S. civilian noninstitutionalized population were collected using computer-assisted personal interviews (CAPI). This report is based on 31,044 interviews of adults age 18 years and over. Statistics shown in this report were age adjusted to the year 2000 U.S. standard population.

Results—Sixty-two percent of adults used some form of CAM therapy during the past 12 months when the definition of CAM therapy included prayer specifically for health reasons. When prayer specifically for health reasons was excluded from the definition, 36 percent of adults used some form of CAM therapy during the past 12 months. The 10 most commonly used CAM therapies during the past 12 months were use of prayer specifically for one's own health (43.0 percent), prayer by others for one's own health (24.4 percent), natural products (18.9 percent), deep breathing exercises (11.6 percent), participation in prayer group for one's own health (9.6 percent), meditation (7.6 percent), chiropractic care (7.5 percent), yoga (5.1 percent), massage (5.0 percent) and diet-based therapies (3.5 percent).

Use of CAM varies by sex, race, geographic region, health insurance status, use of cigarettes or alcohol, and hospitalizaton. CAM was most often used to treat back pain or back problems, head or chest colds, neck pain or neck problems, joint pain or stiffness, and anxiety or depression. Adults age 18 years or over who used CAM were more likely to do so because they believed that CAM combined with conventional medical treatments would help (54.9 percent) and/or they thought it would be interesting to try (50.1 percent). Most adults who have ever used CAM have used it within the past 12 months, although there is variation by CAM therapy.

Introduction

Complementary and alternative medicine (CAM) is a group of diverse medical and health care systems, therapies, and products that are not presently considered to be part of conventional medicine. The U.S. public's use of CAM increased substantially during the 1990's (1–11). This high rate of use translates into large out-of-pocket expenditures by CAM. It has been estimated that the U.S. public spent between $36 billion and $47 billion on CAM therapies in 1997 (5). Of this amount, between $12.2 billion and $19.6 billion was paid out-of-pocket for the services of professional CAM health care providers such as chiropractors, acupuncturists and massage therapists. These fees are more than the U.S. public paid out-of-pocket for all hospitalizations in 1997 and about half that paid for all out-of-pocket physician services (12).

Explanations for this growth in CAM use have been proposed, including marketing forces, availability of information on the Internet, the desire for patients to be actively involved in medical decision making, and dissatisfaction with conventional (western) medicine (13). This dissatisfaction may be related to the inability of conventional medicine to adequately treat many chronic diseases and their symptoms such as debilitating pain (1). Rates of CAM use are also exceptionally high among individuals with life threatening illnesses such as cancer (14) or HIV (15). It appears that the majority of people use CAM as a complement to conventional medicine, not as an alternative (1, 3.5).

As used by the U.S. public, CAM consists of many heterogenous systems of medicine as well as numerous stand-alone therapies (16). Several systems of CAM are practiced as part of the health care system in U.S. immigrants' countries of origins (17). For example, Ayurveda is practiced in India at a national level within the Federal health system. Traditional Chinese medicine, which includes acupuncture, acupressure, herbal medicine, tai chi and qi gong, is often practiced in the same hospitals or clinics as conventional medicine in China. Kampo, the system of traditional herbal medicine in Japan, is covered by the national health insurance plan and is practiced by many medical doctors (18). Immigrants from these and other countries of origin may continue to rely on CAM as part of their medical treatment in the United States even as they seek care from conventional health care providers. Some of these systems may eventually prove to be low cost health care options for use by the U.S. public.

Despite the diverse ways in which these systems and therapies developed, they appear to have several characteristics in common: the use of complex interventions, often involving the administration of many medications or medicinal substances at the same time; individualized diagnosis and treatment of patients; an emphasis in maximizing the body's inherent healing ability; and treatment of the "whole" person by addressing their physical, mental and spiritual attributes rather than focusing on a specific pathogenic process as emphasized in conventional medicine (19).

Notwithstanding the growing scientific evidence that some CAM therapies may be effective for specific conditions (20, 21), the public's wide use of many untested CAM therapies might have unanticipated negative consequences. For example, the

U.S. Department of Health and Human Services banned the sale of the herbal supplement ephedra in 2003 after concluding the risks associated with the use of the product by the general public outweighed any potential benefit (22). It has been found that other herbal products interact or interfere with the normal pharmacology of some pharmaceutical drugs with potentially fatal consequences (23). CAM users often do not share information about such use with their conventional health care providers (5), thereby increasing the possibility of serious interactions. Even when conventional health care providers are aware that their patients are taking herbal products, serious interactions could result if providers are unfamiliar with the scientific literature on CAM. Understanding the prevalence and reasons for CAM use is the first step toward improving communication between health care providers and their patients.

This report is based on a CAM supplement that was administered as part of the sample adult questionnaire of the 2002 NHIS. The report focuses on who uses CAM, what is used, and why it is used. It also examines the relationship between the use of CAM and the use of conventional medical practices. In particular, the report examines the relationship of CAM use and demographic and health behaviors among groups not previously studied in detail, including race and ethnic groups, the economically disadvantaged, and the elderly. The 2002 NHIS included questions that asked respondents about their use (ever and during the past 12 months) of 27 different CAM therapies. This report defines CAM broadly by including therapies or practices that may not be considered CAM, such as prayer specifically for health purposes and high-dose vitamin therapy, and examines the use of these practices in specific populations.

Methods

Data Source   The statistics shown in this report are based on the data from the Alternative Health/Complementary and Alternative Medicine supplement, the Sample Adult Core component, and the Family Core component of the 2002 NHIS (24). The NHIS, one of the major data collection systems of CDC's NCHS, is a survey of a nationally representative sample of the civilian noninstitutionalized household population of the United States. Basic health and demographic information were collected on all household members. Adults present at the time of the interview are asked to respond for themselves. Proxy responses are accepted for adults not present at the time of the interview and for children. Additional information is collected on one randomly selected adult age 18 years or over (sample adult) per family. Information on the sample adult is self-reported except in rare cases when the sample adult is physically or mentally incapable of responding, and information on the sample child is collected from an adult family member who is knowledgeable about the child's health.

The Alternative Health/Complementary and Alternative Medicine supplemental questionnaire included questions on 27 types of CAM therapies commonly used in the United States (table 1). These 27 CAM therapies included 10 types of provider-based CAM therapies (e.g., acupuncture, chiropractic care, folk medicine), as well as 17 other CAM therapies for which the services of a provider are not necessary (e.g., natural products, special diets, megavitamin therapy). The

CAM supplement, unlike earlier surveys, includes specific types of CAM diets, such as Atkins, Macrobiotic, Ornish, Pritikin, and Zone; a comprehensive range of mind-body therapies, including biofeedback, deep breathing techniques, guided imagery, hypnosis, progressive relaxation, qi gong, tai chi and yoga and the use of prayer for health purposes. Inclusion and development of the 2002 supplement was supported, in part, by the National Center for Complementary and Alternative Medicine (NCCAM), National Institutes of Health (NIH).

Statistical Analysis   This report is based on data from 31,044 completed interviews with sample adults age 18 years and over, representing a conditional sample adult response rate of 74.3 percent. Procedures used in calculating response rates are described in detail in "Appendix I" of the Survey Description of the NHIS data files (24). Because the CAM questions were administered as part of of the Sample Adult questionnaire and only about 1.4 percent of the sample adults did not answer any questions in the CAM supplement, a separate response rate for the CAM questions was not calculated.

All estimates (percents and frequencies) and associated errors shown in this report were generated using SUDAAN, a software package designed to account for the complex sample design such as that used by the NHIS (25). All estimates were weighted using the sample adult record weight, to represent the U.S. civilian noninstitutionalized population age 18 years and over.

Most estimates presented in this report were age adjusted to the year 2000 U.S. standard population age 18 years and over (26, 27). The SUDAAN procedure PROC DESCRIPT was used to produce age-adjusted percentages and their standard errors. Age adjustment was used to allow comparison of various sociodemographic subgroups that have different age structures. The estimates found in the report were age adjusted using the age groups 18–24 years, 25–44 years, 45–64 years and 65 years and over, unless otherwise noted. (See "Technical Notes" for details.)

Age-adjusted estimates were compared using two-tailed statistical tests at the 0.05 level. No adjustments were made for multiple comparisons. Terms such as "greater than" and "less than" indicate a statistically significant difference. Terms such as "similar" or "no difference" indicate that the statistics being compared were not significantly different. Lack of comment regarding the difference between any two statistics does not mean the difference was tested and found to be not significant.

Most statistics presented in this report can be replicated using NHIS public use data files and accompanying documentation available for downloading from the NCHS web site at: http://www.cdc.gov/nchs/nhis.htm. Variables identifying metropolitan statistical area (MSA), urban/rural residence, and State, which was used to create the category "Pacific States," are not included in the public use data files to protect respondent confidentiality. Therefore, corresponding estimates cannot be replicated. Many of the references cited in this report are also available via the NCHS web site at: http://www.cdc.gov/nchs.

Strengths and Limitations of the Data   A major strength of the data on complementary and alternative medicine in the NHIS is that they were collected for a nationally

Table 1. Frequencies and age-adjusted percents of adults 18 years and over who used complementary and alternative medicine, by type of therapy: United States, 2002

Therapy	Ever used		Used during past 12 months	
	Number in thousands	Percent (standard error)	Number in thousands	Percent (standard error)
Any CAM[1] use	149,271	74.6 (0.37)	123,606	62.1 (0.40)
Alternative medical systems				
Acupuncture.	8,188	4.0 (0.13)	2,136	1.1 (0.07)
Ayurveda.	751	0.4 (0.04)	154	0.1 (0.02)
Homeopathic treatment.	7,379	3.6 (0.14)	3,433	1.7 (0.09)
Naturopathy	1,795	0.9 (0.07)	498	0.2 (0.03)
Biologically based therapies				
Chelation therapy	270	0.1 (0.02)	66	*0.0 (0.01)
Folk medicine	1,393	0.7 (0.05)	233	0.1 (0.02)
Nonvitamin, nonmineral, natural products. . .	50,613	25.0 (0.32)	38,183	18.9 (0.28)
Diet-based therapies[2]	13,799	6.8 (0.18)	7,099	3.5 (0.12)
Vegetarian diet.	5,324	2.6 (0.11)	3,184	1.6 (0.08)
Macrobiotic diet	1,368	0.7 (0.06)	317	0.2 (0.03)
Atkins diet.	7,312	3.6 (0.13)	3,417	1.7 (0.09)
Pritikin diet	580	0.3 (0.04)	137	0.1 (0.02)
Ornish diet	290	0.1 (0.02)	76	*0.0 (0.01)
Zone diet	1,062	0.5 (0.05)	430	0.2 (0.03)
Megavitamin therapy	7,935	3.9 (0.13)	5,739	2.8 (0.11)

Manipulative and body-based therapies

Chiropractic care	40,242	19.9 (0.33)	15,226	7.5 (0.19)
Massage	18,899	9.3 (0.22)	10,052	5.0 (0.16)
Mind-body therapies				
Biofeedback	1,986	1.0 (0.06)	278	0.1 (0.02)
Meditation	20,698	10.2 (0.23)	15,336	7.6 (0.20)
Guided imagery	6,067	3.0 (0.12)	4,194	2.1 (0.10)
Progressive relaxation	8,518	4.2 (0.14)	6,185	3.0 (0.12)
Deep breathing exercises	29,658	14.6 (0.27)	23,457	11.6 (0.24)
Hypnosis	3,733	1.8 (0.10)	505	0.2 (0.03)
Yoga	15,232	7.5 (0.19)	10,386	5.1 (0.16)
Tai chi	5,056	2.5 (0.11)	2,565	1.3 (0.08)
Qi gong	950	0.5 (0.05)	527	0.3 (0.04)
Prayer for health reasons[3]	110,012	55.3 (0.42)	89,624	45.2 (0.40)
Prayed for own health	103,662	52.1 (0.41)	85,432	43.0 (0.40)
Others ever prayed for your health	62,348	31.3 (0.38)	48,467	24.4 (0.35)
Participate in prayer group	25,167	23.0 (0.46)	18,984	9.6 (0.23)
Healing ritual for own health	9,230	4.6 (0.15)	4,045	2.0 (0.09)
Energy healing therapy/Reiki	2,264	1.1 (0.07)	1,080	0.5 (0.05)

*Estimates preceded by an asterisk have a relative standard error of greater than 30% and should be used with caution as they do not meet the standard of reliability or precision.

0.0 Figure does not meet standard of reliability or precision and quantity more than zero but less than 0.05.

[1]CAM includes acupuncture; ayurveda; homeopathic treatment; naturopathy; chelation therapy; folk medicine; nonvitamin, nonmineral, natural products; diet-based therapies; megavitamin therapy; chiropractic care; massage; biofeedback; meditation; guided imagery; progressive relaxation; deep breathing exercises; hypnosis; yoga; tai chi; qi gong; prayer for health reasons; and energy healing therapy/Reiki. Respondents may have reported using more than one type of therapy.

[2]The totals of the numbers and percents of the categories listed under "Diet-based therapies" are greater than the number and percent of "Diet-based therapies" because respondents could choose more than one diet-based therapy.

[3]The totals of the numbers and percents of the categories listed under "Prayer for health reasons" are greater than the number and percent of "Prayer for health reasons" because respondents could choose more than one method of prayer.

NOTES: CAM is complementary and alternative medicine. The denominators for statistics shown exclude persons with unknown CAM information. Estimates were age adjusted to the year 2000 U.S. standard population using four age groups: 18–24 years, 25–44 years, 45–64 years, and 65 years and over.

DATA SOURCE: National Health Interview Survey, 2002.

representative sample of U.S. adults, allowing estimation of CAM use for a wide variety of population subgroups. The large sample size also facilitates investigation of the association between CAM and a wide range of other self-reported health characteristics included in the NHIS such and health behaviors, chronic health conditions, injury episodes, access to medical care, and health insurance coverage.

The CAM data collected in the 2002 NHIS are a significant improvement over the CAM data collected in the 1999 NHIS. The 1999 NHIS included only one question that asked respondents if they had used (during the past 12 months) any of the 11 listed therapies or some other CAM therapy that they were then asked to name. The 2002 NHIS included questions that asked respondents about their use (ever and during the past 12 months) of 27 different CAM therapies. For therapies used during the past 12 months, respondents were asked more detailed questions such as the health problem or condition being treated with the therapy, the reason (s) for choosing the therapy, whether the costs of the therapy were covered by insurance, their satisfaction with the treatment, and whether any of their conventional medical professionals knew they were using the therapy.

The CAM questions have several limitations. First, they are dependent upon respondents' knowledge of CAM therapies and/or their willingness to report use accurately. Secondly, the collection of CAM data at a single point in time results in an inability to produce consecutive annual estimates for CAM use so that changes cannot be tracked over time, and it reduces the ability to produce reliable estimates of CAM use for small population subgroups as this would require a larger sample and/or more than 1 year of data.

Results
Use of Complementary and Alternative Medicine (Table 1)

- Seventy-five percent of adults age 18 and over have ever used CAM when prayer specifically for health reasons was included in the definition (figure 1).
- Sixty-two per cent of adults have used CAM during the past 12 months when prayer specifically for health reasons was included in the definition (figure 1).
- The 10 CAM therapies most commonly used within the past 12 months measured in terms of the percentage of U.S. adults were prayer specifically for one's own health (43.0 percent), prayer by others for one's own health (24.4 percent), natural products (18.9 percent), deep breathing exercising (11.6 percent), participation in prayer group for one's own health (9.6 percent), meditation (7.6 percent), chiropractic care (7.5 percent), yoga (5.1 percent), massage (5.0 percent) and diet-based therapies (3.5 percent).
- Of the 10 CAM therapies most commonly used within the past 12 months, most were mind-body interventions.
- Forty-five percent of adults used some method of prayer for health reasons within the past 12 months.
- The two most widely used diet-based therapies by U.S. adults were the Atkins diet (1.7 percent) and the vegetarian diet (1.6 percent).

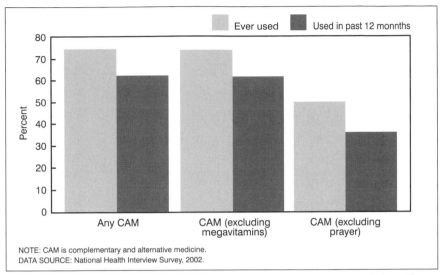

Figure 1. Age-adjusted percent of adults who have used complementary and alternative medicine: United States, 2002

Use of Selected Natural Products

- Nineteen percent of adults used natural products, including herbal medicine, functional foods (garlic), and animal-based (glucosamine) supplements during the past 12 months (table 1).
- The most commonly used natural products were echinacea (40.3 percent), ginseng (24.1 percent), ginkgo biloba (21.1 percent) and garlic supplements (19.9 percent) (table 2).

Medical Conditions Treated with CAM (Table 3)

- CAM was most often used to treat back pain or problems, head or chest colds, neck pain or problems, joint pain or stiffness, and anxiety or depression.
- Approximately 1 percent of adult CAM users utilized it to treat sinusitis (1.2 percent), cholesterol (1.1 percent), asthma (1.1 percent), hypertension (1.0 percent) and/or menopause (0.8 percent).

Use of CAM by selected characteristics (Table 4)

- Women were more likely than men to use CAM. The largest sex differential is seen in the use of mind-body therapies including prayer specifically for health reasons.
- For all therapies combined, CAM use was more likely among older adults than younger adults. However, the positive relationship between age and CAM use is primarily due to the inclusion of prayer specifically for health reasons. When specific types of CAM therapies are

Table 2. Frequencies and age-adjusted percents of adults 18 years and over who used selected types of nonvitamin, nonmineral, natural products during the past 12 months for health reasons: United States, 2002

Nonvitamin, nonmineral, and natural products	Used selected nonvitamin, nonmineral, natural products[1]	
	Number in thousands	Percent[2] (standard error)
Echinacea	14,665	40.3 (0.80)
Ginseng	8,777	24.1 (0.67)
Ginkgo biloba	7,679	21.1 (0.65)
Garlic supplements	7,096	19.9 (0.63)
Glucosamine with or without chondroitin	5,249	14.9 (0.58)
St. John's wort	4,390	12.0 (0.53)
Peppermint	4,308	11.8 (0.52)
Fish oils/omega fatty acids	4,253	11.7 (0.53)
Ginger supplements	3,768	10.5 (0.51)
Soy supplements	3,480	9.4 (0.49)
Ragweed/chamomile	3,111	8.6 (0.44)
Bee pollen or royal jelly	2,755	7.4 (0.41)
Kava kava	2,441	6.6 (0.41)
Valerian	2,131	5.9 (0.38)
Saw palmetto	2,054	5.8 (0.35)

[1]Respondents may have used more than one nonvitamin, nonmineral, natural product.
[2]The denominators used in the calculation of percents are the estimated number of adults who used nonvitamin, nonmineral, natural products within the past 12 months, excluding persons with unknown information for usage of the specified nonvitamin, nonmineral, natural product.

NOTE: Estimates were age adjusted to the year 2000 U.S. standard population using four age groups: 18–24 years, 25–44 years, 45–64 years, and 65 years and over.

DATA SOURCE: National Health Interview Survey, 2002

Table 3. Frequencies and age-adjusted percents of adults 18 years and over who used complementary and alternative medicine (excluding megavitamin therapy and prayer) during the past 12 months by diseases and conditions for which it was used: United States, 2002

Disease or condition[1]	Used CAM as treatment	
	Number in thousands	Percent[2] (standard error)
Back pain or problem	11,965	16.8 (0.45)
Head or chest cold.	6,924	9.5 (0.34)
Neck pain or problem	4,756	6.6 (0.29)
Joint pain or stiffness	3,420	4.9 (0.26)
Anxiety/depression	3,249	4.5 (0.22)
Arthritis, gout, lupus, or fibromyalgia	3,216	4.9 (0.24)
Stomach or intestinal illness	2,656	3.7 (0.20)
Severe headache or migraine	2,307	3.1 (0.19)
Recurring pain	1,762	2.4 (0.16)
Insomnia or trouble sleeping	1,595	2.2 (0.16)
Sinusitis	900	1.2 (0.13)
Cholesterol	797	1.1 (0.13)
Asthma.	788	1.1 (0.11)
Hypertension	714	1.0 (0.11)
Menopause	657	0.8 (0.08)

[1]Respondents may have used more than one CAM therapy to treat a condition, but were counted only once under each condition treated.
[2]The denominators used in the calculation of percents are the estimated number of adults who used CAM (excluding megavitamin therapy and prayer) within the past 12 months, excluding persons with unknown information about whether CAM was used to treat the specified condition.

NOTES: CAM is complementary and alternative medicine. Estimates were age adjusted to the year 2000 U.S. standard population using four age groups: 18–24 years, 25–44 years, 45–64 years, and 65 years and over.

DATA SOURCE: National Health Interview Survey, 2002.

153

Table 4. Age-adjusted percents of adults 18 years and over who used selected complementary and alternative medicine categories during the past 12 months, by selected characteristics: United States, 2002

Selected characteristic	Any use of—								
	CAM including megavitamin therapy and prayer[1]	Biologically based therapies including megavitamin therapy[2]	Mind-body therapies including prayer[3]	CAM excluding megavitamin therapy and prayer[4]	Biologically based therapies excluding megavitamin therapy[5]	Mind-body therapies excluding prayer[6]	Alternative medical systems[7]	Energy therapies[7]	Manipulative and body-based therapies[8]
				Percents (standard error)					
Total[9,10]	62.1 (0.40)	21.9 (0.30)	52.6 (0.42)	35.1 (0.38)	20.6 (0.29)	16.9 (0.31)	2.7 (0.12)	0.5 (0.05)	10.9 (0.24)
Sex[10]									
Male	54.1 (0.54)	19.6 (0.41)	43.4 (0.54)	30.2 (0.49)	18.2 (0.40)	12.5 (0.36)	2.2 (0.15)	0.3 (0.06)	9.5 (0.30)
Female	69.3 (0.49)	24.1 (0.40)	61.1 (0.51)	39.7 (0.50)	22.9 (0.39)	21.1 (0.42)	3.2 (0.17)	0.7 (0.08)	12.2 (0.33)
Age									
18–29 years	53.5 (0.84)	19.6 (0.63)	44.2 (0.87)	32.9 (0.80)	18.8 (0.62)	17.7 (0.62)	2.3 (0.25)	0.4 (0.09)	9.5 (0.47)
30–39 years	60.7 (0.75)	23.2 (0.64)	49.8 (0.75)	37.8 (0.76)	22.1 (0.63)	18.3 (0.57)	3.3 (0.28)	0.6 (0.11)	12.8 (0.49)
40–49 years	64.1 (0.68)	24.7 (0.64)	53.3 (0.75)	39.4 (0.73)	23.3 (0.62)	18.9 (0.59)	3.2 (0.25)	0.7 (0.12)	13.0 (0.51)
50–59 years	66.1 (0.85)	26.2 (0.72)	56.1 (0.90)	39.6 (0.82)	24.7 (0.71)	19.6 (0.67)	3.3 (0.29)	0.8 (0.16)	11.3 (0.52)
60–69 years	64.8 (0.97)	21.3 (0.81)	56.3 (1.04)	32.6 (0.93)	19.6 (0.79)	14.4 (0.70)	2.1 (0.29)	*0.4 (0.13)	9.8 (0.62)
70–84 years	68.6 (0.94)	15.3 (0.68)	63.3 (1.00)	25.1 (0.85)	13.3 (0.63)	9.4 (0.58)	1.4 (0.22)	*0.1 (0.06)	7.7 (0.52)
85 years and over	70.3 (2.05)	9.1 (1.35)	66.0 (2.16)	14.9 (1.58)	8.4 (1.32)	6.4 (1.14)	*0.9 (0.33)	*0.3 (0.18)	2.1 (0.52)
Race[10]									
White, single race	60.4 (0.44)	22.3 (0.33)	50.1 (0.46)	35.9 (0.42)	20.9 (0.32)	17.0 (0.35)	2.8 (0.13)	0.5 (0.06)	12.0 (0.28)
Black or African American, single race.	71.3 (0.98)	16.5 (0.71)	68.3 (0.98)	26.2 (0.85)	15.2 (0.68)	14.7 (0.69)	1.4 (0.22)	*0.3 (0.11)	4.4 (0.37)
Asian, single race	61.7 (1.94)	29.5 (1.87)	48.1 (1.99)	43.1 (2.03)	28.9 (1.83)	20.9 (1.67)	4.5 (0.74)	*0.6 (0.27)	7.2 (0.90)
Hispanic or Latino origin[10,11]									
Hispanic or Latino	61.4 (0.94)	20.6 (0.74)	55.1 (0.98)	28.3 (0.86)	19.8 (0.73)	10.9 (0.57)	2.4 (0.28)	*0.4 (0.14)	5.8 (0.43)
Not Hispanic or Latino.	62.3 (0.43)	22.3 (0.32)	52.4 (0.45)	36.1 (0.40)	20.9 (0.31)	17.7 (0.33)	2.8 (0.12)	0.6 (0.05)	11.6 (0.26)

154

Education[10]

Less than high school	57.4 (0.88)	12.5 (0.57)	52.0 (0.89)	20.8 (0.72)	11.7 (0.55)	8.0 (0.46)	1.3 (0.19)	*0.2 (0.06)	5.1 (0.40)
High school graduate/GED[12] recipient	58.3 (0.68)	17.8 (0.47)	49.6 (0.70)	29.5 (0.61)	16.8 (0.46)	12.4 (0.46)	1.6 (0.16)	0.3 (0.08)	9.4 (0.39)
Some college - no degree	64.7 (0.76)	24.1 (0.64)	54.8 (0.81)	38.8 (0.77)	22.6 (0.63)	19.1 (0.60)	2.7 (0.23)	0.7 (0.12)	12.5 (0.54)
Associate of arts degree	64.1 (1.18)	24.6 (1.01)	53.8 (1.24)	39.8 (1.14)	23.1 (0.99)	20.2 (0.92)	3.0 (0.37)	*0.5 (0.17)	12.6 (0.79)
Bachelor of arts or science degree	66.7 (0.82)	29.8 (0.80)	54.9 (0.89)	45.9 (0.89)	27.7 (0.78)	25.0 (0.79)	4.6 (0.37)	0.9 (0.17)	15.3 (0.65)
Masters, doctorate, professional degree	65.5 (1.92)	31.5 (1.45)	52.7 (1.81)	48.8 (1.87)	29.8 (1.44)	26.5 (1.55)	5.2 (0.79)	*1.6 (0.67)	12.8 (0.78)

Family income[10,13]

Less than $20,000	64.9 (0.84)	18.9 (0.65)	58.8 (0.84)	29.6 (0.78)	18.0 (0.64)	14.8 (0.58)	2.4 (0.23)	0.4 (0.12)	6.7 (0.38)
$20,000 or more	61.6 (0.44)	23.1 (0.34)	51.2 (0.46)	37.0 (0.43)	21.6 (0.34)	17.9 (0.35)	2.9 (0.14)	0.6 (0.06)	12.1 (0.28)
$20,000-$34,999	63.5 (0.80)	21.1 (0.70)	55.3 (0.82)	34.1 (0.83)	19.9 (0.67)	16.9 (0.66)	2.0 (0.25)	0.5 (0.15)	10.0 (0.53)
$35,000-$54,999	62.8 (0.83)	22.6 (0.72)	52.8 (0.86)	36.6 (0.84)	21.2 (0.68)	17.9 (0.64)	2.9 (0.28)	0.6 (0.11)	11.8 (0.55)
$55,000-$74,999	60.9 (1.09)	22.7 (0.84)	50.1 (1.12)	37.4 (1.04)	21.2 (0.81)	18.2 (0.84)	2.4 (0.26)	0.4 (0.13)	11.0 (0.65)
$75,000 or more	61.9 (0.94)	27.1 (0.85)	48.7 (0.97)	43.3 (0.94)	25.6 (0.84)	20.7 (0.74)	4.0 (0.33)	0.7 (0.12)	15.2 (0.66)

See footnotes at end of table.

Table 4. Age-adjusted percents of adults 18 years and over who used selected complementary and alternative medicine categories during the past 12 months, by selected characteristics: United States, 2002—Con.

Selected characteristic	Any use of—								
	CAM including megavitamin therapy and prayer[1]	Biologically based therapies including megavitamin therapy[2]	Mind-body therapies including prayer[3]	CAM excluding megavitamin therapy and prayer[4]	Biologically based therapies excluding megavitamin therapy[5]	Mind-body therapies excluding prayer[6]	Alternative medical systems[7]	Energy therapies	Manipulative and body-based therapies[8]
	Percents (standard error)								
Poverty status[10,14]									
Poor.	65.5 (1.10)	17.9 (0.81)	60.8 (1.13)	28.2 (1.02)	17.0 (0.81)	14.1 (0.79)	2.0 (0.29)	*0.3 (0.13)	5.9 (0.52)
Near poor.	64.3 (0.91)	19.1 (0.68)	57.1 (0.98)	30.4 (0.83)	18.3 (0.67)	14.7 (0.63)	1.9 (0.25)	*0.4 (0.13)	7.7 (0.52)
Not poor.	62.6 (0.49)	24.7 (0.41)	51.2 (0.52)	39.8 (0.49)	23.2 (0.40)	19.5 (0.42)	3.2 (0.17)	0.6 (0.07)	13.1 (0.33)
Health insurance[15]									
Under 65 years:									
Private.	61.4 (0.47)	24.6 (0.40)	50.0 (0.49)	39.4 (0.48)	23.2 (0.39)	19.3 (0.38)	3.0 (0.15)	0.6 (0.07)	13.1 (0.33)
Public.	65.1 (1.21)	17.9 (0.88)	59.8 (1.22)	31.1 (1.10)	16.5 (0.85)	18.0 (0.92)	2.3 (0.36)	*0.4 (0.20)	7.3 (0.64)
Uninsured.	57.7 (1.00)	21.1 (0.74)	49.5 (1.01)	31.2 (0.89)	20.4 (0.74)	14.7 (0.69)	3.1 (0.34)	0.7 (0.15)	8.0 (0.49)
65 years and over:									
Private.	68.2 (0.96)	16.0 (0.72)	61.9 (1.04)	27.2 (0.86)	14.0 (0.67)	10.6 (0.59)	1.4 (0.23)	*0.2 (0.09)	9.4 (0.54)
Public.	65.9 (1.18)	14.6 (0.83)	61.1 (1.26)	21.3 (1.00)	13.4 (0.81)	8.4 (0.70)	1.3 (0.26)	*0.1 (0.07)	4.5 (0.55)
Uninsured.	74.4 (8.33)	18.2 (4.64)	73.2 (8.31)	19.7 (4.73)	18.2 (4.64)	*3.0 (1.52)	*0.7 (0.74)	*–	*0.7 (0.74)

156

Marital status[10]									
Never Married	60.2 (1.01)	21.0 (0.76)	52.0 (1.04)	33.0 (0.90)	19.7 (0.73)	18.0 (0.74)	2.6 (0.28)	0.7 (0.16)	9.4 (0.53)
Married	62.4 (0.55)	21.8 (0.43)	52.7 (0.57)	35.0 (0.51)	20.5 (0.42)	15.6 (0.39)	2.7 (0.17)	0.4 (0.08)	11.1 (0.32)
Cohabiting	59.4 (1.86)	25.9 (1.47)	47.7 (1.91)	37.9 (1.87)	24.6 (1.46)	20.4 (1.50)	2.9 (0.46)	*1.3 (0.44)	11.1 (1.15)
Divorced or Separated	65.4 (1.20)	23.5 (0.94)	57.5 (1.21)	38.8 (1.15)	22.2 (0.93)	22.1 (1.00)	2.6 (0.22)	0.6 (0.11)	11.1 (0.70)
Widowed	72.8 (2.39)	22.6 (3.90)	65.5 (2.52)	33.9 (4.05)	21.0 (3.87)	18.5 (3.68)	*2.0 (0.86)	*0.1 (0.07)	8.4 (1.86)
Urban/rural[10]									
Urban	62.6 (0.43)	22.9 (0.34)	53.2 (0.44)	36.0 (0.41)	21.5 (0.33)	18.0 (0.33)	2.9 (0.14)	0.6 (0.06)	10.8 (0.27)
Rural	60.4 (0.80)	19.3 (0.55)	50.9 (0.86)	32.6 (0.76)	18.3 (0.54)	13.9 (0.60)	2.1 (0.21)	0.4 (0.09)	11.1 (0.48)
Place of residence[10]									
MSA,[16] central city	63.5 (0.66)	22.5 (0.55)	55.3 (0.68)	34.9 (0.67)	21.1 (0.54)	18.3 (0.55)	3.1 (0.23)	0.6 (0.09)	9.9 (0.41)
MSA,[16] not central city	61.2 (0.52)	23.2 (0.42)	50.9 (0.55)	36.5 (0.49)	21.8 (0.41)	17.4 (0.40)	2.7 (0.15)	0.6 (0.07)	11.1 (0.32)
Not MSA[16]	62.1 (1.09)	18.2 (0.66)	53.1 (1.17)	31.9 (0.97)	17.2 (0.63)	13.9 (0.76)	2.1 (0.24)	0.3 (0.07)	11.6 (0.63)
Region[10]									
Northeast	57.9 (0.91)	22.6 (0.70)	46.9 (0.91)	35.7 (0.84)	21.1 (0.69)	16.9 (0.69)	3.1 (0.27)	0.7 (0.12)	10.9 (0.53)
Midwest	61.4 (0.80)	20.9 (0.60)	52.0 (0.82)	37.0 (0.77)	19.7 (0.57)	18.2 (0.59)	2.2 (0.20)	0.5 (0.10)	13.2 (0.57)
South	64.6 (0.65)	19.3 (0.45)	57.2 (0.66)	29.9 (0.61)	18.0 (0.44)	14.0 (0.45)	1.9 (0.15)	0.3 (0.07)	7.9 (0.33)
West	62.1 (0.91)	27.7 (0.70)	50.3 (1.08)	42.2 (0.82)	26.4 (0.69)	21.1 (0.82)	4.6 (0.36)	0.8 (0.13)	13.8 (0.55)
Pacific States[17]	64.0 (1.08)	27.7 (0.86)	52.4 (1.22)	43.0 (1.00)	26.4 (0.86)	22.4 (0.98)	4.8 (0.47)	0.8 (0.16)	13.3 (0.65)
Body weight status[10,18]									
Underweight	62.0 (2.55)	18.4 (2.00)	55.1 (2.57)	33.6 (2.38)	17.6 (1.96)	20.4 (2.08)	3.0 (0.74)	*0.5 (0.25)	8.9 (1.38)
Healthy weight	62.7 (0.60)	23.3 (0.49)	53.2 (0.61)	37.2 (0.57)	21.9 (0.47)	19.5 (0.49)	3.4 (0.21)	0.7 (0.10)	11.6 (0.39)
Overweight	60.1 (0.64)	21.9 (0.50)	49.6 (0.66)	34.8 (0.58)	20.6 (0.50)	15.8 (0.44)	2.6 (0.18)	0.5 (0.09)	11.2 (0.38)
Obese	64.6 (0.73)	21.1 (0.56)	56.3 (0.75)	33.4 (0.71)	19.8 (0.55)	15.3 (0.54)	1.9 (0.17)	0.4 (0.09)	10.3 (0.46)

See footnotes at end of table.

Table 4. Age-adjusted percents of adults 18 years and over who used selected complementary and alternative medicine categories during the past 12 months, by selected characteristics: United States, 2002—Con.

Selected characteristic	Any use of—								
	CAM including megavitamin therapy and prayer[1]	Biologically based therapies including megavitamin therapy[2]	Mind-body therapies including prayer[3]	CAM excluding megavitamin therapy and prayer[4]	Biologically based therapies excluding megavitamin therapy[5]	Mind-body therapies excluding prayer[6]	Alternative medical systems[7]	Energy therapies	Manipulative and body-based therapies[8]
	Percents (standard error)								
Lifetime cigarette smoking status[10,19]									
Current smoker	57.2 (0.81)	19.7 (0.56)	47.6 (0.78)	32.9 (0.70)	18.7 (0.55)	16.8 (0.55)	2.0 (0.17)	0.5 (0.10)	9.2 (0.42)
Former smoker	66.6 (0.81)	27.0 (0.78)	55.6 (0.87)	41.9 (0.88)	25.3 (0.76)	21.1 (0.77)	4.0 (0.32)	0.8 (0.14)	13.6 (0.60)
Never smoker	62.8 (0.50)	21.2 (0.38)	54.3 (0.53)	34.1 (0.46)	20.0 (0.37)	16.1 (0.37)	2.6 (0.15)	0.5 (0.06)	10.7 (0.30)
Lifetime alcohol drinking status[10,20]									
Lifetime abstainer	61.6 (0.79)	14.9 (0.54)	56.9 (0.82)	24.3 (0.66)	14.0 (0.52)	10.8 (0.47)	1.5 (0.18)	*0.2 (0.06)	6.1 (0.33)
Former drinker	69.2 (0.96)	20.5 (0.82)	62.3 (0.99)	33.4 (0.97)	19.0 (0.79)	16.6 (0.74)	2.3 (0.27)	0.5 (0.13)	9.4 (0.57)
Current infrequent/light drinker	62.2 (0.56)	24.3 (0.45)	51.6 (0.58)	39.7 (0.55)	23.0 (0.46)	19.6 (0.45)	3.1 (0.18)	0.7 (0.08)	13.3 (0.37)
Current moderate/heavier drinker	57.0 (0.83)	25.5 (0.65)	43.5 (0.84)	38.5 (0.76)	24.0 (0.64)	18.4 (0.64)	3.4 (0.28)	0.6 (0.11)	12.1 (0.51)
Hospitalized in the last year[10]									
Yes	75.9 (0.97)	22.1 (0.91)	70.4 (1.04)	37.4 (1.14)	20.5 (0.89)	19.5 (0.91)	3.1 (0.40)	*0.5 (0.16)	11.2 (0.71)
No	60.6 (0.42)	22.0 (0.31)	50.8 (0.44)	34.9 (0.39)	20.7 (0.30)	16.7 (0.32)	2.7 (0.12)	0.5 (0.05)	10.9 (0.25)

*Estimates preceded by an asterisk have a relative standard error of greater than 30% and should be used with caution as they do not meet the standard of reliability or precision.
– Quantity zero.
[1]CAM including megavitamins and prayer includes acupuncture; ayurveda; homeopathic treatment; naturopathy; chelation therapy; folk medicine; nonvitamin, nonmineral, natural products; diet-based therapies; megavitamin therapy; chiropractic care; massage; biofeedback; meditation; guided imagery; progressive relaxation; deep breathing exercises; hypnosis; yoga; tai chi; qi gong; prayer for health reasons; and energy healing therapy/Reiki.
[2]Biologically based therapies including megavitamin therapy includes chelation therapy; folk medicine; nonvitamin, nonmineral, natural products; diet-based therapies; and megavitamin therapy.
[3]Mind body therapies including prayer includes biofeedback; meditation; guided imagery; progressive relaxation; deep breathing exercises; hypnosis; yoga; tai chi; qi gong; and prayer for health reasons.
[4]CAM excluding megavitamins and prayer includes acupuncture; ayurveda; homeopathic treatment; naturopathy; chelation therapy; folk medicine; nonvitamin, nonmineral, natural products; diet-based therapies; chiropractic care; massage; biofeedback; meditation; guided imagery; progressive relaxation; deep breathing exercises; hypnosis; yoga; tai chi; qi gong; and energy healing therapy/Reiki.
[5]Biologically based therapies excluding megavitamin therapy includes chelation therapy; folk medicine; nonvitamin, nonmineral, natural products; and diet-based therapies.
[6]Mind-body therapies excluding prayer includes biofeedback; meditation; guided imagery; progressive relaxation; deep breathing exercises; hypnosis; yoga; tai chi; and qi gong.
[7]Alternative medical systems includes acupuncture; ayurveda; homeopathic treatment; and naturopathy.
[8]Manipulative and body-based therapies includes chiropractic care and massage.
[9]Total includes other races not shown separately and persons with unknown education, family income, poverty status, health insurance status, marital status, body weight status, lifetime smoking status, alcohol consumption status, and hospitalization status
[10]Estimates were age adjusted to the year 2000 U.S. standard population using four age groups: 18–24 years, 25–44 years, 45–64 years, and 65 years and over.

158

[11]Persons of Hispanic or Latino origin may be of any race or combination of races. Similarly, the category "Not Hispanic or Latino" refers to all persons who are not of Hispanic or Latino origin, regardless of race.

[12]GED is General Education Development high school equivalency diploma.

[13]The categories "Less than $20,000" and "$20,000 or more" include both persons reporting dollar amounts and persons reporting only that their incomes were within one of these two categories. The indented categories include only those persons who reported dollar amounts.

[14]Poverty status is based on family income and family size using the Census Bureau's poverty thresholds for 2001. "Poor" persons are defined as below the poverty threshold. "Near poor" persons have incomes of 100% to less than 200% of the poverty threshold. "Not poor" persons have incomes that are 200% of the poverty threshold or greater.

[15]Classification of health insurance coverage is based on a hierarchy of mutually exclusive categories. Persons with more than one type of health insurance were assigned to the first appropriate category in the hierarchy. Persons under age 65 years and those age 65 years and over were classified separately due to the prominence of Medicare coverage in the older population. The category "Uninsured" includes persons who had no coverage as well as those who had only Indian Health Service coverage or had only a private plan that paid for one type of service such as accidents or dental care (see "Definition of terms" for more details). Estimates are age-adjusted to the 2000 U.S. standard population using three age groups: 18–24 years, 25–44 years, and 45–64 years for persons under age 65, and two age groups: 65–74 years and 75 years and over for persons aged 65 years and over.

[16]MSA is metropolitan statistical area.

[17]Pacific states includes California, Oregon, Washington, Alaska, and Hawaii.

[18]Body weight status was based on Body Mass Index (BMI) using self-reported height and weight. The formula for BMI is kilograms/meters^2. Underweight is defined as a BMI of less than 18.5; healthy weight is defined as a BMI of at least 18.5 and less than 25; overweight, but not obese, is defined as a BMI of at least 25 and less than 30; and obese is defined as a BMI of 30 or more.

[19]Lifetime cigarette smoking status: Current smoker: smoked at least 100 cigarettes in lifetime and currently smoked cigarettes every day or some days; Former smoker: smoked at least 100 cigarettes in lifetime but did not currently smoke; Never smoker: never smoked at all or smoked less than 100 cigarettes in lifetime.

[20]Lifetime alcohol drinking status: Lifetime abstainer is less than 12 drinks in lifetime; former drinker is 12 or more drinks in lifetime, but no drinks in past year; current infrequent/light drinker is defined as at least 12 drinks in lifetime and 1–11 drinks in past year (infrequent) or 3 drinks or fewer per week, on average (light); current moderate/heavier is defined as at least 12 drinks in lifetime and more than 3 drinks per week up to 14 drinks in past week up to 7 drinks per week on average for men and more than 3 drinks per week up to 14 drinks per week on average for men and more than 7 drinks per week on average for women (heavier).

NOTES: CAM is complementary and alternative medicine. The denominators for statistics shown exclude persons with unknown CAM information.

DATA SOURCE: National Health Interview Survey, 2002.

considered, only mind-body therapies including prayer specifically for health reasons show a positive correlation with age.

- If prayer specifically for health reasons is excluded from the definition of CAM, all the CAM categories demonstrated inverse "U" relationships with age, with the youngest and oldest groups reporting the least use of CAM.
- Black adults (68.3 percent) were more likely to use mind-body therapies including prayer specifically for health reasons than white adults (50.1 percent) or Asian adults (48.1 percent).
- Asian adults were more likely (43.1 percent) to use CAM (excluding megavitamin therapy and prayer specifically for health reasons) than white adults (35.9 percent) or black adults (26.2 percent).
- White adults (12.0 percent) were more likely to use manipulative and body-based therapies than Asian adults (7.2 percent) or black adults (4.4 percent).
- Non-Hispanic adults were more likely than Hispanic adults to use mind-body therapies excluding prayer specifically for health reasons and less likely to use mind-body therapies including prayer specifically for health reasons.
- Except for the groups of therapies that included prayer specifically for health reasons, use of CAM increased as education levels increased.
- Poor adults were more likely than not to use CAM including megavitamin therapy and prayer specifically for health reasons, while not poor adults were more likely than poor adults to use CAM if megavitamin therapy and prayer specifically for health reasons were excluded.
- Adults who live in urban areas were more likely than adults who live in rural areas to use alternative medical systems, biologically based therapies (including and excluding prayer specifically for health reasons).
- Adults who were former smokers were more likely to use CAM than adults who were current smokers or those who had never smoked.
- Adults who were hospitalized in the last year were more likely than adults who were not hospitalized in the last year to use CAM when the definition included prayer specifically for health reasons.

Selected Reasons for Using CAM (Table 5)

- Adult CAM users were most likely to utilize CAM because they believed that CAM combined with conventional medical treatments would help (54.9 percent).
- About one-half of adult CAM users initially utilized CAM because they thought it would be interesting to try (50.1 percent).
- Twenty-six percent of adult CAM users utilized it because a conventional medical professional suggested they try it.
- Twenty-eight percent of adult CAM users used CAM because they felt that conventional medicine was too expensive.

Table 5. Age-adjusted percents of adult users of complementary and alternative medicine specifying selected reasons for using it, by types of therapy: United States, 2002

Therapy	Sample size	Reason[1]				
		Conventional medical treatments would not help	Conventional medical treatments were too expensive	Therapy combined with conventional medical treatments would help	Suggested by a conventional medical professional	Thought it would be interesting to try
		Percents (standard error)				
Any CAM[2] use	6,619	27.7 (0.67)	13.2 (0.46)	54.9 (0.78)	25.8 (0.66)	50.1 (0.76)
Alternative medical systems						
Acupuncture	276	44.2 (3.52)	7.4 (1.62)	56.2 (3.30)	24.8 (3.28)	51.6 (3.69)
Ayurveda	10	60.6 (16.01)	*43.2 (17.29)	*52.6 (16.98)	*17.4 (13.73)	100.0 (0.00)
Homeopathic treatment	416	36.7 (3.01)	19.4 (2.34)	43.1 (2.94)	14.2 (2.01)	45.8 (3.06)
Naturopathy	66	53.1 (7.23)	28.3 (6.31)	62.4 (6.50)	16.5 (4.95)	43.9 (6.96)
Biologically based therapies						
Chelation therapy	6	28.5 (5.72)	*–	84.6 (10.64)	76.4 (8.72)	*18.7 (9.08)
Folk medicine	32	43.1 (8.65)	47.6 (9.79)	53.5 (9.73)	*7.5 (4.45)	49.3 (9.47)
Nonvitamin, nonmineral, natural products	3,315	19.2 (0.80)	14.4 (0.67)	47.5 (1.08)	15.3 (0.77)	51.7 (1.03)
Diet-based therapies	418	22.4 (2.55)	11.3 (2.02)	38.1 (2.92)	26.3 (2.65)	52.6 (2.97)
Megavitamin therapy	360	27.5 (2.84)	13.5 (2.19)	55.0 (3.09)	38.3 (2.94)	37.7 (2.96)
Manipulative and body-based therapies						
Chiropractic care	1,869	39.6 (1.35)	9.5 (0.75)	52.9 (1.40)	20.2 (1.11)	31.8 (1.27)
Massage	703	33.9 (2.05)	12.6 (1.46)	59.6 (2.17)	33.4 (2.01)	44.1 (2.33)
Mind-body therapies						
Biofeedback	37	*22.9 (7.08)	*8.0 (5.07)	61.0 (8.82)	62.7 (7.17)	45.5 (7.86)
Relaxation techniques	1,406	20.6 (1.30)	12.5 (1.01)	56.1 (1.63)	36.3 (1.61)	54.5 (1.69)
Hypnosis	74	30.0 (6.84)	*10.4 (3.44)	22.9 (4.98)	21.1 (4.83)	65.2 (7.38)
Yoga, tai chi, qi gong	315	30.9 (3.37)	14.4 (2.56)	52.3 (3.57)	21.0 (3.09)	59.2 (3.47)
Healing ritual for own health	419	19.1 (2.34)	13.6 (2.02)	66.9 (2.95)	8.4 (1.56)	34.1 (2.86)
Energy healing therapy/Reiki	86	46.5 (6.48)	22.9 (5.25)	60.6 (6.03)	18.0 (5.02)	50.4 (5.92)

*Estimates preceded by an asterisk have a relative standard error of greater than 30% and should be used with caution as they do not meet the standard of reliability or precision.

– Quantity zero.

[1]Respondents may select more than one reason for using a CAM therapy.

[2]CAM includes acupuncture; ayurveda; homeopathic treatment; naturopathy; chelation therapy; folk medicine; nonvitamin, nonmineral, natural products; diet-based therapies; megavitamin therapy; chiropractic care; massage; biofeedback; meditation; guided imagery; progressive relaxation; deep breathing exercises; hypnosis; yoga; tai chi; qi gong; healing ritual for own health; and energy healing therapy/Reiki.

NOTES: CAM is complementary and alternative medicine. The denominators for statistics shown exclude persons with unknown CAM information. Estimates were age adjusted to the year 2000 U.S. standard population using four age groups: 18–24 years, 25–44 years, 45–64 years, and 65 years and over.

DATA SOURCE: National Health Interview Survey, 2002.

Discussion

Overall, in 2002, about 62 percent of U.S. adults used some form of CAM in the past 12 months. Subgroup differences were noted in the use of CAM; women were more likely than men to use CAM; black adults were less likely than white adults or Asian adults to use CAM when megavitamin therapy and prayer specifically for health reasons were included in the definition; persons with higher educational attainment were more likely than persons with lower educational attainment to use CAM; and those who had been hospitalized in the past year were more likely than those who had not been in the hospital in the past year to use CAM. However, when specific CAM therapies were examined, different patterns of use were noted, indicating the importance of the relationship between respondent characteristics and CAM therapy. The findings that gender, education, and health status are associated with CAM use are consistent with earlier reports. (1,2,5,9,11). However, this is the first observation that black adults (71.3 percent) and Asian adults (61.7 percent) are substantial users of CAM. Additional surveys are needed to explore use within minority groups.

The survey also revealed that most people who have ever used CAM have used it within the past 12 months and provided national confirmation of an observation seen in a single State (9). These results are surprising given the lack of definitive evidence supporting the efficacy of most CAM interventions. Research-based information on CAM therapies is available to the public from sources such as the National Library of Medicine's "CAM on PubMed" and "MedLine Plus" or the Cochrane Collaboration Database (28–30).

The data confirm most earlier observations that most people use CAM to treat and/or prevent musculoskeletal conditions or other conditions associated with chronic or recurring pain (1,5,9,10). The high prevalence of CAM use for these conditions is not surprising when one considers that one-quarter to one-third of the adult population might be suffering from one of these disorders in any given year (31,32), yet many forms of chronic pain are resistant to conventional medical treatment (33,34).

The high prevalence of CAM use for colds has not been reported previously for the U.S. adult population (35) and is consistent with the observation that 40.3 percent of individuals who use natural products use the herbal product echinacea, which is widely used for diseases of the upper respiratory tract.

About 1.0 percent of adult CAM users utilized CAM to treat each of the following three conditions: high cholesterol (1.1 percent); asthma (1.1 percent); and hypertension (1.0 percent). These results are interesting given that there are many effective ways to manage these conditions using both normal lifestyle changes and conventional pharmaceutical drugs. Further analyses will need to clarify the specific populations with these conditions using CAM, the types of CAM they employ, and the reasons why they use CAM.

Compared with earlier surveys, the NHIS CAM supplement has several important characteristics. These include questions about use of an extensive list of CAM therapies, a wide variety of health conditions and diseases for which they may be used, and questions about reasons for use and satisfaction with treatment. In addition, unlike earlier surveys, the NHIS yielded CAM data that are representative of the adult U.S. population. Also, the NHIS has a large sample size so that subgroups can be examined. and data from the CAM component can be linked to a wide variety of respondent characteristics, enriching the analytic potential.

In the population-based surveys conducted in the United States on CAM use since 1990, CAM has been operationally defined in a variety of ways (1–11). Most surveys asked participants to indicate whether they used one or more items from a list of CAM interventions/therapies, but the lists varied considerably among the surveys. The most common CAM intervention/therapies included in the surveys, in order of most common inclusion, were chiropractic care, acupuncture, herbal medicine, hypnosis, massage therapy, relaxation techniques, biofeedback, and homeopathic treatment. CAM interventions/therapies such as chelation therapy, energy therapies, qi gong, tai chi, yoga, high-dose vitamins, and spirituality-prayer for health purposes were less commonly used. In addition to differences in the definition of CAM, the previous population-based surveys varied from the NHIS survey in several other ways that might affect estimates of CAM use in the adult population. Few of the previous surveys were conducted using extensive, in-person interviews with participants randomly chosen to reflect the U.S. population (2, 3, 8, 10). Instead, most relied on telephone interviews with random-digit dialing used to select households or a mail survey with recipients randomly chosen from an existing database of individuals who had previously agreed to respond to such surveys. Telephone and mail surveys tend to exclude lower income individuals who might not have access to a telephone or a stable mailing address and thus impair the representativeness of the data. Most previous surveys were small, with only two having sample sizes about a few thousand individuals (2,3,8). This limited the ability to estimate CAM use among minority populations of interest such as adults of Hispanic or Asian heritage. Only six of the previous surveys identified the diseases and/or conditions associated with CAM use (1,2,4,5,9,10), and only four collected information on participant satisfaction with their CAM treatment (1,6,9,11). Most of the earlier surveys did not include questions about health insurance coverage, and only one included a question about reasons for CAM use (1).

Comparison of estimates derived from the NHIS CAM supplement using approximations of the CAM selection criteria from six of those earlier studies are shown in table 6. The estimates of CAM use range from 20.3 percent to 48.8 percent. The NHIS estimates of total CAM use are higher than those from earlier studies, partly because of differences in operational definitions of CAM and differences in survey design described above. Given the breadth of CAM therapies queried in the NHIS, it is not surprising the NHIS estimates of CAM use (62.1 percent) are greater than previously reported in the literature. The inclusion of detailed questions on prayer for health purposes, items are rarely queried in previous surveys of CAM use, accounted for most

Table 6. Frequencies and age-adjusted percents of adults 18 years and over who used complementary and alternative medicine during the past 12 months, using the combination of complementary and alternative medicine therapies included in previous surveys: United States, 2002

CAM therapies[1]	Population	
	Number in thousands[2]	Percent (standard error)[2]
Acupuncture; Ayurveda; biofeedback; chelation therapy; chiropractic care; deep breathing exercises; diet-based therapies; energy healing therapy/Reiki; folk medicine; guided imagery; homeopathic treatment; hypnosis; massage therapy; meditation; megavitamin therapy; naturopathy; nonvitamin, nonmineral, natural products; prayer for health reasons; progressive relaxation; qi gong; tai chi; and yoga[3]	123,606	62.1 (0.40)
Acupuncture; Ayurveda; biofeedback; chelation therapy; chiropractic care; deep breathing exercises; diet-based therapies; energy healing therapy/Reiki; folk medicine; guided imagery; homeopathic treatment; hypnosis; massage therapy; meditation; naturopathy; nonvitamin, nonmineral, natural products; prayer for health reasons; progressive relaxation; qi gong; tai chi; and yoga[4]	122,804	61.6 (0.40)
Acupuncture; Ayurveda; biofeedback; chelation therapy; chiropractic care; deep breathing exercises; diet-based therapies; energy healing therapy/Reiki; folk medicine; guided imagery; homeopathic treatment; hypnosis; massage therapy; meditation; naturopathy; nonvitamin, nonmineral, natural products; progressive relaxation; qi gong; tai chi; and yoga[5]	72,401	36.0 (0.38)
Acupuncture; Ayurveda; biofeedback; chelation therapy; chiropractic care; energy healing therapy; folk medicine; hypnosis; massage therapy; meditation; and naturopathy[6]	23,955	11.8 (0.25)
Acupuncture; Ayurveda; biofeedback; chiropractic care; deep breathing exercises; diet-based therapies; energy healing therapy; folk medicine; guided imagery; massage therapy; meditation; naturopathy; progressive relaxation; and prayer by others (5)	97,253	48.8 (0.40)
Acupuncture; biofeedback; chiropractic care; deep breathing exercises; diet-based therapies; energy healing therapy; folk medicine; guided imagery; nonvitamin, nonmineral, natural products; megavitamin therapy; homeopathic treatment; hypnosis; massage therapy; progressive relaxation; and prayer by others (1,4)	95,921	48.1 (0.40)
Acupuncture; biofeedback; chiropractic care; deep breathing exercises; diet-based therapies; energy healing therapy; guided imagery; nonvitamin, nonmineral, natural products; homeopathic treatment; hypnosis; massage therapy; progressive relaxation; and prayer by others (8)	94,671	47.4 (0.40)
Biofeedback; chiropractic care; deep breathing exercises; diet-based therapies; energy healing therapy; folk medicine; guided imagery; nonvitamin, nonmineral, natural products; homeopathic treatment; hypnosis; massage therapy; progressive relaxation; and prayer by others (9)	90,299	45.3 (0.39)
Acupuncture; biofeedback; chiropractic care; diet-based therapies; energy healing therapy; guided imagery; nonvitamin; nonmineral; natural products; megavitamin therapy; hypnosis; and meditation (11)	60,425	30.0 (0.35)
Acupuncture; chiropractic care; deep breathing exercises; massage therapy; and progressive relaxation (10)	40,984	20.3 (0.31)

[1]The combinations of CAM are based on selected studies.

[2]Numbers and percents are calculated using data from the 2002 NHIS.

[3]This definition of CAM comes from the study on which this report is based and consists of all the CAM therapies included in the 2002 NHIS questionnaire.

[4]This definition of CAM comes from the study on which this report is based and consists of all the CAM therapies included in the 2002 NHIS questionnaire excluding megavitamin therapy.

[5]This definition of CAM comes from the study on which this report is based and consists of all the CAM therapies included in the 2002 NHIS questionnaire excluding prayer for health reasons.

[6]This definition of CAM comes from the study on which this report is based and consists of all the CAM therapies included in the 2002 NHIS questionnaire that are practitioner-based therapies.

NOTES: CAM is complementary and alternative medicine. The denominators for statistics shown exclude persons with unknown CAM information.

DATA SOURCE: National Health Interview Survey, 2002.

of the differences. About 45 percent of adults used prayer specifically for health reasons during the past 12 months. Excluding prayer specifically for health reasons is a therapy reduced by NHIS estimates of CAM use from 62.1 percent to 36.0 percent.

Table 6 also presents the percentage of U.S. adults who use practitioner-based therapies. The fact that only 11.8 percent of adults sought care from a licensed or certified practitioner suggests that most individuals who use CAM self-prescribe and/or self medicate, as suggested by another study (5). This practice could increase the chance of inappropriate use of a given CAM therapy and result in negative consequences.

Consistent with previous studies (1,3,5), the present study found that the majority of individuals used CAM in conjunction with conventional medicine (54.9 percent). About one-quarter of U.S. adults who used CAM during the past 12 months did so because CAM use was suggested by a conventional health care provider, a rate almost identical to that seen in South Carolina (9). More surprising is the finding that 27.7 percent of individuals who use CAM believed that conventional medicine would not help their health problems. These data are contrary to a previous observation that CAM users are not, in general, dissatisfied with conventional medicine (1).

Conclusions

The NHIS survey provides the most comprehensive and reliable current data describing CAM use by the U.S. adult population. Their report adds to the increasing body of evidence about CAM use in the United States. The descriptive statistics and highlights presented in this report are a foundation for future studies of CAM use as it relates to health and disease among various population subgroups. Ongoing analysis of the NHIS dataset by NCHS and NCCAM staff will further explore the relationship of CAM use with various health behaviors, race and gender and the differences between those who use CAM in conjunction with conventional medicine and those who only use CAM or only conventional medicine.

References

1. Astin JA. Why patients use alternative medicine; results of a national study. JAMA 279 (19): 1548–53. May 20, 1998.
2. Bausell RB, Lee WL, Berman BM. Demographic and health-related correlates to visits to complementary and alternative medical providers. Med Care 39 (2): 190–6. Feb 2001.
3. Druss BG, Rosenheck RA. Association between use of unconventional therapies and conventional medical services. JAMA 282 (7): 651–6. Aug. 18, 1999.
4. Eisenberg DM, Kessler RC, Foster C, et al. Unconventional medicine in the United States. Prevalence, costs and patterns of use. N Engl J Med 328 (4): 246–52. Jan 28, 1993.

5. Eisenberg DM, Davis RB, Ettner SL, et al. Trends in alternative medicine use in the United States, 1990-19997: results of a follow-up national survey. JAMA 280 (18): 1569–75. Nov 11, 1998.

6. Landmark Healthcare, Inc. The Landmark Report on Public Perceptions of Alternative Care. Landmark Healthcare, Inc. Sacramento, CA. 1998.

7. Mackenzie ER, Taylor L, Bloom BS, et al. Ethnic minority use of complementary and alternative medicine (CAM); A national probability survey of CAM utilizers. Alternative Therapies in Health and Medicine 9(4): 50–56. 2003.

8. Ni H, Simile C, Hardy AM. Utilization of complementary and alternative medicine by United States adults. Results from the 1999 National Health Interview Survey. Med Care 40 (4): 353–8, April 2002.

9. Oldendick R, Coker AL, Wieland, D et al. Population-based survey of complementary and alternative medicine usage, patient satisfaction, and physician involvement. Southern Medical Journal 93 (4): 375–81. 2000.

10. Paramore LC. Use of alternative therapies: Estimates from the 1994 Robert Wood Johnson Foundation National Access to Care Survey, J Pain Symptom Manage 13 (2): 83–9. Feb 1997.

11. Rafferty, AP, McGee HB, Miller CE, Reyes M. Prevalence of complementary and alternative medicine use: state-specific estimates from the 2001 Behavioral Risk Factor Surveilance System. Am J Public Health 92 (10): 1598–1600. 2002.

12. Center for Medicare and Medicaid Services. 1997 National Health Expenditures Survey. Available at:http://www.cms.hhs.gov/statistics/nhe/.

13. Engel LW, Straus SE. Development of therapeutics: opportunities within complementary and alternative medicine. Nat Rev Drug Discov 1(3): 229–37. Mar 1, 2002.

14. Sparber A, Wootton JC. Surveys of complementary and alternative medicine: Part II use of alternative and complementary cancer therapies. J Altern Complement Med 7(3): 281–7. June 2001.

15. Wootton JC, Sparber A. Surveys of Complementary and alternative medicine: Part III use of alternative and complementary therapies for HIV/AIDS. J Altern Complemt Med 7 (4): 371–7. Aug 2001.

16. NCCAM. Five Year Strategic Plan: 2001–2005. Available at: http://nccam.nih.gov/about/plans/fiveyear/index.htm

17. WHO. Legal status of traditional medicine and complementary/ alternative medicine: A worldwide review. WHO Geneva. 2001.

18. Watanabe S, Imanishi J, Satoh M, Ozasa K. Unique place of Kampo (Japanese traditional medicine) in complementary and alternative medicine: A survey of doctors belonging to the regional medical association in Japan. Tohoku J Exp Med 194 (1): 55–63. May 2001.

19. Jonas WB, Levin JS (eds). Essentials of complementary and alternative medicine. Lippincott, Williams and Wilkins. 1999.

20. NIH Consensus Conference Statement, Acupuncture. JAMA 280 (17): 1518–24. Review. Nov 4, 1998.

21. NIH Technology Assessment Conference Statement, Integration of behavioral and relaxation approaches into treatment of chrnoic pain and insomnia. NIH Technology Assessment Panel on Integration of Behavioral and Relaxation Approaches in the Treatment of Chronic Pain and Insomnia. JAMA 276 (4): 313–8. July 24–31, 1996.

22. DHHS. FDA announces plans to prohibit sales of dietary supplements containing ephedra. Dec 30, 2003. Available at: http://www. hhs.gov/news/press/2003pres/20031230.html

23. Izzo AA, Ernst E. Interactions between herbal medicines and prescribed drugs: a systematic review. Drugs 61 (15): 2163–75. 2001.

24. National Center for Health Statistics. 2002 National Health Interview Survey (NHIS). Public use data release. NHIS survey description. ftp://ftp.cdc.gov/pub/Health_Statistics/NCHS/Dataset_Documentation/NHIS/2002/srvydesc.pdf.

25. Research Triangle Institute. SUDAAN (release 9.0.1) (Computer Software). Research Triangle Park, NC: Research Triangle Institute 2002.

26. Day JC. Population projections of the United States by age, sex, race and Hispanic origin: 1995 to 2050, U.S. Bureau of the Census, Current Population Reports, p. 25–1130, U.S. Government Printing Office, Washington, 1996. (http://www.consus.gov/prod/1/pop/p25–1130/)

27. Klein RJ, Scoenborn CA. Age adjustment using the 2000 projected U.S. population. Heathy People Statistical Notes. no. 20. Hyattsville, MD. National Center for Health Statistics: Jan 2001.

28. CAM on PubMed. http://www./nlm.nih.gov/nccam/camonpubmed. html

29. Medline Plus. http://www.nlm.nih.gov/medlineplus/

30. Cochrane Collaboration Database. http://www.update-software. com/cochrane/

31. Lipton RB, Stewart WF, Diamond S, et al. Prevalence and burden of migraine in the United States: Data from the American Migraine Study II. Headache 41: 646–57. 2002.

32. Yelin E, Herndorf A, Trupin L, Sonneborn D. A national study of medical care expenditures for musculoskeletal conditions: the impact of health insurance and managed care. Arthritis and Rheumatology 44(5): 1160–69. 2001.

33. Deyo RA, Weinstein, JN. Low back pain. N Engl J Med 344 (5): 363–70. 2001.

34. Turk DC. Clinical effectiveness and cost-effectiveness of treatments for patients with chronic pain. Clin J Pain 18: 355–65. 2001.

35. Fendrick AM, Monto AS, Nightengale B, Sarnes M. The economic burden of non-influenza related viral respiratory tract infection in the United States. Arch Intern Med 163: 487–94. 2003.

36. Office of Managemernt and Budget. Revisions to the standards for the classification of Federal data on race and ethnicity. Federal Register 62 (210): 58782–90. 1997.

37. U. S. Census Bureau. http://www.census.gov/population/www/estimates/aboutmetro.html.

Table I. Age distributions used in age-adjusting data shown in tables 1–5 and figure 1

Age	2000 U.S. standard population (in thousands)
18 years and over	203,851
18–24 years	26,258
25–44 years	81,892
45–64 years	60,991
65 years and over.	34,710
Health insurance	
18–64 years.	169,141
18–24 years	26,258
25–44 years	81,892
45–64 years	60,991
65 years and over	34,710
65–74 years	18,136
75 years and over.	16,574

Technical Notes

Sample Design   The National Health Interview Survey (NHIS) is a cross-sectional household survey of the U.S. civilian noninstitutionalized population. Data are collected continuously throughout the year in all 50 states and the District of Columbia. The NHIS uses a multistage, clustered sample design to produce national estimates for a variety of health indicators. Information on basic health topics is collected for all household members by proxy from one family member, if necessary. Additional information is collected for one randomly selected adult and one randomly selected child in each family. Self-response is required for the Sample Adult questionnaire except in rare cases where sample adults are physically or mentally incapable of responding for themselves. Interviews are conducted in the home using a computer-assisted personal interview (CAPI) questionnaire with telephone interviewing permitted for follow-up, if necessary.

Response Rates   In 2002, interviews were completed in 36,161 households and 36,831 families, with 31,044 adults completing the Sample Adult portion of the interview. The final household response rate was 89.6 percent and the final response rate for the 2002 Sample Adult questionnaire was 74.3 percent. Procedures used in calcultating response rates are described in detail in "Appendix I" of the Survey Description of the NHIS data files (24).

Item Nonresponse   Item nonresponse for each of the sociodemographic indicators shown in table 4 was about 1 percent or less, with the exception of poverty status, which is based on detailed family income asked in the family component of the questionnaire. Item nonresponse for the poverty indicator was 29.0 percent. Item nonresponse for the health behavior items ranged from 1.0 percent to

5.2 percent and was less than 1 percent for hospitalization during the past year. For the complementary and alternative medicine items, nonresponse ranged from 1.7 percent to 3.2 percent. The denominators for statistics shown in the tables exclude persons with unknown complementary and alternative medicine information for a given table. In table 4, persons with unknown sociodemographic characteristics, health behavior items, and hospitalization during the past year are not shown separately, but are included in the total. Among the 31,044 interviewed sample adult respondents in the 2002 NHIS, 427 persons were missing data for all the complementary and alternative medicine items.

Age Adjustment   Data shown in this report were age adjusted using the year 2000 U.S. standard population provided by the U.S. Census Bureau (26, 27). Age adjustment was used to allow comparison among various population subgroups that have different age structures. This is particularly important for demographic characteristics such as race and ethnicity, education and marital status. It is also helpful for other characteristics. The following age groups were used for age adjustment: 18–24 years; 25–44 years; 45–64 years and 65 years and over, unless otherwise noted (table 1). Health insurance is restricted to certain age groups and is, therefore, adusted accordingly.

Tests of Significance   Statistical tests performed to assess significance of differences in the estimates were two-tailed with no adjustments for multiple comparisons. The test statistic used to determine statistical significance of differences between two percents was

$$Z = \frac{\left| X_a - X_b \right|}{\sqrt{S_a^2 + S_b^2}}$$

where X_a and X_b are the two percents being compared, and S_a and S_b are the standard errors of those percents. The critical value used for two-sided tests at the 0.05 level of significance was 1.96.

Relative Standard Error   Estimates with a relative standard error greater than 30 percent are considered unreliable and are indicated with an asterik (*). The relative standard errors are calculated as follows:

Relative standard error
(as a percent) = (SE/Est) 100.

where SE is the standard error of the estimate and Est is the estimate.

Definition of Terms

Demographic Terms

   Age—The age recorded for each person is the age at last birthday.

Education—The categories of education are based on the years of school completed or highest degree obtained. Respondents were shown a flash card to chose an appropriate category. Only years completed in a school that advances a person toward a elementary or high school diploma, General Education Development high school equivalency diploma (GED), college, university or professional degree are included. Education in other schools or home schooling is counted only if the credits are accepted in a regular school system.

Family Income—Each member of a family is classified according to the total income of all family members. Family members are all persons within the household related to each other by blood, marriage, cohabitation or adoption. The income recorded is the total income received by all family members in the previous calendar year, income from all sources-including wages, salaries, military pay (when an Armed Forces member lives in the household), pensions, government payments, child support/alimony, dividends, help from relatives-is included. Unrelated individuals living in the same household (e.g., roomates) are considered to be separate families and are classified according to their incomes.

Health Insurance Coverage—NHIS respondents were asked about their health insurance coverage at the time of interview. Respondents reported whether they were covered by private insurance (obtained through the employer or workplace, purchased directly or through a local or community program), Medicare, Medigap (supplemental Medicare coverage), Medicaid, State Children's Health Insurance Program (SCHIP), Indiana Health Service (IHS), military coverage (including VA, TRICARE or CHAMP-VA), a State-sponsored health plan, another government program and/or any single service plans. This information was used to create a health insurance hierarchy that consisted of three mutually exclusive categories. Persons with more than one type of health insurance were assigned to the first appropriate category in the following hierarchy: private coverage; public coverage (includes persons with Medicare, Medigap, Medicaid, SCHIP, military coverage, a state-sponsored health plan and/or another government program) and uninsured (includes persons with only single service plans and/or only IHS).

Hispanic or Latino origin—Hispanic or Latino origin includes persons of Mexican, Puerto Rican, Cuban, Central and South Anerican, or Spanish origins. Persons of Hispanic or Latino origin may be of any race.

In this report, subsets of Hispanic or Latino origin are no shown for reasons of statistical reliability.

Marital Status—Respondents were asked to choose a marital status category most appropriate for their marital situation. In some cases, persons reporting their marital status as "married" may have been living in common-law marital unions. Alternatively, these individuals could have identified their marital status as "living with partner." Adults who were living with a partner were considered to be members of the same family (as if married) and are categorized as "cohabiting" in this report. The distinction between "married" and "living with partner" was made by the respondent.

Race—The 1997 Office of Management and Budget (OMB) Federal guidelines (36) for reporting race require that persons of "single race" be distinguished from persons of "multiple race." Single race refers to persons who indicated only a single race group. Estimates for the smaller subcategories of single race persons and multiple race combinations can only be reported to the extent that the estimates meet the requirements for confidentiality and statistical reliability. In this report, three categories are shown for single race individuals (white, single race; black or African American, single race; and Asian, single race). Other subcategories of single race persons and multiple race persons are not shown due to statistical unreliability as measured by the relative standard errors of the estimates.

The text in this report uses shorter versions of the new OMB race terms for conciseness and the table uses complete terms. For example, the category "Black or African American, single race" in the table is referred to as "Black" in the text.

Place of Residence—Metropolitan statistical area (MSA), a term first used in 1983, was defined by the U.S. Office of Management and Budget and is used by their U.S. Census Bureau to classify geographic areas (37). The categories shown in this report are: (a) "MSA central city," which generally refers to cities with populations of 50,000 or more: (b) "MSA, not central city," which refers to communities adjacent to the central city of an MSA that have a high degree of economic and social integration with the central city; and (c) "Not MSA," which refers to more rural areas of the country. The classification of areas in the 2002 NHIS is based on data from the 1990 decennial census.

Poverty Status—Poverty Status is based on family income and family size using the U.S. Census Bureau's poverty thresholds. "Poor" persons are defined as below the poverty threshold. "Near poor" persons have incomes of 100 percent to less than 200 percent of the poverty threshold or greater.

Region—In the geographic classification of the U.S. population, States are grouped into the following four regions used by the U.S. Census Bureau:

Region	States Included
Northeast	Maine, Vermont, New Hampshire, Massachusetts, Connecticut, Rhode Island, New York, New Jersey and Pennsylvania.
Midwest	Ohio, Illinois, Indiana, Michigan, Wisconsin, Minnesota, Iowa, Missouri, North Dakota, South Dakota, Kansas, and Nebraska.
South	Delaware, Maryland, District of Columbia, West Virginia, Virginia, Kentucky, Tennesee, North Carolina, South Carolina, Georgia, Florida, Alabama, Mississippi, Louisiana, Oklahoma, Arkansas and Texas.
West	Washington, Oregon, California, Nevada, New Mexico, Arizona, Idaho, Utah, Colorado, Montana, Wyoming, Alaska and Hawaii.

For this report, an additional region called "Pacific States" was created. This region is the subset of the West and consists of the following states: Arizona, California, Hawaii, Oregon and Washington. This additional region was created because of the high concentration of immigrants in these states who may be using CAM.

Urban/rural—The assignment of "urban" or "rural" is based on a block's 1990 Census designation.

Health Behavior Terms   Alcohol consumption status

Lifetime abstainer—Adults who had fewer than 12 drinks in entire lifetime.
Former drinker—Adults who had 12 drinks or more in lifetime, but who had no drinks in the past year.
Current infrequent/light drinker—Adults who had at least 12 drinks in their lifetime and more than 3 drinks per week up to 14 drinks per week, on average for men and more than 3 drinks per week up to 7 drinks per week, on average for women (moderate) or more than 14 drinks per week, on average for men and more than 7 drinks, on average for women (heavier).

Body weight status: Body weight status is based on body mass index (BMI), which is calculated from self-reported height and weight without shoes. BMI is calculated as weight divided by height (squared) using metric units (i.e., kilograms/meter [squared]).

Underweight—Adults with a body mass index of less than 18.5.
Healthy Weight—Adults with a body mass index of at least 18.5, but less than 25.
Overweight but not obese—Adults with a body mass index of 30 or more.

Smoking Status

Current—Adults who had smoked at least 100 cigarettes in their lifetime and currently smoked cigarettes every day or some days.
Former—Adults who had smoked at least 100 cigarettes in their lifetime, but did not currently smoke.
Never—Adults who never smoked a cigarette or who smoked fewer than 100 cigarettes in their entire lifetime.

Complementary and Alternative Medicine Terms

Acupuncture—Acupuncture is based on the theory that health is determined by a balanced flow of energy (chi or pi), which is thought to be present in all living organisms. This life energy circulates throughout the body along a series of energy pathways (meridians). Each of these meridians is linked to specific internal organs and organ systems. Within this system of energy pathways, there are over 1,000 acupoints that can be stimulated through the insertion of needles. This is thought to help correct and rebalance the flow of life energy, and restore health. Acupuncture has been used to treat health problems and conditions ranging from the common cold to addiction and chronic fatigue syndrome.

Alternative provider or practitioner—Someone who is knowledgeable about a specific alternative health therapy provides care or advice about its use, and usually receives payment for his or her services.

For some therapies, the provider may have received formal training and may be certified by a licensing board or related professional association. For example, a practitioner of biofeedback (biofeedback therapist) has usually received training in psychology and physiology and may be certified by the Biofeedback Certification Institute of America.

Atkins Diet—A diet emphasizing a drastic reduction in the daily intake of carbohydrates (to 40 grams or less), it is countered by an increase in protein and fat. According to proponents of this diet, obesity results from the overconsumption of carbohydrates and reducing the intake of carbohydrates typically consumed for energy causes the body to lose weight by burning stored fat.

Ayurveda—This comprehensive system of medicine, developed in India over 5,000 years ago, places equal emphasis on body, mind and spirit. The goal is to restore the natural harmony of the individual. An ayurvedic doctor identifies an individual's "constitution" or overall health profile by ascertaining the patient's metabolic body type (Vatta, Pitta or Kapha) through a series of personal history questions. Then the patient's "constitution" becomes a foundation for a specific treatment plan designed to guide the individual back into harmony with his or her environment. This plan may include dietary changes, exercise, yoga, meditation, massage, herbal tonics and other remedies.

Biofeedback—This method teaches clients, through the use of simple electronic devices, how to consciously regulate normally unconscious bodily functions (e.g., breathing, heart rate, blood pressure) to improve overall health. Biofeedback had been used to reduce stress, eliminate headaches, recondition injured muscles, control asthmatic attacks and relieve pain.

Chelation therapy—This therapy involves a series of intravenous injections of a binding (chelating) agent, such as amino acid EDTA, to remove toxic metals and wastes from the bloodstream. Following injection, the binding agent travels through the bloodstream attaching itself to toxic metals and wastes, which are subsequently excreted through the patient's urine. Used initially to treat lead poisoning, chelation therapy is used by a growing number of practitioners to treat and reverse the process of atherosclerosis (hardening of the arteries).

Chiropractic care—This care involves the adjustment of the spine and joints to influence the body's nervous system and natural defense mechanisms to alleviate pain and improve general health. It is primarily used to treat back problems, headaches, nerve inflammation, muscle spasms and other injuries or traumas.

Complementary and alternative medicine—Therapies are not usually taught in U.S. medical schools or generally available in U.S. hospitals, it includes a broad range of therapies and beliefs such as acupuncture, chiropractic care, relaxation techniques, massage therapy and herbal remedies.

Deep breathing—Deep breathing involves slow, deep inhalation through the nose, usually for a count of 10, followed by slow and complete exhalation for a similar count. To help quiet the mind, one generally concentrates fully on breathing and counting through each cycle. The process may be repeated 5 to 10 times, several times a day.

Energy healing therapy/Reiki—This method helps the body's ability to heal itself through the flow and focusing of healing energy (Reiki means universal healing energy). During treatment, this healing energy is channeled through the hands of a practitioner into the client's body to restore a normal balance and health. Energy healing therapy has been used to treat a wide variety of ailments and health problems and is often used in conjunction with other alternative and conventional medical treatments.

Folk medicine—These systems of healing (such as Curanderismo and Native American healing) have persisted since the beginning of culture and have flourished long before the development of conventional medicine. Folk healers usually participate in a training regimen of observation and imitation, with healing often considered a gift passed down through several generations of a family. Folk healers may employ a range of remedies including prayer, healing touch or laying on of hands, charms, herbal teas or tinctures, magic rituals and others. Folk healers are found in all cultures and operate under a variety of names and labels.

Guided imagery—This method involves a series of relaxation techniques followed by the visualization of detailed images, usually calm and peaceful in nature. If used for treatment, the client may visualize his/her body as healthy, strong and free of the specific problem or condition. Sessions, conducted in groups or one-on-one, are typically 20–30 minutes and may be practiced several times a week. Guided imagery has been advocated for a number of chronic conditions, including headaches, stress, high blood pressure and anxiety.

Healing circles—These spiritual gatherings usually occur in informal settings, may involve invocations (calling upon a higher power or authority) and may use other healing approaches such as prayer, energy healing therapy/Reiki, and natural herbs.

High dose or megavitamin therapy—This therapy refers to the use of vitamins in excess of the Recommended Daily Allowance (RDA) established by the National Academy of Sciences, Food and Nutrition Board. Although these therapies have been used for the prevention and treatment of diseases and illnesses such as cancer, heart disease, schizophrenia, and the common cold, some high dose or megavitamin regimens can produce advserse or toxic effects.

Homeopathic treatment—This system of medical practice is based on the theory that any substance that can produce symptoms of disease or illness in a healthy person can cure those symptoms in a sick person. For example, someone suffering from insomnia may be given a homeopathic dose of coffee.

Administered in a diluted form, homeopathic remedies are derived from many natural sources, including plants, metals and minerals. Numbering in the thousands, these remedies have been used to treat a wide variety of ailments including seasonal allergies, asthma, influenza, headaches and indigestion.

Hypnosis—An altered state of consciousness, it is characterized by increased responsiveness to suggestion. The hypnotic state is attained by first relaxing the body, then shifting the client's attention toward a narrow range of objects or ideas as suggested by the hypnotist or hypnotherapist. The procedure is used to access various levels of the mind to effect positive changes in a person's behavior and to treat numerous health conditions. For example, hypnosis has been used to lose weight, improve sleep and reduce pain and stress.

Laying on of hands—This religious ceremony involves the placement of hands, by one or more persons (lay or clergy), on the body of the recipient. Usually including prayer, the ceremony may occur in a church or less formal setting and may be used for minor as well as more serious ailments and illnesses.

Macrobiotic diet—This low fat diet emphasizes whole grains and vegetables and restricts the intake of fluids. Consumption of fresh, unprocessed foods is especially important. Daily intakes break out as follows: 50–60 percent whole grains; 25–30 percent fresh vegetables; 5–10 percent beans; soy-based products; and sea vegetables; and 5–10 percent soups. Meat, poultry, dairy products, eggs, alcohol, coffee, caffeinated tea, sweeets and sugar, and strong spices are to be avoided.

Massage—This therapy involves pressing, rubbing and otherwise manipulating muscles and other soft tissues of the body, causing them to relax and lengthen and allowing pain-relieving oxygen and blood flow to the affected area. Using their hands and sometimes feet, elbows and forearms, massage therapists may use over 75 different methods, such as Swedish massage, deep-tissue massage, neuromuscular massage and manual lymph drainage. Massage is considered effective for relieving any type of pain in the body's soft tissue, including back, neck and shoulder pain, headaches, bursitis and tendonitis.

Meditation—Mental calmness and physical relaxation is achieved by suspending the stream of thoughts that normally occupy the mind. Generally performed once or twice a day for approximately 20 minutes at a time, meditation is used to reduce stress, alter hormone levels and elevate one's mood. In addition, a person experienced in meditation can achieve a reduction in blood pressure, adrenaline levels, heart rate and skin temperature.

Natural products—See nonvitamin, nonmineral, natural products.

Naturopathy—This broad system of medicine is based on the theory that the body is a self-regulating mechanism with a natural ability to maintain a state of health and wellness. Naturopathic doctors, who generally reject invasive techniques and the use of synthetic drugs, try to cure illness and disease by harnessing the body's natural healing powers. This is done with the use of various alternative and traditional techniques, including herbal medicine, homeopathic treatment, massage, dietary supplements and other physical therapies.

Nonvitamin, nonmineral, natural products—These products are taken by mouth and contain a dietary ingredient intended to supplement the diet other than vitamins and minerals. They include herbs or herbal medicine (as single herbs or mixtures), other botanical products, such as soy or flax products, and dietary substances such as enzymes and glandulars. Among the most popular are echinacea, ginkgo biloba, ginseng, feverfew, garlic, kava kava and saw palmetto. Garlic, for example, has been used to treat fevers, sore throats, digestive ailments, hardening of the arteries, and other health problems and conditions.

The text in this report uses a shorter version of the CAM therapy nonvitamin, nonmineral, natural products for conciseness and the tables use the complete term. The therapy nonvitamin, nonmineral, natural products is referred to as natural products in the text.

Ornish diet—This is a high fiber, low-fat vegetarian diet that promotes weight loss and health by controlling what one eats, not by restricting the intake of calories. Fruits, beans, grains and vegetables can be eaten at all meals, and nonfat dairy products such as skim milk, nonfat cheeses, and egg whites are consumed in moderation. Products such as oils, avocados, nuts and seeds, and meats of all kinds are avoided.

Pritikin diet—This diet (or Pritikin Principle) is a low-fat diet (10 percent fat or less) that emphasizes the consumption of foods with a large volume of fiber and water (low in caloric density), including many vegetables, fruits, beans and natural, unprocessed grains. According to this diet, weight loss will occur if the average caloric density of a meal is kept below 400 calories per pound.

Progressive relaxation—This therapy involves the successive tensing and relaxing of each of the 15 major muscle groups. Performed lying down, one generally begins with the head and progresses downward, tensing each muscle as tightly as possible for a count of 5 to 10 and then releasing it completely. Often combined with deep breathing, progressive relaxation is particularly useful for reducing stress, relieving tension and inducing sleep.

Qi gong—This ancient Chinese discipline combines the use of gentle, physical movements, mental focus, and deep breathing designed to integrate the mind, body and spirit and to stimulate the flow of vital life energy (qi). Directed toward specific parts of the body, qi gong exercises are normally performed two or more times a week for 30 minutes at a time and have been used to treat a variety of ailments including asthma, arthritis, stress, lower back pain, allergies, diabetes, headaches, heart disease, hypertension and chronic pain.

Reiki—See Energy healing therapy/Reiki.

Tai chi—This Chinese self-defense discipline and low intensity, low-impact exercise regimen is used for health, relaxation and self-exploration. Usually performed daily, tai chi exercises include a set of forms, with each form comprising a series of body positions connected into one continuous movement. A single form may include up to 100 positions and may take as long as 20 minutes to complete. Some of the proposed benefits of tai chi include improved concentration, circulation, and posture, reduction of stress and prevention of osteoporosis.

Vegetarian diets—These diets are devoid of meat. there are, however, numerous variations on the nonmeat theme. For example, some vegetarian diets are restricted to plant products only, and others may include eggs and dairy products. Another variation limits food consumption to raw fruit, sometimes supplemented with nuts and vegetables. Some vegetarian diets prohibit alcohol, sugar, caffeine, or processed foods.

Yoga—This combination of breathing exercises, physical postures, and meditation, practiced for over 5,000 years, calms the nervous system and balances body, mind and spirit. It is thought to prevent specific diseases and maladies by keeping the energy meridians (see acupuncture) open and life energy (qi) flowing. Usually performed in classes, sessions are conducted at least once a week and for approximately 45 minutes. Yoga has been used to lower blood pressure, reduce stress, and improve coordination, flexibility, concentration, sleep and digestion. It has also been used as supplementary therapy for such diverse conditions as cancer, diabetes, asthma and AIDS.

Zone diet—Each meal in this diet consists of a small amount of low-fat protein (30 percent) fats (30 percent) and carbohydrates in the form of fiber-rich fruits and vegetables (40 percent). The basic goal is to alter the body's metabolism by controlling the production of key hormones. According to proponents, this will aid in weight loss, help prevent heart disease, high blood pressure, diabetes and enhance athletic performance.

Complementary and alternative medicine questions   The 2002 National Health Interview Survey Sample Adult questionnaire included questions on complementary and alternative medicine (CAM). Each question is preceded by its question number, beginning with ALT. ALT is the acronym for the CAM section of the Sample Adult questionnaire. Due to the unusually large number of questions used to produce the data used in this report and the complexity of the question skip patterns, CAM questions have not been included in this report. The CAM questions, which are located in the Sample Adult questionnaire, and information about other components of the NHIS are available at www.cdc.gov/nchs/nhis.htm.

Suggested Citation

Barnes, PM Powell-Griner, E, McFann, K, Nahin RL. Complementary and alternative medicine use among adults: United States, 2002. Advance data from vital and health statistics; no 343. Hyattsville, Maryland: National Center for Health Statistics. 2004.

Copyright Information

National Center for Health Statistics
Director: Edward J. Sondick, Ph.D.
Deputy Director: Jack R. Anderson

APPENDIX ITEM IV: IMPORTANT EVENTS IN NCCAM HISTORY

October 1991

- The U.S. Congress passes legislation (P.L. 102–170) that provides $2 million in funding for fiscal year 1992 to establish an office within the National Institutes of Health (NIH) to investigate and evaluate promising unconventional medical practices.
- Stephen C. Groft, Pharm.D. is appointed acting director to the new office: the Office of Alternative Medicine (OAM).

September 1992

- A Workshop on Alternative Medicine is convened in Chantilly, Virginia, to discuss state-of-the-art of the major areas of alternative medicine and to direct attention to priority areas for future research activities.

October 1992

- Joseph Jacobs, M.D., M.B.A., is appointed first Director of the OAM.

June 1993

- The National Institutes of Health Revitalization Act of 1993 (P.L. 103–43) formally establishes the OAM within the Office of the Director, NIH, to facilitate study and evaluation of CAM practices and to disseminate the resulting information to the public.

September 1993

- The first OAM research project grants are funded through the National Center for Research Resources.

December 1993

- The Alternative Medicine Program Advisory Council is established.

September 1994

- Alan I. Trachenberg, M.D., M.P.H., is appointed acting director of the OAM.

January 1995

- Wayne B. Jonas, M.D. is appointed as the second Director of the OAM.

October 1995
- A Research Centers Program is established to provide a nationwide focus for interdisciplinary CAM research in academic institutions.

October 1996
- A Public Information Clearinghouse is established.

November 1996
- The OAM is designated as a World Health Organization Collaborating Center in Traditional Medicine.

September 1997
- The first OAM Phase III clinical trial is funded, a study of St. John's Wort for depression. The trial is co-sponsored by OAM, the National Institute of Mental Health, and the NIH Office of Dietary Supplements.

October 1998
- NCCAM is established by congressional mandate under provisions of the Omnibus Appropriations Bill (P.L. 105-277). This bill amends Title IV of the Public Service Act and elevates the status of the OAM to an NIH Center.

January 1999
- William R. Harlen, M.D., is named Acting Director of NCCAM.

February 1999
- A charter creating NCCAM and making it the 25th independent component of the NIH is signed. This law gives the NCCAM Director contro of the Center's day-to-day financial and administrative management, as well as broad decision-making authority, fiscal and review responsibility for grants and contracts. Donna Shalala, Secretary for Health and Human Services, is present on the Center's first official day, February 1, 1999.

May 1999
- NCCAM independently awards its first research project grant.
- The NCCAM Trans-Agency CAM Corrdinating Committee (TCAMCC) is established by NCCAM Director to foster the Center's collaboration across DHHS and othe federal agencies. This committee supersedes a trans-agency committee established by the NIH Director in 1997.

June 1999
- A Special Emphasis Panel is chartered to enable NCCAM to conduct peer review of mission specific CAM applications.

August 1999
- The National Advisory Council on Complementary and Alternative Medicine (NCCAM) is chartered.

September 1999
- NCCAM awards two multicenter research studies, on ginkgo biloba for dementia, co-funded with the National Institute on Aging, and on glucosamine/chondroitin sulfate for knee osteoarthritis, co-funded with the National Institute of Arthritis and Musculoskeletal and Skin Diseases.

October 1999
- Stephen E. Straus, M.D., is appointed as the first Director of NCCAM.
- NCCAM and the NIH Office of Dietary Supplements establish the first Dietary Supplements Research Centers with an emphasis on botanicals.

June 2000
- NCCAM collaborates with the National Heart, Lung and Blood Institute to sponsor a workshop on complementary and alternative medicine in cardiovascular, lung and blood research.

September 2000
- NCCAM's first strategic plan is published, Expanding Horizons of Healthcare: Five Year Strategic Plan 2001–2005.
- "The Science of the Placebo: Toward an Interdisciplinary Research Agenda," a workshop examining the many aspects of the placebo effect, is organized and sponsored by NCCAM, in conjunction with a group of other NIH Institutes and Centers and Department of Health and Human Services agencies.

January 2001
- NCCAM holds its first international conference, in London England, co-sponsored with the Royal College of Physicians.

February 2001
- CAM on PubMed, a comprehensive Internet csource of research-based information on CAM, is launched by NCCAM and the National Library of Medicine.

April 2001
- The Division of Intramural Research is established.

May 2001
- NCCAM holds a colloquium to foster dialogue with and among key groups in the CAM therapeutic products industry.
- The first draft Strategic Plan to Address Racial and Ethnic Health Disparities is published.

June 2001
- The Office of Scientific Review is established.

NCCAM, National Institute of Health
9000 Rockville Pike
Bethesda, Maryland 20892 USA

APPENDIX ITEM V: *GET THE FACTS: 10 THINGS TO KNOW ABOUT EVALUATING MEDICAL RESOURCES ON THE WEB*

The number of Web sites offering health-related resources grows every day. Many sites provide valuable information, while others may have information that is unreliable or misleading. This short guide contains important questions you should consider as you look for health information online. Answering these questions when you visit a new site will help you evaluate the information you find.

1. Who runs the site?
2. Who pays for the site?
3. What is the purpose of the site?
4. Where does the information come from?
5. What is the basis of the information?
6. How is the information selected?
7. How current is the information?
8. How does the site choose links to the other sites?
9. What information does the site collect and why?
10. How does the site manage interactions with visitors?

1. Who Runs the Site?

Any good health-related Web site should make it easy for you to learn who is responsible for the site and its information. On this site, for example, the National Center for Complementary and Alternative Medicine (NCCAM) is clearly marked on every major page of the site, along with a link to the NCCAM homepage.

2. Who Pays for the Site?

It costs money to run a site. The source of a Web site's funding should be clearly stated or readily apparent. For example, Web addresses ending in ".gov" denote a Federal Government-sponsored site. You should know how the site pays for its existence. Does it sell advertising? Is it sponsored by a drug company? The source of funding can affect what content is presented, how the content is presented and what the site owners want to accomplish on the site.

3. What is the Purpose of the Site?

The question is related to who runs and pays for the site. An "About This Site" link appears on many sites; if it's there, use it. The purpose of the site should be clearly stated and should help you evaluate the trustworthiness of the information.

4. Where Does the Information Come From?

Many health/medical sites post information collected from other Web sites or sources. If the person or organization in charge of the site did not create the information, the original source should be clearly labeled.

5. What is the Basis of the Information?

In addition to identifying who wrote the material you are reading, the site should describe the evidence that the material is based on. Medical facts and figures should have references (such as articles in medical journals). Also, opinions or advice should be clearly set apart from information that is evidence-based (that is, based on reasearch results).

6. How Is the Information Selected?

Is there an editorial board? Do people with excellent professional and scientific qualifications review the material before it is posted?

7. How Current Is the Information?

Web sites should be reviewed and updated on a regular basis. It is particularly important that medical information be current. The most recent update or review date should be clearly posted. Even if the information has not changed, you want to know whether the site owners have reviewed it recently to ensure that it is still valid.

8. How Does the Site Choose Links to Other Sites?

Web sites have a policy about how they establish links to other sites. Some medical sites take a conservative approach and don't link to any other sites. Some link to any site that asks, or pays, for a link. Others only link to sites that have met certain criteria.

9. What Information about You Does the Site Collect and Why?

Web sites routinely track the paths visitors take through their sites to determine what pages are being used. However, many health Web sites ask for you to "subscribe" or "become a member." In some cases, this may be so that they can collect a user fee or select information for you that is relevant to your concerns. In all cases, this will give the site personal information about you.

Any credible site asking for this kind of information should tell you exactly what they will and will not do with it. Many commercial sites sell "aggregate" (collected) data about their users to other companies-information such as what percentage of their users are women with breast cancer, for example. In some cases they may collect and reuse information that is "personally identifiable," such as your zip code, gender and birth date. Be certain that you read and understand any privacy policy or similar language on the site, and don't sign up for anything that you are not sure you fully understand.

10. How Does the Site Manage Interactions with Visitors?

There should always be a way for you to contact the site owner if you run across problems or have questions or feedback. If the site hosts chat rooms or other online discussion areas, it should tell visitors what the terms of using this service are. Is it moderated? If so, by whom and why? It is always a good idea to spend time reading the discussion without joining in, so that you feel comfortable with the environment before becoming a participant.

The NCCAM Clearinghouse provides information about CAM and about NCCAM. Services include fact sheets, other publications and searches of Federal databases of scientific and medical literature. The Clearinghouse does not provide medical advice, treatment recommendations or referrals to practitioners.

This publication is adapted from a fact sheet produced by the National Cancer Institute. It is not copyrighted and it is in the public domain.
NCCAM Publication No. D142
February 19, 2002.

APPENDIX VI: COMMITTEE ON THE USE OF COMPLEMENTARY AND ALTERNATIVE MEDICINE BY THE AMERICAN PUBLIC, *EXECUTIVE SUMMARY: COMPLEMENTARY AND ALTERNATIVE MEDICINE IN THE UNITED STATES*

Americans' use of complementary and alternative medicine (CAM)—approaches such as chiropractic or acupuncture—is widespread. More than a third of American adults report using some form of CAM, with total visits to CAM providers each year now exceeding those to primary-care physicians. An estimated 15 million adults take herbal remedies or high-dose vitamins along with prescription drugs. It all adds up to annual out-of-pocket costs for CAM that are estimated to exceed $27 billion.

Friends confer with friends about CAM remedies for specific problems, CAM-related stories appear frequently in the print and broadcast media, and the Internet is replete with CAM information. Many hospitals, managed care plans and conventional practitioners are incorporating CAM therapies into their practices, and schools of medicine, nursing, and pharmacy are beginning to teach about CAM.

CAM's influence is substantial yet much remains unknown about these therapies, particularly with regard to scientific studies that might convincingly demonstrate the value of individual therapies. Against this background the National Center for Complementary and Alternative Medicine (NCCAM), 15 other centers and institutes of the National Institutes of Health (NIH) and the Agency for Healthcare Research and Quality commissioned the Institute of Medicine (IOM) to covene a committee that would

- Describe the use of CAM therapies by the American public and provide a comprehensive overview, to the extent that data are available, of the therapies in widespread use, the populations that use them, and what is known about how they are provided.
- Identify major scientific, policy and practice issues related to CAM research and to the translation of validated therapies into conventional medical practice.
- Develop conceptual models or frameworks to guide public and private-sector decisionmaking as research and practice communities increasingly conduct research on CAM, translate the research findings into practice, and address the barriers that may impede such translation.

Toward Common Research Ground

Decisions about the use of specific CAM therapies should primarily depend on whether they have been shown to be safe and effective. But this is easier said then done, as there are extremes of belief about what counts as evidence. For some individuals, evidence limited to their own experience or knowledge is all that is necessary as proof that a CAM therapy is successful; for others, no amount of evidence is sufficient. This report will please neither of those extremes.

There are unproven ideas of all kinds, stemming from CAM and conventional medicine alike, and the committee believes that the same principles and standards of evidence should apply regardless of a treatment's origin. Study results may then move useful therapies from unproven ideas into evidence-based practice.

The goal should be the provision of comprehensive care that respects contributions from all sources. Such care requires decisions based on the results of scientific inquiry, which in turn can lead to new information that results in improvements in patient care.

This report's core message is therefore as follows: The committee recommends that the same principles and standards of evidence of treatment effectiveness apply to all treatments, whether currently labeled as conventional medicine or CAM. Implementing this recommendation requires that investigators use and develop as necessary common methods, measures and standards for the generation and interpretation of evidence necessary for making decisions about the use of CAM and conventional therapies.

The committee acknowledges that the characteristics of some CAM therapies—such as variable practitioner approaches, customized treatments, "bundles" (combinations) of treatments, and hard-to-measure outcomes—are difficult to incorporate into treatment-effectiveness studies. These characteristics are not unique to CAM, but they are more frequently found in CAM than in conventional therapies. The effects of mass-produced, essentially identical prescription drugs, for example, are somewhat easier to study than those of Chinese herbal medicines tailored to the needs of individual patients.

But while randomized controlled trials (RCT's) remain the "gold standard" of evidence for treatment efficacy, other study designs can be used to provide information about effectiveness when RCT's cannot be done or when the results may not be generalizable to the real world of CAM practice. These innovative designs include:

- Preference RCT's: trials that include randomized and non-randomized arms, which then permit comparisons between patients who chose a particular treatment and those who were randomly assigned to it.
- Observational and cohort studies, which involve the identification of patients who are eligible for study and who may receive a specified treatment, but are not randomly assigned to the specified treatment as part of the study.
- Case-control studies, which involve identifying patients who have good or bad outcomes, when "working back" to find aspects of treatment associated with those different outcomes.
- Studies of bundles of therapies: analyses of the effectiveness, as a whole, of particular packages of treatments.
- Studies that specifically incorporate, measure or account for placebo or expectation effects: patients' hopes, emotional states, energies and other self-healing processes are not considered extraneous but are included as part of the therapy's main "mechanisms of action."
- Attribute-treatment interaction analyses: a way of accounting for differences in effectiveness outcomes among patients within a study and among different studies of varying design.

Given limited available funding, prioritization is necessary regarding CAM therapies to evaluate. The following criteria could be used to help make this determination.

- A biologically plausible mechanism exists for the intervention, but the science base on which plausibility is judged is a work in progress.
- Research could plausibly lead to the discovery of biological mechanisms of disease or treatment effect.

- The condition is highly prevalent (e.g., diabetes mellitus).
- The condition causes a heavy burden of suffering.
- The potential is great.
- Some evidence that the intervention is effective already exists.
- Some evidence exists that there are safety concerns.
- The research design is feasible, and research will likely yield an unambiguous result.
- The target condition or the intervention is important enough to have been detected by existing population-surveillance mechanisms.

A therapy should not be excluded from consideration because it does not meet any one particular criterion—say, biological plausibility. However, the absence of such a mechanism will inevitably raise the level of skepticism about the potential effectiveness of the treatment (whether conventional or CAM). Moreover, the amount of basic research needed to justify funding for clinical studies of the treatment, and the level of evidence from those studies that is needed to consider the treatment as "established," will both increase under those circumstances.

A New Position on Dietary Supplements

The committee has taken a similarly pragmatic approach to dietary supplements, which have become a prominent part of American popular health culture but continue to present unique regulatory, safety and efficacy challenges.

Under the Dietary Supplement Health and Education Act of 1994—the capstone, thus far of herbal-medicine regulation—the Food and Drug Administration (FDA) was authorized to establish good-manufacturing-practice regulations specific to dietary supplements. But the Act did not subject supplements to the same safety precautions that apply to prescription and over-the-counter medications. Instead, it designated that supplements be regulated like foods, a crucial distinction that exempted manufacturers from conducting premarket safety and efficacy testing. Similarly, FDA's regulatory-approval process—which would be standard operating procedure if supplements had been classified as drugs—was eliminated, thereby limiting the agency to a reactive, postmarketing role.

The committee is concerned about the quality of dietary supplements in the United States. Product reliability is low, and because patent protection is not available for natural substances there is little incentive for manufacturers to invest resources in improving product standardization. Yet reliable and standardized supplements are needed not only for consumer protection but also for research on safety and efficacy. Without consistent products, research is extremely difficult to conduct or generalize. And without high-quality research, medical practitioners cannot make evidence-based recommendations to help guide patients.

Therefore, the committee recommends that the U.S. Congress and federal agencies, in consultation with industry, research scientists, consumers and other stakeholders, amend the Dietary Supplement Health and Education Act of 1994, and the current regulatory scheme for dietary supplements, with emphasis on strengthening:

- Seed-to-shelf quality-control (based on standards for each step of the manufacturing process—from planting to growth, harvest, extraction, and screening for impurities).
- Accuracy and comprehensiveness in labeling and other disclosures.
- Enforcement efforts against inaccurate and misleading claims.
- Research into how consumers use supplements.
- Incentives for privately funded research into the efficacies of products and brands.
- Consumer protection against all potential hazards.

Filling the Gaps

Evidence of the safety and efficacy of individual CAM treatments is essential, but it represents just one facet of the research that is needed. For example, there is a paucity of clinical research that compares CAM therapies with each other or other conventional interventions. Very little research has been done on the cost-effectiveness of CAM. And although there is great opportunity for scientific discovery in the study of CAM treatments, it is an opportunity largely missed.

Such investigations are hindered by shortages of established scientists engaged in CAM research, which tends to involve subject matter beyond the conventional scientist's knowledge base. CAM also needs a cadre of new junior researchers. While major U.S. health-sciences campuses have long offered training in basic and clinical research for conventional medicine, the challenge to induce these schools to embrace CAM research as well. One approach might be to add specific CAM content to conventional-medicine postdoctoral training programs.

Furthermore, CAM research will benefit from the contributions of more than one discipline. In addition to providers who have specialized knowledge of CAM treatments and methodologists who can address the challenges inherent in CAM study design, investigators with backgrounds in fields such as psychology, sociology, anthropology, economics, genetics, pharmacology, neuroscience, health services, and health policy can make important contributions. Interdisciplinary teams, grouped into "critical masses" at various locations, will be favorably positioned to probe the many factors that influence individuals to use CAM treatments and that determine the outcomes of those treatments.

Research on CAM is extricably linked to practice. CAM therapies are already in widespread use today; it is reasonable to attempt to evaluate the outcomes of that use, and in the practice setting one can focus on research that answers questions about how therapies function in the "real world" where patients vary, often have a number of health problems, and are using multiple therapies. Practice-based research addresses real world practice issues and facilitates adoption of practice changes that are based on research results.

To address these gaps, the committee recommends that the National Institutes of Health (NIH) and other public agencies provide the support necessary to:

- Develop and implement a sentinel surveillance system (composed of selected sites able to collect and report data on patterns of use of CAM and conventional medicine); practice-based research networks (defined by the Agency for Healthcare Research and Quality as "a group of ambulatory practices devoted principally to the primary care of patients, affiliated with each other (and often with academic or professional organizations) in order to investigate questions related to community-based practice"; and CAM research centers to facilitate the work of the networks (by collecting and analyzing information from national surveys, identifying important questions, designing studies, coordinating data collection and analysis, and providing training in research and other areas.
- Include questions relevant to CAM on federally funded health care surveys (e.g., the National Health Interview Survey) and in ongoing longitudinal cohort studies (e.g., the Nurse's Health Study and Framingham Heart Study).
- Implement periodic comprehensive, representative national surveys to assess the changes in prevalence, patterns, perceptions and costs of therapy use (both CAM and conventional), with oversampling of ethnic minorities.

Integrating CAM and Conventional Medicine

Even as CAM and conventional medicine each maintain their identities, traditions and practitioners, integration of CAM and conventional medicine is occurring in many settings. Hospitals are offering CAM therapies, a growing number of physicians are using them in their private practices, integrative-medicine centers (many with close ties to medical schools and teaching hospitals) are being established, and health maintenance organizations and insurance companies are covering CAM.

Cancer treatment centers in particular often use CAM therapies in combination with conventional approaches. For example, the Memorial Sloan-Kettering Cancer Center has developed an Integrative Medicine Service that offers music therapy, massage, reflexology, and mind-body therapies. As the Website of the Dana Farber Cancer Institute's own Zakim Center for Integrated Therapies explains, "When patients integrate these therapies into their medical and surgical care, they are creating a more comprehensive treatment plan and helping their own bodies to regain health and vitality."

In response to the growing recognition of CAM therapies by conventional-medicine practitioners for their patients' care, the Federation of State Medical Boards of the United States has developed *Model Guidelines for the Use of Complementary and Alternative Therapies in Medical Practice.*

Other tools are also needed to add to conventional practitioners' decision making, about offering or recommending CAM, where patients might be referred, and what organizational structures are most appropriate for the delivery of integrated care. The committee believes that the overarching rubric for guiding the development of these tools should be the goal of providing comprehensive care that is safe, effective, interdisciplinary and collaborative; is based on the best scientific evidence available; recognizes the importance of compassion and caring; and encourages patients to share in the choices of therapeutic options.

Studies show that patients frequently do not limit themselves to a single modality of care—they do not see CAM and conventional medicine as being mutually exclusive—and this pattern will probably continue and may even expand as evidence of therapies' effectiveness accumulates. Therefore it is important to understand how CAM and conventional medical treatments (and providers) interact with each other and to study models of how the two kinds of treatments can be provided in coordinated ways.

In that spirit, there is an urgent need for health systems research that focuses on identifying the elements of these integrative-medicine models, their outcomes, and whether they are cost-effective when compared to conventional practice.

The committee recommends that NIH and other public and private agencies sponsor research to compare:

- The outcomes and costs of combinations of CAM and conventional medical treatments and models that deliver such care.
- Models of care delivery involving CAM practitioners alone, both CAM and conventional medical practitioners, and conventional practitioners alone. Outcome measures should include reproducibility, safety, cost effectiveness and research capacity.

Additionally, the committee recommends that the Secretary of the U.S. Department of Health and Human Services and the Secretary of the U.S. Department of Veteran Affairs support research on integrated medical care delivery, as well as the development of a research infrastructure within such organizations and clinical training programs to expand the number of providers able to work in integrated care.

The pursuit of such goals requires examination of the ethics of medicine, both in the provision of personal health services and the profession's advocacy for public health. Medicine is continuously shaped by larger social, cultural and political forces, and the integration of CAM therapies is another juncture in this evolutionary process.

The ethical principles that guide conventional biomedical research should also be applied to CAM research. Legal and ethical principles often arise and sometimes conflict with use of CAM therapies because the decision facing a conventional practitioner or institution may engender a conflict between medical paternalism (the desire to protect patients from foolish or ill-informed, though voluntary decisions) and patient autonomy. The Model Guidelines noted above seek to establish greater balance between physician and patient preferences. In addition, a number of legal rules—including state licensure laws, precedents regarding malpractice liability and professional discipline, state and federal food and drug laws, and statutes on health care fraud—protect patients by enhancing quality assurance, offering enhanced access to therapies, and honoring medical pluralism in creating models of integrative care.

Without rejecting what has been of great value and service in the past, it is important that these ethical and legal norms be brought under critical scrutiny and evolve along with medicine's expanding knowledge base and larger aims and meanings of medical practice. The integration of CAM therapies with conventional medicine requires that practitioners and researchers be open to diverse intepretations of health and healing, to finding innovative ways of obtaining evidence, and to expanding the medical knowledge base.

Educating for Improved Care

Essential to conventional and CAM practitioners alike is education about the others' field. Conventional professionals in particular need enough CAM-related training, the committee believes, so that they can counsel patients in a manner consistent with high-quality comprehensive care. Therefore the committee recommends that health profession schools (e.g., schools of medicine, nursing, pharmacy, and allied health) incorporate sufficient information about CAM into the standard curriculum at the undergraduate, graduate and postgraduate levels to enable licensed professionals to competently advise their patients about CAM.

Executive Summary

Because the content and organization of an education initiative on CAM will vary from institution to institution, depending on the objectives of each program, there is no consensus on what should be taught and how to fit it into an already crowded set of courses. At Brown University School of Medicine, for example, the program includes didactic sessions in acupuncture, chiropractic and massage therapy and an elective clinical experience and variations exist at many of the other leading schools. Some of these initiatives have been aided by NCCAM's education projects, which aim to develop new ways of incorporating CAM into health-professional curricula and training programs.

CAM practitioners, for their part, need training that will enable them to participate as full partners and leaders in research so that studies may accurately reflect how CAM therapies are practiced. But many CAM institutions do not have the infrastructure for research of the financial resources to develop them. Training in research has not traditionally been part of the CAM curricula, nor for the mot part have practitioners' careers been dependent on publishing research findings. CAM institutions focus primarily on training for practice.

Strategic partnerships between CAM institutions, NIH and health-sciences universitites would help foster development of the necessary infrastructure; and NCCAM has already begun funding such partnerships. In addition, lessons can be learned from other fields, such as geriatrics and HIV/AIDS research, which have gone through processes relevant to CAM's current need to develop qualified researchers. In geriatrics, for instance, the establishment of centers of excellence at major academic health centers, foundation support for the development of curricula and partnerships, and continuing-education mechanisms such as summer institutes illustrate the importance of using multiple strategies to create an environment in which new science has been able to flourish.

The committee recommends that federal and state agencies, and private and corporate foundations, alone and in partnership, create models of research training for CAM practitioners.

Furthermore, both CAM research and the quality of CAM treatment would be fostered by the development of practice guidelines—what a 1992 IOM Report defines as "systematically developed statements to assist practitioner and patient decisions about appropriate health care for specific clinical circumstances." Key to guideline development is the participation of those who will be most directly affected. This means that CAM practitioners, possibly through their own professional organizations, should formulate guidelines for their own therapies.

The committee recommends that national professional organizations for all CAM disciplines ensure the presence of training standards and develop practice guidelines. Health care professional licensing boards and accrediting and certifying agencies (for both CAM and conventional medicine) should set compentency standards in the appropriate use of both conventional medicine and CAM therapies, consistent with practitioners' scope of practice and standards of referral across health professions.

Knowns and Unknowns about CAM Use

Prevalence estimates for CAM use range from 30 percent to 62 percent of U.S. adults, depending on the definition of CAM. Women are more likely than men to seek CAM therapies, use appears to increase as educational level increases, and there are varying patterns of use by race. Adults who undergo CAM therapies usually draw on more than one type, and they tend to do so in combination with conventional medical care-though a majority do not disclose CAM use to their physicians, thereby incurring the risk, for example, of potential interactions between prescription drugs and CAM-related herbs. Studies of specific illnesses have documented the popularity of CAM for health problems that lack definitive cures, have unpredictable courses and prognoses and are associated with substantial pain, discomfort or medicinal side effects.

Existing surveys tell us little, however, about how CAM treatment is initiated (Does the patient unilaterally decide to use a therapy? Does a CAM or a conventional provider recommend the therapy?), and we have scant data about how the American public makes decisions about accessing CAM options. While there is an extensive literature on adherence to conventional treatment, there are virtually no data available on adherence to CAM treatment. This is an important issue given that any therapy, even if efficacious, may place users at risk of harm, or cause them to experience little or no effect, when used in the wrong way. Similarly, we have virtually no information about the extent to which the use of CAM may interfere with compliance in the use of conventional therapies, how people's self-administration of CAM therapies changes over time, and the factors that influence such change.

Moreover, there is little research on the public's perception of information as alternately credible, marginal or spurious; how people understand such information in terms of risks and benefits; and what they expect their providers to tell them. Because the few small studies that have occurred suggest that considerable misinformation is dispensed by vendors and on the Web, a closer monitoring of Websites, enhanced enforcement of the Dietary Supplement Health and Education Act as well as the Federal Trade Commission Regulations, and the creation of a user-friendly authoritative Website on CAM modalities are needed.

As a means of remedying the dearth of information noted above, the committee recommends that the National Institutes of Health and other public or private agencies sponsor quantitative and qualitative research to examine:

- The social and cultural dimensions of illness experiences, health care-seeking processes and preferences, and practitioner-patient interactions.
- How often users of CAM, including patients and providers, adhere to treatment instructions and guidelines.
- The effects of CAM on wellness and disease-prevention.
- How the American public accesses and evaluates information about CAM modalities.
- Adverse events associated with CAM therapies and interactions between CAM and conventional treatments.

Further, the committee recommends that the National Library of Medicine and other federal agencies develop criteria to assess the quality and reliability of information about CAM.

We are in the midst of an exciting time of discovery, when evidence-based approaches to health bring opportunities for incorporating the best from all sources of care, be they conventional medicine or CAM. Our challenge is to keep an open mind and to regard each treatment possibility with an appropriate degree of skepticism. Only then will we be able to ensure that we are making informed and reasoned decisions.

APPENDIX B

Alternative Medicine Timelines

"Alternative and complementary medicine" refers to health practices outside the scope of conventional, or allopathic, medicine, which includes tests, surgical procedures, and prescription medications. Alternative therapies are identified as those therapies used in lieu of conventional medical practices, whereas complementary medicine includes medical practices that are used in tandem with conventional medical practices.

The National Center for Complementary and Alternative Medicine (NCCAM), part of the National Institutes of Health, lists five types of alternative and complementary medicine: alternative medical systems, mind–body interventions, biologically based therapies, manipulative and body-based methods, and energy therapies. Timelines of historical significance for each of these five categories follow.

According to the NCCAM, alternative medical systems encompass a broad range of integrated medical systems that have both theoretical and practical applications; these are discussed in Chapter 2. Two of the primary systems, which hail from Eastern cultures, are traditional Chinese medicine (TCM) and ayurvedic medicine, from India.

ALTERNATIVE MEDICAL SYSTEMS

1065–771 BC *Chinese Materia Medica*, a reference guide utilizing herbs and botanical compounds to remedy various ailments. Botanicals used in TCM are multiple and varied, with frequent use of combinations in differing strengths.

520 BC Ayurvedic medicine, drawing from Vedic culture in India. It has been used for more than 5000 years in the Eastern world. Ayurvedic medicine emphasizes diet, herbal compounds, exercise, and meditation.

460–377 BC Hippocrates of Cos, referred to as the "Father of Medicine." Hippocrates dismissed the teaching of primitive medicine and was the first to focus on medicine as a scientific endeavor. Two of the most important contributions of Hippocrates were (1) the importance of confidentiality in treatment of the patient and the documenting of medical records to promote continuity of care for the patient, and (2) the well-known "Hippocratic Oath": "First, do no harm," or *primum non nocere.*

430 BC–AD 200 Most of the work defined as the "Hippocratic Corpus" was thought to have been written during this period by a variety of individuals under the name of Hippocrates. The most important contribution was the "Hippocratic Oath," *primum non nocere* ("First, do no harm").

BOTANICAL MEDICINE

340 BC Theophrastus, philosopher and natural scientist often referred to as the "Father of Botany," wrote the treatise "Inquiry into Plants."

200 BC Traditional Chinese medicine first published in the *Yellow Emperor's Classic of Internal Medicine.* According to the NCCAM's "Whole Medical Systems: An Overview," there are three treatment approaches in Chinese medicine: acupuncture (needles applied to key pressure points throughout the body), moxibustion (applied heat and herbal remedy, moxa, to key pressure points), and massage/manipulation.

TCM also includes *Chinese Materia Medica*, which is the reference guide for the use of substances in herbal remedies.

First century AD Dioscorides, a physician who traveled with the ruler Nero in Asia Minor, Italy, Greece, Gaul, and Spain. Dioscorides studied and recorded the effects of plants as sources of healing and published *De Materia Medica.*

130–200 Claudius Galen, a healer who served as an associate to Aeskulapius, received the "Prince of Physicians" award for healing a Roman scholar named Eudemus through adjustment of the vertebrae in his neck.

480 The herbal manuscript "Herbarium Apuleius," which continued to be expanded up to AD 1050 and covered the applied use of over 100 herbal remedies.

925 "The Leechbook of Bald" provided herbal applications.

980–1037 Avicenna, a well-known physician and botanist, expanded Galen's work, and his work was reportedly widely used for six hundred years.

1197–1248 Jami-Ibnal-Baitar, physician and botanist, included the use of more than 2000 medicinal plants and their applications in a treatise.

1493–1554 Swiss alchemist and physician Paracelsus was referred to as the "Father of the science of pharmacology." His views on medicine were unorthodox; he believed that the role of the doctor was to help the body fulfill its capacity to heal itself.

1498 The *Nuovo Receptario* was published in Italy. The book was considered the official Western reference guide for the compounding of herbal formulas and their applications.

1518 The *Nuovo Receptario* was translated into Latin and disseminated throughout Western Europe.

1596–1650 Rene Descartes, French mathematician, scientist, and philosopher, argued that mind and body are separate and distinct.

1870–1955 Henri Leclerc, a physician from France, played a critical role in the expansion of herbal remedies in the clinical setting. He published the text *Precis de Phytotherapie*, for which he became known as the "Father of Phytomedicine."

THOMSONIANISM

1769–1843 Life span of Samuel Thomson, namesake of the "Thomsonian system" of medicine. Thomson's beliefs stemmed from his experiences with conventional medical practice in the unsuccessful treatment of his ailing wife. Ultimately, the correction of his wife's medical problem was initiated by an herbalist, making Thomson a believer. Thomson was known for his recommendation of lobelia, an herb used as an emetic to purge the body of toxins and restore health. Thomson believed in the restorative value of body heat, and many of his botanical remedies focused on the induction of heat within the body as a result of the ingestion of cayenne pepper or lobelia or immersion in steam baths.

1822 Thomson authored *New Guide to Health*, and began selling patented cures to those in need for $20.

HOMEOPATHY

Homeopathy, or the "law of similars," was introduced by Christian Friedrich Samuel Hahnemann (1755–1843). The underlying theory regarding its effectiveness was that the symptoms induced by a certain homeopathic mixture given to the sick would produce the cure. A modern-day version is "a little hair of the dog that bit you." Homeopathy tends to be used more widely in the European countries than in the United States.

1789 Hahnemann translated Dr. William Cullen's *A Treatise on Materia Medica*. In that book, Hahnemann first noted Cullen's report that certain substances in diluted concentrations could reverse malaria.

1796 Hahnemann published his first book on homeopathy.

1810 Hahnemann published the first text on homeopathy, titled *Organon of Rational Medical Science*, with the revised title *Organon of the Art of Healing*.

1835 A student of Hahnemann, Dr. Constantine Hering, established the first homeopathic school in the United States in Allentown, Pennsylvania. Hering was known for developing the "law of cure," which states that healing extends downward from the top of the body, that healing originates from the inside out and from the large to the small organs, and that symptomatology resolves itself in reverse order from that in which it appeared.

1844 The American Institute of Homeopathy was founded.

HYDROTHERAPY

1697 John Floyer's *The History of Hot and Cold Bathing* was published.

1747 Reverend John Wesley, founder of the Methodist religion, wrote one of the first books on water therapy, *Primitive Physik*.

1816 An Austrian physician by the name of Vincent Priessnitz first utilized what came to be known as "water wraps" to expedite the healing of an injured wrist.

1829 Hydrotherapy is recognized as a formal system of medical treatment. Hydrotherapy includes the use of water to reduce pain and resolve medical problems.

1830 The Austrian government gave official authorization to Vincent Priessnitz to use the "Priessnitz compress" as a therapeutic treatment for a wide range of health conditions.

1842 Sebastian Kneipp, a German, was the first to use hydrotherapy to restore his health. After completing his religious training, he was ordained a priest and assigned to the village of Worishofen, outside of Munich.

NATUROPATHY

1872–1945 The life span of Benedict Lust, founder of what came to be known as the "nature cure," or naturopathy.

1892   Lust began to add to Sebastian Kneipp's philosophy of hydro-therapy with therapies that included exercise, diet, and sun-bathing, with a focus on drugless options. With nature viewed as the cure, the emphasis was on correcting the root cause of the problem, treating the person in his or her entirety, and prevention.

1901   The first school of naturopathy was opened in New York, New York.

1910   The Flexner Report led to the closure of U.S. medical schools practicing forms of alternative medicine.

1919   Lust founded the Naturopathic Society of America.

CHRISTIAN SCIENCE

1821–1910   Life span of Christian Science founder Mary Baker Eddy. Christian Science is a philosophy that employs religious beliefs in the healing process, through prayer.

1866   Mary Baker Eddy founded Christian Science and wrote the book *Science and Health with Key to the Scriptures*, on which Christian Science is based. Followers of Christian Science believe that all healing involves a spiritual solution, namely prayer. The development of Christian Science resulted from Eddy herself being healed in 1866 after reading scripture.

OSTEOPATHY

1828–1917   Life span of Andrew Taylor Still, the founder of osteopathy, a type of healing that focuses on the whole person. Osteopathic medicine is based on the interplay of various parts of the body and the capacity of the body to restore itself to health. The name *osteopath* stems from the root *osteon*, meaning "skeletal structure" or "bone," which was thought to be at the core of the healing process.

CHIROPRACTIC

1845–1913   Life span of Daniel David Palmer, author of *The Chiropractor's Adjuster: Text-Book of the Science, Art and Philosophy of Chiropractic*, published in 1910. Chiropractic is a type of healing therapy that focuses on the misalignment of the musculoskeletal system, which is thought to have an impact on the central nervous system and to be the source of ailments throughout the body.

1896 Reverend Samuel H. Weed coined the term *chiropractic*, based on the Greek root *cheir*, meaning "hand," and *praktikos*, meaning "practice." It was thought that the manipulation of the musculoskeletal system resulted in improvement of the body's ability to regulate itself.

Glossary

Academic medical centers Teaching hospitals affiliated with research universities.

Acupuncture A Chinese method of treatment that involves needle insertion at various pressure points and is used to alleviate pain.

Allopathic medicine Conventional medicine, incorporating traditional forms of healthcare practices, including procedures, tests, surgery, radiation, and prescription drugs.

Ayurvedic medicine A healing system that originated in India some 5000 years ago and views the incorporation of mind–body–spirit as the pathway to health.

Bilateral oophorectomy Removal of both ovaries, typically done in conjunction with a hysterectomy.

CAM Acronym for "complementary and alternative medicine."

Clinical outcomes Health outcomes of patients undergoing various procedures.

Doshas Body types or body constitutions identified in ayurvedic medicine, including *vata, pitta*, and *kapha*.

Efficacy The effectiveness of a given treatment protocol.

Evidenced-based medicine Diagnostic and treatment protocols based on scientific underpinnings of proven effectiveness.

Homeopathy A healing philosophy originated by Dr. Samuel Hahnemann and based on the "law of similars," the belief that substances that create illness in a healthy person have the ability to cure a sick person with similar symptoms.

Hysterectomy Removal of the uterus.

Insulin resistance The body's inability to metabolize refined carbohydrates and sugar properly.

Naturopathy A healing philosophy whose advocates claim that the body has the ability to heal itself and incorporates the mind–body–spirit connection in health restoration.

NIH Abbreviation for the National Institutes of Health

NCCAM Abbreviation for the National Center for Complementary and Alternative Medicine, a division of the National Institutes of Health whose task is to evaluate complementary and alternative forms of healthcare.

Orthomolecular medicine A type of medicine, coined by Linus Pauling, Ph.D., in 1968 that is based on providing "the right molecules in the right concentrations" for optimal functioning.

Pharmacoepidemiology The analysis of prescription medications and their impacts on public health.

Protocol Standardized set of practices used in the diagnosis and treatment of particular health conditions.

Risk-benefit analysis A type of analysis utilized in business and economics that provides a breakdown of the risks and benefits of various actions. Applied to the healthcare arena, it involves the analysis of the risks and the benefits of a given health intervention.

APPENDIX D

Bibliography

Abelson, Reed. 2003 (October 26). "Hospitals Fight for Heart Patients Paid For by Medicare," *Lexington Herald-Leader*, A1.

Adams, Karen, Cohen, Michael, Eisenberg, David, and Jonsen, Albert. 2002. "Ethical Considerations of Complementary and Alternative Medical Therapies in Conventional Medical Settings," *Annals of Internal Medicine* 137(8), 660–64.

Agency for Healthcare Research and Quality (AHRQ). 2000. *Medical Errors: The Scope of the Problem.* Publication No. AHRQ 00-P037. Rockville, MD: AHRQ, http://www.ahrq.gov/qual/errback.htm

American Holistic Medical Association (AHMA). 2005 (January). "Principles of Holistic Practice." Permission to utilize revised definition and ten principles received in personal communication by Dr. Robert Ivker, former president of the American Holistic Medical Association.

Atkins, Robert. 1981. *Dr. Atkins' Nutrition Breakthrough: How to Treat Your Medical Condition without Drugs.* New York: Bantam Books.

Avorn, Jerry. 2004. *Powerful Medicines: The Benefits, Risks and Costs of Prescription Drugs.* New York: Alfred A. Knopf.

Balas, E. A. 2001. "Information Systems Can Prevent Errors and Improve Quality," *Journal of the American Medical Informatics Association* 8(4), 398–99.

Barlett, Donald L., and Steele, James B. 2004. *Critical Condition: How Health Care Became Big Business and Bad Medicine.* New York: Doubleday.

Barnes, Patricia, Powell-Griner, Eve, McFann, Kim, and Nahin, Richard L. 2004 (May 27). *Complementary and Alternative Medicine Use Among Adults: United States, 2002 (Advance Data from Vital and Health Statistics, No. 343).* Hyattsville, MD: National Center for Health Statistics.

Barrett, Bruce. 2003. "Alternative, Complementary and Conventional Medicine: Is Integration upon Us?" *Journal of Alternative and Complementary Medicine* 9(3), 417–27.

Bates, D. W., Spell, N., Cullen, D. J., Burdick, E., Laird, N., Paterson, L. A., Small, S. D., Sweitzer, B., and Leape, L. L. 1997. "The Costs of Adverse Drug Events in Hospitalized Patients: Adverse Drug Events Prevention Study Group," *JAMA* 277(4), 307–11.

Benson, Herbert. 2000. *The Relaxation Response.* New York: HarperCollins.

Berliner, Uri. 2005 (November 28). *How General Motors Got Stuck in Reverse.* npr.org

Berwick, Donald. 2004. *Escape Fire: Designs for the Future of Healthcare.* San Francisco: Jossey-Bass.

Beyerstein, Barry. 2001. "Alternative Medicine and Common Errors of Reasoning," *Academic Medicine* 76, 230–37.

Broder, Michael S., Kanouse, David E., Mittman, Brian S., and Bernstein, Steven J. 2000 (February). "The Appropriateness of Recommendations for Hysterectomy," *Obstetrics and Gynecology* 95(2), 199–205.

Burton, Thomas. 2006a (February 22). "Amid Alarm Bells, a Blood Substitute Keeps Pumping," *Wall Street Journal*, A1.

Burton, Thomas. 2006b (March 6). "Grassley Accuses FDA of Laxity in Study of Blood Substitute," *Wall Street Journal*, D5.

Carey, John. 2006 (May 29). "Medical Guesswork," *BusinessWeek*, 72–79.

Cassileth, B. R., Lusk, E. J., Strouse, T. B., and Bodenheimer, B. J. 1984. "Contemporary Unorthodox Treatments in Cancer Medicine," *Annals of Internal Medicine* 101, 105–12.

Centers for Disease Control and Prevention (CDC). 2002 (July 12). *Hysterectomy Surveillance—United States, 1994–1999.* http://www.cdc.gov/mmwr/preview/mmwrhtml/ss5105a1.htm?

Challem, Jack, Berkson, Burton, and Smith, Melissa Diane. 2000. *Syndrome X: The Complete Nutritional Guide to Prevent and Reverse Insulin Resistance.* New York: John Wiley & Sons.

Cheraskin, Emanuel, Ringsdorf, W. M., and Brecher, A. 1974. *Psychodietetics: Food as the Key to Emotional Health.* New York: Bantam Books.

Chopra, Deepak. 2000. *Perfect Health: The Complete Mind/Body Guide*, rev. ed. New York: Three Rivers Press.

Chopra, Deepak. 2001. *Grow Younger, Live Longer: 10 Steps to Reversing Aging.* New York: Harmony Books.

Cleary-Guida, M. B., Okvat, H. A., Oz, M. C., and Ting, W. 2001 (June). "A Regional Survey of Health Insurance Coverage for Complementary and Alternative Medicine: Current Status and Future Ramifications," *Journal of Alternative and Complementary Medicine* 7(3), 269–73.

Cohen, Michael, Hrbek, Andrea, Davis, Roger, Schacter, Sten, and Eisenberg, David. 2005 (February 14). "Emerging Credentialing Practices, Malpractice Liability Policies, and Guidelines Governing Complementary and Alternative Medical Practices and Dietary Supplement Recommendations," *Archives of Internal Medicine* 165(3), 289–95.

Colgate, M. A. 1995. "Gaining Insurance Coverage for Alternative Therapies: Lessons Can Be Learned from the Distinct Marketing Strategies Used by

Chiropractic, Acupuncture and Biofeedback," *Journal of Healthcare Marketing* 15, 24–28.

Collinge, William. 1987. *The American Holistic Health Association's Complete Guide to Alternative Medicine.* New York: Warner Books.

Cousins, Norman. 1989. *Head First: The Biology of Hope and the Healing Power of the Human Spirit.* New York: Penguin Books.

Cox News Service. 2006 (May 29). "Medicine 'More Guesswork than Science,'" *Lexington Herald-Leader.*

Curtis, Peter, and Gaylord, Susan. 2005. "Safety Issues in the Interaction of Conventional, Complementary and Alternative Health Care," *Complementary Health Practice Review* 10(1), 3–31.

Dartmouth Atlas Project. 2006 (May 16) *The Care of Patients with Severe Chronic Illness: A Report on the Medicare Program by the Dartmouth Atlas Project.* http://www.dartmouthatlas.org/atlases/2006_Chronic_Care_Atlas.pdf

Davidson, Eleanor. 2004 (November/December). "A Whole New Way of Thinking about Healthcare," *Journal of American College Health* 53(3), 141.

Dossey, Larry. 1996. *Prayer Is Good Medicine: How to Reap the Healing Benefits of Prayer.* San Francisco: HarperCollins.

Dossey, Larry. 1998. *Be Careful What You Pray For . . . You Just Might Get It: What We Can Do about the Unintentional Effects of Our Thoughts, Prayers, and Wishes.* San Francisco: HarperCollins.

Dossey, Larry. 2001a. *Healing Beyond the Body: Medicine and the Infinite Reach of the Mind.* Westminster, MD: Shambala.

Dossey, Larry. 2001b. *Healing Words: The Power of Prayer and the Practice of Medicine.* Boston: Shambala.

Dyer, Wayne. 1969. *You'll See It When You Believe It.* New York: William Morrow.

Dyer, Wayne. 1999. *Manifest Your Destiny: The Nine Spiritual Principles for Getting Anything You Want.* New York: Harper.

Eisenberg, David. 1993. "Unconventional Medicine in the United States: Prevalence, Costs and Patterns of Use," *New England Journal of Medicine* 328, 246–52.

Eisenberg, David. 1997 (July). "Advising Patients Who Seek Alternative Medical Therapies," *Annals of Internal Medicine* 127(1), 61–69.

Eisenberg, David, Davis, Roger, Ettner, Susan, Appel, Scott, Wilkey, Sonja, Van Rampay, Maria, and Kessler, Ronald. 1998. "Trends in Alternative Medicine Use in the United States, 1990–1997: Results of a Follow-up National Survey," *JAMA* 280, 1569–75.

Erikson, Erik. 1980. *Identity and the Life Cycle.* New York: W. W. Norton.

Fisher, Elliott S., and Welch, H. Gilbert. 1999 (February 3). "Avoiding the Unintended Consequences of Growth in Medical Care: How Might More Be Worse?" *JAMA* 281(5), 446–53.

Foster, Harold. 1988. "Lifestyle Changes and the 'Spontaneous' Regression of Cancer: An Initial Computer Analysis," *International Journal of Biosocial Research* 10(1), 17–33.

Frankl, Victor E. 2000. *Man's Search for Meaning.* Boston: Beacon Press.

Gardner, Amanda. 2006 (February 7). *Low-Fat Diets Don't Protect Postmenopausal Women.* National Women's Health Resource Center, healthywomen.org

Gibbs, Nancy, and Bower, Amanda. 2006 (May 1). "Q: What Scares Doctors Most? A: Being the Patient," *Time*, 43–52.

Gross, David. 1998 (June 27). "How Will America Stay Healthy? The Future U.S. Healthcare System: Who Will Care for the Poor and Uninsured?" *The Lancet* 351(9120), 1971.

Heller, Richard, Heller, Rachel, and Vagnini, Fredric. 1999. *The Carbohydrate Addict's Healthy Heart Program: Break Your Carbo-Insulin Connection to Heart Disease.* New York: Ballantine Books.

Horrobin, David. 2001. *The Madness of Adam and Eve: How Schizophrenia Shaped Society.* London: Transworld.

Hulley, S., Grady, D., Bush, T., et al. 1998. "Randomized Trial of Estrogen Plus Progestin for Secondary Prevention of Coronary Heart Disease in Post-menopausal Women," *JAMA* 280, 605–13.

Illich, Ivan. 1976. *Medical Nemesis: The Expropriation of Health.* New York: Random House.

Institute of Medicine. 1999. *To Err Is Human: Building a Safer Health System.* L. T. Kohn, J. M. Corrigan, and M. S. Donaldson, eds. Washington, DC: National Academies Press.

Institute of Medicine. 2000. *Crossing the Quality Chasm: The IOM Health Care Quality Initiative: The Chasm in Quality: Select Indicators from Recent Reports.* Washington, DC: National Academies Press.

Johnson, Carla K., and Stobbe, Mike. 2006 (May 3). "Study: Americans Sicker than Brits: U.S. Spends Twice as Much on Health Care for Its Citizens," *Lexington Herald-Leader*, A3.

Jores, Andrew. 1961. *Medicine in the Crisis of Our Time* (in German). Bern, Switzerland: Huber.

Kirka, Danica. 2006 (March 6). "Child Obesity Becomes 'Truly a Global Epidemic,'" *Lexington Herald-Leader*, A3.

Langreth, Robert. 2004 (November 29). "Just Say No," *Forbes*, 103–12.

Langreth, Robert, and Herper, Matthew. 2006 (May 8). "Pill Pushers: How the Drug Industry Abandoned Science for Salesmanship," *Forbes*, 94–102.

Lauer, Charles. 2005. "The Place to Be: Naysayers Are Wrong about the State of the Healthcare Industry," *Modern Healthcare* 35(7), 40.

Legorreta, A. P., Liu, X., Zaher, C. A., and Jatulis, D. E. 2000. "Variation in Managing Asthma: Experience at the Medical Group Level in California," *American Journal of Managed Care* 6(4), 445–53.

Mate, Gabor. 2003. *When the Body Says No: Understanding the Stress-Disease Connection.* New York: John Wiley & Sons.

McBride, P., Schrott, H. G., Plane, M. B., Underbakke, G., and Brown, R. L. 1998. "Primary Practice Adherence to National Cholesterol Education Program Guidelines for Patients with Coronary Heart Disease," *Archives of Internal Medicine* 158(11), 1238–44.

McGlynn, Elizabeth, Asch, S. M., Adams, J., Keesey, J., Hicks, J., and DeCristofaro, A. 2003. "The Quality of Health Care Delivered to Adults in the United States," *New England Journal of Medicine* 348(26), 2635–45.

Millman, Joel. 2006 (March 6). "Amish Bargain with Hospital for Lower Rates," *Lexington Herald-Leader*, C1, C3.

Morrow, Monica. 2002 (October 17). "Rational Local Therapy for Breast Cancer," *New England Journal of Medicine*, 347(16), 1270–71.

Moss, Ralph. 1989. *The Cancer Industry.* New York: Paragon House.

Murphy, Joseph. 2000. *The Power of Your Subconscious Mind.* Rev. by Ian McMahan. New York: Bantam Books.

Myss, Carolyn. 1996. *Anatomy of the Spirit: The Seven Stages of Power and Healing.* New York: Harmony Books.

Myss, Carolyn, and Shealy, C. Norman. 1993. *The Creation of Health: The Emotional, Psychological, and Spiritual Responses That Promote Health and Healing.* Walpole, NH: Stillpoint.

National Center for Complementary and Alternative Medicine. 2002 (May 2). *Get the Facts: What Is Complementary and Alternative Medicine?* Publication D156. http://nccam.nih.gov/health/whatiscam

National Center for Complementary and Alternative Medicine. 2004 (October). *Backgrounder: Whole Medical Systems: An Overview.* Publication D236. http://nccam.nih.gov/health/backgrounds/wholemed.htm

National Center for Complementary and Alternative Medicine. 2004. *More Than One-Third of U.S. Adults Use Complementary and Alternative Medicine, According to New Government Survey.* http://nccam.nih.gov/news/2004/052704.htm

National Center for Complementary and Alternative Medicine. 2005 (October). *Backgrounder: What Is Ayurvedic Medicine?* Publication D287. http://nccam.nih.gov/health/ayurveda

Neergaard, Lauran. 2006 (August 17). "Breast Cancer Chemo Side Effects: Younger Patients Appear to Suffer More Than Thought," *Lexington Herald-Leader,* B12.

Ni, H., Nauman, D. J., and Hershberger, R. E. 1998. "Managed Care and Outcomes of Hospitalization among Elderly Patients with Congestive Heart Failure," *Archives of Internal Medicine* 158(11), 1231–36.

Null, Gary. 1987. "Medical Genocide, Part 16," *Penthouse.* Quoted in Lynes, Barry. 1989. *The Healing of Cancer.* Queensville, ON: Marcus Books.

Null, Gary. 2005a. *The Complete Encyclopedia of Natural Healing.* Revised and updated. New York: Kensington.

Null, Gary. 2005b. Presentation at the American Academy of Anti-Aging conference, Chicago, August.

Null, Gary, Rasio, D., and Feldman, M. 2002. *Women's Health Risks Associated with Orthodox Medicine—Part 2.* http://www.garynull.com/documents/womenriskorthodoxmedpt2.htm.

Nussbaum, Samuel. 2003. Presentation to the Disease Management Congress.

Ornish, Dean. 1990. *Dr. Dean Ornish's Program for Reversing Heart Disease.* New York: Ballantine Books.

Orthomolecular Medicine Hall of Fame. 2005. http://orthomolecular.org/hof/index.shtml

Orthomolecular Medicine Hall of Fame. 2006. http://orthomolecular.org/hof/index.shtml

Parker, William, Broder, M. S., Lin, Z., Shoupe, D., Farquar, C., and Berek, J. S. 2005 (August). "Ovarian Conservation at the Time of Hysterectomy for Benign Disease," *Journal of Obstetrics and Gynecology* 106(2), 219–26.

Parsons, Talcott. 1951. *The Social System.* Boston: Routledge.

Patton, Laura. 1997. "The Role of the Consumer in Coverage Decisions." Paper presented at the 1997 Washington Health Policy Forum with the Group Health Cooperative of Puget Sound. Survey results published in Weeks, John. 2001 (May 1). "Charting the Mainstream: A Review of Trends in the Dominant Medical System," *Townsend Letter for Doctors and Patients* 177.

Pauling, Linus. 1968 (April 19). "Orthomolecular Psychiatry: Varying the Concentrations of Substances Normally Present in the Human Body May Control Mental Disease," *Science* n.s. 160(3825), 265–71.

Pauling, Linus. 2004. *The 2004 Orthomolecular Medicine Hall of Fame.* http://orthomolecular.org

Payer, Lynn. 1988. *Medicine and Culture: Varieties of Treatment in the United States, England, West Germany, and France.* New York: Penguin Books.

Pelletier, Kenneth. 2000. *The Best Alternative Medicine: What Works? What Does Not?* New York: Simon & Schuster.

Perez-Stable, E. J., and Fuentes-Afflick, E. 1998. "Role of Clinicians in Cigarette Smoking Prevention," *Western Journal of Medicine* 169(1), 23–29.

Pert, Candace. 1999. *Molecules of Emotion: The Science behind Mind–Body Medicine.* New York: Simon & Schuster.

Plaza, Carla L. 2005 (March). "States Focus on Health Issues to Minimize Future Healthcare Costs," *Healthcare Financial Management* 59(3), 20.

Radley, David C., Finkelstein, Stan N., and Stafford, Randall S. 2006. "Off-Label Prescribing among Office-Based Physicians," *Archives of Internal Medicine* 166(9), 1021–26.

Ritter, Malcolm. 2006 (March 31). "Strangers' Prayers Don't Help Patients Recover, Study Finds," *Lexington Herald-Leader*, A4.

Ross, Emma. 2005 (July 30). "Hormone Pills Put on Cancer List: Health Agency Reclassifies Them as Carcinogenic," *Lexington Herald-Leader*, A1, A6.

Rubin, Rita. 2004 (October 12). "How Did the Vioxx Debacle Happen?" *USA Today*, http://www.usatoday.com/news/health/2004-10-12-vioxx-cover_x.htm

Sampson, Wallace. 2001. "The Need for Educational Reform in Teaching about Alternative Therapies," *Academic Medicine* 76, 248–50.

Saul, Andrew. 2000. Review of *Vitamin C and Cancer: Discovery, Recovery and Controversy.* DoctorYourself.com.

Saul, Andrew. 2005. "The 2005 Orthomolecular Medicine Hall of Fame," *Journal of Orthomolecular Medicine* 20(2), 113–17.

Schuitemaker, Gert. *The 2005 Orthomolecular Medicine Hall of Fame.* http://orthmolecular.org

Schultz, Johannes, and Luthe, Wolfgang. 1969. *Autogenic Training.* New York: Grune and Stratton.

Selye, Hans. 1978. *The Stress of Life.* New York: McGraw-Hill.

Shames, Richard, and Shames, Kara Lee. 2002. *Thyroid Power: 10 Steps to Total Health.* New York: HarperCollins.

Sheehan, George. 1978. *Running and Being: The Total Experience.* Red Bank, NJ: Second Wind II.

Sinatra, Stephen. 1996a. *Heartbreak and Heart Disease: The Mind/Body Prescription for Healing the Heart.* New Canaan, CT: Keats.

Sinatra, Stephen. 1996b. *Optimum Health: A Natural Lifesaving Prescription for Your Body and Mind.* New York: Lincoln-Bradley.

Sinatra, Stephen. 2000. *Heart Sense for Women: Your Plan for Natural Prevention and Treatment.* Washington, DC: Lifeline Press.

Sinatra, Stephen. 2003. *Lower Your Blood Pressure in Eight Weeks: A Revolutionary Program for a Longer, Healthier Life.* New York: Random House.

Sinatra, Stephen. 2005. Presentation at the American Academy of Anti-Aging conference, Chicago, August.

Sinatra, Stephen. 2005. *The Sinatra Solution: Metabolic Cardiology.* Laguna Beach, CA: Basic Health Publications.

Sinatra, Stephen. 2006 (January). Personal communication.

Smith, Richard. 1991. "Where Is the Wisdom . . . ? The Poverty of Medical Evidence," *British Medical Journal* 303(6806), 709–99.

Stein, Rob. 2005 (November 4). "Americans Pay More, Get Less for Health Care: Survey Looks at U.S. and Other Western Nations," *Lexington Herald-Leader*, A5.

Stenstrom, Ulf. 1997. "Psychological Factors and Metabolic Control in Insulin-Dependent Diabetes Mellitus." Ph.D. dissertation, Lund University, Lund, Sweden.

Stobbe, Mike. 2006 (June 2). "U.S. Trails in 2nd Health Survey: Uninsured Canadians Say They're Better Off than American Counterparts," *Lexington Herald-Leader*, B10.

Studdert, David M., Eisenberg, David, Miller, Frances, Curto, Daniel, Kaptchuk, Ted, and Brennan, Troyen A. 1998 (November 11). "Medical Malpractice Implications of Alternative Medicine," *JAMA* 280(18), 1610–15.

"Study Outlines Three Scenarios for the Future of Healthcare Financing." 2003 (September 8). *Health and Medicine Week*, 510.

Sturm, R., and Unutzer, J. 2000–2001. "State Legislation and the Use of Complementary and Alternative Medicine," *Inquiry* 37(4), 423–39.

Tindle, H. A., Davis, R. B., Phillips, R. S., and Eisenberg, D. M. 2005 (January–February). "Trends in Use of Complementary and Alternative

Medicine by U.S. Adults: 1997–2002," *Alternative Therapies in Health and Medicine* 11(1), 42–49.

Walters, Richard. 1993. *Options: Alternative Cancer Therapy Book.* New York: Avery.

Weick, Karl. 1995. *Sensemaking in Organizations (Foundations for Organizational Science).* Thousand Oaks, CA: Sage.

Weil, Andrew. 1983. *Health and Healing: Understanding Conventional and Alternative Medicine.* Boston: Houghton Mifflin.

Weil, Andrew. 1998. *8 Weeks to Optimal Health.* New York: Ballantine Books.

Whorton, James. 2002. *Natural Cures: The History of Alternative Medicine.* New York: Oxford University Press.

Women's Health Initiative. 2002 (July 17). "Risks and Benefits of Estrogen Plus Progestin in Healthy Postmenopausal Women: Principal Results from the Women's Health Initiative Randomized Controlled Trial," *JAMA* 288(3), 321–33.

Women's Health Initiative. 2006a. Ross, L. et al. 2006 (February 8). "Low-Fat Dietary Pattern of Risk of Invasive Breast Cancer: The Women's Health Initiative Randomized Controlled Dietary Modification Trial," *JAMA* 295(6), 629–642.

Women's Health Initiative. 2006b. Shirley, A., et al. 2006 (February 8). "Low-Fat Dietary Pattern and Risk of Colorectal Cancer: The Women's Health Initiative Randomized Controlled Dietary Modification Trial," *JAMA* 295(6), 645–654.

Women's Health Initiative. 2006c. Barbara, V. et al. 2006 (February 8). "Low-Fat Dietary Pattern and Risk of Cardiovascular Disease: The Women's Health Initiative Randomized Controlled Dietary Modification Trial," *JAMA* 295(6), 655–666.

Won Tesoriero, Heather. 2006 (March 14). "In Vioxx Case Plaintiff Outlines His Disabilities," *Wall Street Journal,* D5.

World Health Organization (WHO). 2000. *World Health Report 2000. Health Systems: Improving Performance.* http://www.who.int/whr/2000/media_centre/dgmessage/en/index.html

Vergano, Dan. 2006 (April 20). "Study: Medical Manual's Authors Often Tied to Drugmakers," *USA Today,* 6A.

INDEX

SIMPLY SANE

SIMPLY SANE

Stop Fixing Yourself
and
Start Really Living

by

GERALD G. MAY, M.D.

PAULIST PRESS
New York, N.Y./Ramsey, N.J.

Library of Congress
Catalog Card Number: 76-24436

ISBN: 0-8091-0215-3

Published by Paulist Press
Editorial Office: 1865 Broadway, N.Y., N.Y. 10023
Business Office: 545 Island Rd., Ramsey, N.J. 07446

Printed and bound in the
United States of America

CONTENTS

IN APPRECIATION

There is no idea in this book which could rightly be called "original." The lineage of searching expressed herein arises from scriptures of the world's great religions, from the deep mystery of silence, from my parents and teachers, and from countless other people who have shared their insights and legacies. Some of those who have had particular impact could be mentioned with the deepest appreciation. Rev. Richard Geib and Rev. Myron Ebersole; Rev. Tilden Edwards; Rinpoches Tarthang Tulku and Chogyam Trungpa; Roshi Shunryu Suzuki; the written riches of pilgrims such as Thomas Merton, Teilhard de Chardin and the medieval Christian mystics; and all the modern women and men who cut themselves on the edges of psychology and religion in attempting to discover the basic unity and sanity they know is there. I also wish to thank Richard Payne of Paulist Press who began as editor, became teacher, and grew into friend. Above all, the most helpful contributions have come from the honest searching of those who would call themselves clients, students and colleagues. And from the eyes of my children.

To Betty

1

DEATH AND RESURRECTION

For all things born in truth must die,
and out of death in truth comes life.
Face to face with what must be,
Cease thou from sorrow.

Bhagavad-Gita 2:27

The world is filled with newness. And it has been for years. This new product, that new invention, this revolutionary idea. Always something new and, presumably, better. We are a people of progress. For years the new and the novel have captured the energy of our culture. But fatigue is beginning to set in. The novelty of novelty is wearing off.

That doesn't mean we simply want the good old days back again. For many people, the good old days don't look so great either. It's something else, something in a different kind of dimension that is being sought. There is a sense that one can't just go on forever discovering new and better things, nor can one comfortably go back to the old. There is now a desire for some kind of attitude, some way of perceiving existence which undercuts and undergirds both the old and the new. Something giving meaning to the old and the new. Something giving meaning to *us*. Some way of freely, fully and *simply* being. Nearly everyone has a nagging sense of this, for from time to time, in fleeting moments of abandonment, *it* is experienced. "Just being" happens. But exactly what it is or how to get it or

whether we really want it or what it might do to us if we did
get it are all unanswered questions.

So most people return to the tried and trustworthy world of
doing. The world of progress, growth, advancement, achievement and mastery. Learning things. Creating new ideas. Ac-
tualizing ourselves. Encountering penetrating insights into the
depths of individual and cultural psychology. Learning how to
become assertive. How to use and acquire power. How to
amass wealth. How to become liberated from oppression. How
to act as if we'd overcome our basic feelings of inferiority and
inadequacy. We practice hard and become proficient at the
games of politics, management, economics, security, morality,
social fitness and human relations. And we become very good
at it all.

But if by chance we have a moment with nothing to do, if
by mistake we get just a little quiet for a while, the nagging
sense comes back.

Sanity speaks in those moments.

"What for?" it says "Why?" it asks. "O. K., you've learned
and accomplished and grown. But so what? What's the meaning
of it? Where is it getting you? What is it worth?" That in-
trusive voice of sanity is most disquieting, so one tends to
move, rather quickly, to shut it up. Most of the time this is
accomplished by just becoming very busy. Busy on something
else. "I've got work to do. Can't sit around here contemplating
my navel." And if that doesn't work, one can say, "Oh, that's
just my sense of insecurity talking." One can label one's sanity
as insanity. See it as representing inadequate self-confidence,
a lack of self-esteem. Or even laziness. When that most sensible
part of ourself begins to ask, "Why are you struggling so hard?"
we can handle it by labeling it as a problem.

"Well, maybe I need a little more therapy in order to
overcome my uncertainties."

"It must be time to go on another weekend workshop to

put me in touch with my feelings. Then I will return to the world more confidently. Without all these self-doubts.'' Never stopping to realize that perhaps those self-doubts are the most honest, most sincere voice we can hear.

And if *that* doesn't work, if the nagging questions remain after even more work at self-improvement, then one can always drink. Or eat. Or sleep a lot. Or drug oneself in a myriad other ways. Anything to kill the nagging sanity.

Periodically, certain identifiable groups of people discover how they've been murdering their sanity. A young woman who "used to be a housewife" recently told me her experience. "For years I saw myself as Bob's wife. The mother of his children. The keeper of the house. The preparer of food. I took pride, real legitimate pride in these things. The women's lib business always seemed kind of crazy to me, and in a way it still does. But one day, when I'd watched that TV thing about being proud of your clean bathroom for the thousandth time, something sort of cracked inside of me. I mean, what was I doing trying so hard to be the wife and mother and cook, as if that's all there was? I suddenly remembered all the moments in the past when I'd felt sort of angry or depressed, and perhaps I just didn't *want* to do the dishes and I'd say, 'Hey now, you shouldn't feel that way. We all have to do things we don't want to do. What's wrong with you? Everybody else you know and respect finds great meaning in being a wife and mother. You've got to get yourself together and shape up. There's something wrong with you if you feel this way.'

"And so I'd go ahead and do what needed to be done. And I'd try so *hard* to have it make me feel good. But sometimes I couldn't get to sleep at night, and I didn't feel like I had much energy, and I'd get these headaches. Then it *really* seemed as if something was wrong with me. 'Why can't I be happy?' Well, after that last TV commercial something changed. Just because everybody else looked so happy with

their clean bathrooms didn't necessarily mean *I* had to. And as time went on, it became clearer and clearer to me that what I had always thought was something wrong with me—all those doubts and resistances and stuff—was really something that was *right* with me. Now I still am a wife and a mother and a cook, but I don't feel that I have to love it all. I don't feel I must make it my nirvana. And it's O.K. to love some of it and hate some of it. And thank God, though my bathroom may be clean, I'm not in the least bit proud of it."

A very familiar and encouraging story. That kind of thing happens to many groups of people at certain times in their lives. Slaves discovered that maybe it made more sense to want to be free than to try to be comfortable as slaves. Workers found out that perhaps sanity lay in asking for their due rather than in finding ways of putting up with unfair management practices. Oppressed minorities began to entertain the idea that maybe they weren't *really* inferior. In many areas, little bits of sanity which had been labeled as insanity have become liberated.

But the sad thing about this process is that as soon as one becomes liberated from one way of stifling sanity, one tends to move immediately into another more sophisticated way of doing the same thing. The woman who overcame bathroom pride was left with a bit of a question. She never formed it into words, but it went something like, "Well, now that I know I don't have to get the meaning of my life out of being a good housewife, where *do* I get my meaning?" Lots of nice, entertaining, enticing possibilities. A career, maybe. Not noticing how men and women whose meaning lies in a career tend to have increasing numbers of martinis when they get home from work. Get rich, perhaps. Forgetting the anguish of the wealthy. Join a consciousness-raising group? Some deeply meaningful encounter with other human beings? Not even suspecting the empty pit in the hearts of those who have learned well all the

techniques for relating to others in deeply meaningful ways.

And what do the "oppressed masses" do when they permit themselves not to feel inferior? They sweat, harder than slaves, forging their way "upward" into good jobs and high-class neighborhoods, wracking brains to learn how to sound sophisticated and what kind of drinks to serve and how to frequent the best restaurants. Tremendous energy to get there. And then tremendous energy to try to convince oneself that it was worth the struggle. After all, one seeks out the good life. And if one finds that one doesn't really enjoy the good life very much once it's been achieved, what is left?

The bathroom woman did join a consciousness-raising group. She went on weekend workshops where she established contact with other people. She learned how to touch them and respond to them and trust them and be trusted by them. She learned how to ask for her needs to be met, how to express her anger. She learned how to communicate "straight." And how to take risks. And each time she'd come back all warm and glowing and full of vitality, ready to tackle life with all the gusto of her being. For a while. The energy itself would last for a day or two. Then she'd pretend she still had it for another week or two. And then she'd begin to admit that she was running down a bit and that her existence wasn't quite as meaningful as she'd like it to be. So she'd say, "I'm falling back into my old patterns again. I'm still basically inhibited and not spontaneous. I need to do some more work on myself. Grow a little more. Get in touch with more of my feelings. Move along the cutting edge of my personal development."

There is a creeping insidious odor of similarity here. She might as well have been watching another TV commercial. She'd adopted another set of standards to which she felt she must adhere in order to be all right. And her natural, sensible being was drifting back somewhere far, out of sight. And she was, again, saying that there was something wrong with her.

Something needing to be fixed. Some immaturity to be out-
grown. Some hang-up to be overcome.

The entire process can be very exciting and entertaining.
But the problem is there's no end to it. The fantasy is that if
one heads in the right direction and just works hard enough
and learns enough new things and grows enough and gets ac-
tualized, one will be *there*. None of us is quite certain exactly
where "there" is, but it obviously has something to do with
resting. As Joseph Conrad put it,

> What all men are really after is some form, or perhaps
> only some formula, of peace.

"There" has something to do with being able to stop all
the existential struggling, and finally, just being able to let
one's self be. Just to be. Fully and freely, unfettered and with
wholeness. To be able to relax and be all right. To take a deep
breath and lean back and sigh and *be* and have it somehow
be just fine. To rest.

But always it seems this "there," this place of peace, is
someplace *else*, somewhere or sometime other than the here
and now of immediate experience. So in one way or another,
many lives are saturated with a frantic struggle to "get there."
To arrive at it. To achieve it. After I get out of college I can
rest. When I land this new job. If we can just close the deal on
that house. When the last kid is through school. If we can just
resolve this marital problem. When my therapy is completed.

But there's no end to this kind of searching. What appears
to be a destination winds up being an empty promise. There's
always someplace else to go, something more to learn. And
one's awareness is locked somewhere in the future, looking for
the promised land that never seems to come; or in the past,
saying, "Look how far I've come" or "My God how awfully
deranged I used to be!" And in those very few moments when
now is perceived, awareness becomes trapped in judgement. A

judgement which is always made in terms of past and future. "How am I doing?" "Are they going to approve of this?" "Will this get me what I want?"

And all the time there's the buried, stifled, bare potential of sanity feebly trying to ask "Why?" In the slightest of moments when this voice is heard, it is stomped out. Heavy boot grinding it back into the ground. "I must not doubt myself this way. Not so deeply. That's not what healthy, well-adjusted people do." And then one goes on to something "new."

Now and then this cycle explodes within the soul of some unsuspecting individual. Sanity bursts forth like the Phoenix and fire rains. It all comes crashing down. The point. The point of total despair. The point where giving up happens. There is no further choice. Nothing new worth doing. No more hope for the future. No more aspiration. There is some deep factor in people that makes a difference here. Something beyond the realm of predictability that determines *how* one gives up.

Some people give up *away* from life. In one last pitiful attempt to remain in control, they commit suicide. Either outright with pills or gun, or masochistically with alcohol or crime, or finally and ultimately all-in-all committing themselves to work, country, church, or value systems. It doesn't matter what form it takes. It's suicide.

But others will give up *into* life. Realizing that all the intelligence, all the learning, all the strategies, all the loving and hating and giving and taking will bring absolutely nothing, one finally gives up and lets one's self be. What we were "after" all along. What we worked for and sweated about and suffered and bled for we are finally given. But as no result of all the effort. Only as a result of having driven ourselves so far and fatigued ourselves so much that we stop the effort altogether. And then freely being is given. Not as a result of effort, but as a result of stopping the effort. Quitting.

It is a magnificent paradox. One seeks peace and fulfill-

ment by ever-increasing effort at self-determination, self-improvement and self-control. But it is when self-manipulation and self-control are given up that peace and fulfillment are found. They were there all along.

In recent years it has become quite popular to write about the "death of psychotherapy." And in a sense this book is also about the death of psychotherapy. But it is not, I hope, another bitter attack. Nor is it an attempt to kill anything. It is rather a description of a death-and-resurrection cycle. What is dying is a mistaken attitude toward life, of which psychotherapy is but a part. A part with which I happen to be quite familiar. And what is being reborn, I hope, is sanity.

The mistaken attitude is that people have come to see themselves as things. Things to be built when they are young. Things to be fixed, altered and improved upon when they are older. Psychotherapy, along with many other cultural institutions, has fallen prey to this myth. And in its own way psychotherapy has helped to keep the myth alive. Inherent in the very idea of psychotherapy is the assumption that the human mind is an object which can and should be fixed. And that people must somehow willfully manipulate themselves in order to be "healthy." Psychotherapy has come to mean that some persons do something to other persons to fix them.

Many recent antipsychotherapy books attack the attitude of one person fixing another. They say that one person should not have this kind of power over another. They say that one should be free to fix one's self, in whatever way one deems best. But in saying this, it is obvious that the antipsychotherapy writings have also fallen prey to the delusion. They are concerned about who fixes whom. The question which still remains to be asked is "Why do we need to be fixed at all?"

There is nothing wrong in one person helping another with a problem. And there is no injury in wanting to grow or

heal. The problem is that growth and healing have become building and fixing, and this distortion of reality has led us into a despairing endless struggle for self-improvement. The idea of effecting repairs and improvements upon this thing which is "myself" has so blocked our awareness of the natural processes of growth and healing that simple living has become an incredibly hard job.

But this attitude may now be dying. At this moment in time, the delusion which sees people-as-things and therapy-as-fixing is experiencing some significant symptoms of illness. There are some serious cracks in its foundation, and its death may not be far off. If death occurs, we can hope to see sanity growing from the bones of delusion. A sanity which will allow clear perception of the natural processes of healing and growth within each person. A sanity which will bring us home to our vital, dynamic, elemental roots. A sanity which will allow us to be rather than try to be; to live rather than strive to live; to be in the process of healing rather than to be the healer or the healed.

I do not advocate hastening the death of delusion by any willful means—even to put it out of its misery. Nor do I advocate wrenching the seeds of sanity from the ground before their time of birth has come. But on the other hand, if it is indeed time for delusion to die, I hope we will not take any heroic measures to keep it alive.

The current illness of self-fixing and self-building is caused by sanity struggling for rebirth. People are becoming deeply dissatisfied with the fact that in a world overfilled with self-improvement methods, fulfillment has not been found. Having tried this method of self-enrichment and that technique for personal growth, and still not finding peace, people are beginning to experience a wave of disillusionment.

As a race and as a culture, we human beings have learned so much we're beginning to wonder what the value of learning

is. Many of us have become so affluent that we're beginning to
wonder what it means to have power and luxury. We've been
developing doubts about the importance of wealth. And we've
become so sophisticated at analyzing every aspect of ourselves,
our hopes and impulses, fears and faiths, that we're beginning
to ask, "What for?" These questions come from the voice of
sanity. And as troublesome as these questions may be, it is just
possible that they will mark the beginning of salvation.

2

BEYOND SELF-CONTROL

He got the better of himself,
and that's the best kind of
victory one can ask for.

Cervantes, *Don Quixote*

Mary Jo had a sexual fantasy. It was an ugly fantasy, filled
with pain and blood. Mary Jo hated herself for having the
fantasy. She felt guilty, sinful and terribly defective. She wanted to be fixed. She could not see the *fantasy* as the problem,
but had to see her *self* as the problem because she was the one
who had the fantasy. In this, she reflected a quixotic attitude
which is civilization-wide. "I'm not happy so *I* need to
change." "I'm not efficient enough so *I* need to be improved
upon." "I'm not functioning well so *I* need to be fixed."

When Mary Jo came into my office to be fixed, I took a
furtive little stab at sanity. "Why," I asked, "do you need to
feel badly about your*self* because of this fantasy? I know it
hurts you, but is there any reason to belittle yourself because of
it?"

"Because it's me thinking it," she said, as if I'd asked a
dumb question. "Can't you do something for me to get rid of
it? Maybe hypnosis?"

I tried again. "Sure the fantasy makes you feel bad. Sure

11

it's a lot of trouble. But maybe if you could relax a little and let yourself be who you are . . ."

"You don't understand. I can't control it. I can't control myself. How can I relax when I can't control myself?"

There's the rub. She's laid it out clearly. She wants to be fixed so she can control herself. Her self. Once she feels she has mastered her self, then she can relax. Only then.

I succumbed to Mary Jo's conviction that self-control is the only way out, and we got into psychotherapy. On my part it was a try for second best. At least I was trying to support her attempts to control herself *by* herself and fend off her desire for me to control her through pills, hypnosis or magical medical wisdom. And, as might be expected, psychotherapy worked. Somewhere along the line the fantasy became less strong. Later it seemed to disappear entirely. But by then Mary Jo had discovered many "underlying psychodynamics" which needed to be taken care of. We were on the road, she and I. Toward the ultimate fix.

From time to time I kept trying to say, "Relax and be who you are. The fact that your impulses need to be controlled doesn't mean that you as a person have to be controlled, by yourself or by anybody else." But she didn't hear. And one of the reasons she didn't hear was because while my words were saying "Be fully, freely yourself," many of my actions were saying, "O.K., Mary Jo, let's get you fixed."

Finally psychotherapy stopped. "I've come a long way," she said. "I understand myself now. I'm stronger. I've got confidence. I'm no longer weak and helpless. Sure I've still got problems, but I can handle them. I've got control of myself now." That's where we stopped. That's where psychotherapy stops. That's even where the antipsychotherapy writings stop. That is where the entire culture seems to stop. Self-control.

The quixotic cultural myth is that in self-control, self-determination, self-direction, self-identity and self-confidence lies

the good life. Nearly every cultural institution reflects this belief. There's nothing special about psychotherapy, or about antipsychotherapy, or about politics or education. All are children of the same craziness, the insanity which says self-determination is utopia. Even art, with all its possibilities for going beyond self-importance, is trampled by analysis of symbolism and refinement of technique so that "better" art can be made. And so that you and I can be "better" artists or appreciators of art. Even religion, the one great timeless gate to beyond-the-self, becomes a technique. A means to an end for self-improvement. To create better behavior, to make more abiding happiness, to manufacture holiness. There are times when through religion one comes close to turning over self-control. Offering it up. Giving up. Sacrificing the delusion. But even then, most often, it becomes the turning over of a defective self to the ultimate fixer in the sky, in the hopes of getting a rebuilt and perfected self in return. This is not going beyond self, nor is it giving up. It's using God to help one get back in control. "Thy will be done" are the words. "I will let your will be done, for now," is the meaning.

The core of this myth lies in the very idea of self. If asked to think about it, most people might say they see themselves as being made up of body and mind. And perhaps soul. Fine, so far. If one could go about life sensing that one's self is simply the name given to a particular collection of body, mind and soul, there would be no great craziness. The three parts could be seen as functioning together, influencing each other, playing out their dance of life in varying degrees of harmony.

But somehow an elaboration of this idea keeps creeping in. An elaboration which is crazy. One comes to feel that the self is something else. Something very real and substantial, which exists *behind* body, mind and soul. One senses that the self somehow "posesses" or "has" the body, mind and soul, and that it is somehow responsible for controlling them. From

this rather goofy assumption, people say things like "I need to control my impulses," or "I want to improve my mind." It makes sense that impulses need to be controlled and that a mind can grow in intelligence and creativity, but who or what is this "I" which is somehow supposed to *do* the controlling or improvement?

If we were to make an object of the mind and break it into parts, it might make some sense to say that impulses, which are one part of the mind, are controlled by conscience, another part of the mind. Or that various parts of the mind control various parts of the body. But the insidious idea keeps coming up that behind mind-controlling-mind and behind mind-controlling-body, there is this "self" which somehow engineers the entire process. It might even make sense to see that the soul, a representation of some ultimate engineer, is really the self. But in action, the soul too becomes an object for the self to handle. People say things like "I wish I could get in touch with my soul," or "I need to develop the spiritual side of my life," or "My soul is thirsting for God." Who is this "I" who wants to get in touch with its soul or to develop the spiritual side of its life? Who is this "me" who possesses "my" soul which is thirsting for God? The elusive self creeps behind all things. Behind the body, behind the mind, behind the soul. Even behind our vision of God, the sense of self crawls in. God said "Thou shalt have no other gods before me." He should have looked behind Him.

Belief in "self" is far more than a simple mistake in logic or an expediency of language. It does real damage. Sensing a self which somehow possesses and manipulates body, mind and soul, these must become objects. They become *things*, and lose their wonder. Even that might be tolerable if we stopped there, but we don't. Sensing that the "self" is ultimately responsible for controlling the rest of the person, what happens when some part gets out of control? When a mistake is made?

When one fails to get what one wants? Then we begin to feel that our "self" is somehow deficient because it didn't do a good job. Then comes a veritable avalanche of delusion. If the self isn't working right, *it* needs to be controlled or improved upon. A self, which can't be found, sets out to control that very same self. Incredible, but it goes even further. When one *is* successful, when one *does* get what one wants, when things *are* "under control," who takes the credit? Who swells with pride and glory? That same elusive self. "I did a good job." Who did? "I am in control of myself." Who is?

To give credit and pride to the self somehow feels good. But of course it also sets the self up to take the blame next time if things don't go well. All serving to keep the self going. To keep it substantial. To keep it important. To keep the delusion alive. The highest values of our society have bowed to this insanity. What is more revered than self-control? Or self-determination? What enterprise holds more respect than that of self-improvement?

Mary Jo, in asking for help with her mind, was living in accordance with these values. Ideally, according to the myth, she'd have fixed herself by herself. But finding this impossible, she'd taken the next best road. She had sought out someone to fix her. She didn't simply want relief from the pain of her symptom. She wanted to become a better person. It sounds very noble. But nobility and insanity often run together, and Mary Jo's driving need for self-control is no exception.

The very words "self-control" reflect an almost indescribable insanity. Do they mean that the self is controlling some thing? Or do they mean that some thing is controlling the self? Do they mean that the self is controlling the self? Perhaps there is more than one self? A self behind the self which controls the first self? And maybe one behind that? Perhaps it is like a hall of mirrors, a never-ending series of nonidentifiable selves, reflecting each other, observing each other, and at-

tempting to control each other? The mind boggles, of course. Because it's absolutely crazy.

How often people feel "I wish I could just let myself be." "I wish I could just be myself." "Why can't I relax and just be who I am?" These feelings are almost always accompanied by a sigh. As if people sense, deeply but unclearly, that freely being would bring relaxation, rest and peace. As if they realize that *not* freely being requires a lot of work. As if they know that *trying* to live and *working* at self-control are burdens one longs to set down. All of these perceptions are correct. They are the voice of sanity. It takes incredible effort to maintain craziness. Self-control is exhausting. And the work of trying to live saps the lifeblood of living. No wonder one longs for rest.

It is a very difficult job to grasp the steering wheel of one's life and operate all the controls when one has no real idea of who's driving, where the controls are, or even where one ultimately wants to go. But being-beyond-self-control is a very threatening prospect. Being "out of control" sounds horrifying. It seems that like Hamlet, we would "rather bear those ills we have than fly to others that we know not of." One would rather drive his machine blindly than give up the driving. The self, as elusive and erratic as it is, as untrustworthy and in need of fixing as it may appear to be, has become very precious. So precious that no matter what price "it" may extract from us, we will not let "it" go.

Mary Jo described her own fear of losing herself. "There have been times, you know, when I did let myself be. Through no special doing on my part. They crept up on me. I remember once when I was doing the dishes. Bill had gone to work and I'd gotten the kids off to school and the day was going to be my own. I had nothing special to do—just the usual routine. I started to wash the dishes, and my mind suddenly became very quiet. I watched my hands as they moved. I felt the water, was aware of its warmth, the softness of the suds. For some reason I wasn't thinking about anything in particular. I was just very

brightly aware of everything. I could hear the birds singing outside, and I sensed the silence of the house. It was a beautiful experience. There was something incredibly wonderful about it. I don't know how long it lasted, but I know I suddenly got scared. Deeply frightened. And the fear killed the experience. It wasn't until long afterwards that I realized what had frightened me. It was that *I* wasn't really there. I mean I was, of course, but I wasn't aware of *me* like I usually am. I was aware of everything, and it was gorgeous, but I wasn't sensing *me*. That's what scared me." The sense of self seems so precious, is held so tightly, that even moments of ecstasy are cut short in its absence.

Humankind is now at the point where the self cannot be given up. There is no way to do it. The self cannot be killed, for it cannot be found. One may kill one part or another of one's self, but always there is another reflection, taking its place, and taking responsibility for the killing. The self cannot be willfully forgotten. Nothing can be willfully forgotten. The only way to be with one's self is to let one's self be. To accept it, as a given. A part of the human condition. Even find love for it. With acceptance and love, relaxation is possible, and one can rest for a while. And with relaxation and rest, a trust can begin to build. A trust that whatever the self is, it will take care of itself. A trust that behavior can remain responsible if one eases one's grip on the elusive steering wheel. A trust that deep and clear living happens when one ceases trying to live. And a trust that aspiration, love, caring, justice and redemption are already given. That they've been there all along, unseen because of a vision clouded by efforts at self-control.

Five Levels of Control

There are many different levels of control. Some are sane and some are crazy. One is a very basic, natural, universal

kind. Most plants will not send their roots into the air. Most animals will not search for water in a stone. Most stones will not roll uphill. This is the control of the-way-things-are. People clearly share this level with the rest of the cosmos. It is simply the way things happen.

A second level of control is that which a creature exerts over its environment. Animals do this kind of controlling when they build their nests or prey on other animals. People, in turn, control animals and plants, rivers and mountains, energy and matter. Much of this is necessary in order to live. But sometimes people get carried away with it. Sometimes the desire to control the environment exceeds our wisdom to know what to do with power. And serious ecological problems arise.

A third level of control is that which some human beings exert over other human beings. It may be the kind which is simple and loving, the kind we share with animals. Like a mother pulling her child away from a fire. Or it may be as complex and nasty as Nazi genocide.

A fourth level is the control which takes place within the minds and bodies of human beings. This is the control of conscience over impulse, of decision over ambivalence, of direction over chaos.

These four levels of control are basically natural and necessary. As one moves through them, human values and ethics become increasingly important. What gets controlled, and how, and by whom, becomes more complex and significant. Good and evil take on great meaning and raise very difficult questions. What *are* we doing to the ecology? Who has the right to control other people, and in what ways? How should thoughts and behavior be directed? Within these four levels of control lie most of humanity's truly sane efforts. Love and hate, joy and sadness, aspiration and failure, creativity and destruction; the very meat and blood of human existence take place within these natural, necessary levels of control. Would that that were enough.

The problem is that human beings, intoxicated with power, try to press on. To a fifth level of control. A level which is neither natural nor necessary. A level which doesn't even really exist.

This is the level of control of the self. Control of the very being of one's life. Control of the very essence of one's existence. *To be in charge not only of what one does, but of who one is.* Humankind's movement through greater and greater levels of control created a momentum which catapulted us into the search for ultimate self-determination. Humanity seems to be saying "If only we could master this one, we could rule all, determine all . . . and then, finally, gratefully, proudly, safely, rest." The awesomeness of the task is seldom a deterrent. And failure only results in intensified effort. There is a tragic heroism to this quest. "We can handle it. If we can handle rivers and oceans, if we can handle disease and pain, if we can handle outer space and nuclear energy, we can handle anything. We can handle our selves."

The agony of the quest is that there is no end. The more that is learned, the more there is to know. And the more desire to know. The absurdity is that the struggle promises final rest and peace, but leads only into greater and greater effort.

The insanity is that in humanity's driving, arrogant search for self-control, it is searching everywhere to find its self, and its self exists only within the very searching. But humankind has made an object of everything it has controlled or desired to control, and so it feels that this "self" must also be an object. A thing. Only where to find it? How to grasp it? How to catch it?

Finally, the despair of this search, the unspoken, unadmitted awful reality of it, is that if we did ultimately discover the self and gain absolute control over it, we wouldn't have the slightest, vaguest idea of what to do with it.

There is then blessing in the midst of this agony. Our very inability to catch and control our selves is what continues to make life worth living. But why then can't we rest with that?

When Mary Jo came in to be fixed, I said, "O.K., you've got an awful problem. But why can't you still relax and appreciate your *self*? Why can't you let your *self* be? Why can't you be, with all the pain and the fighting of pain, with all the ugliness and the struggling for beauty, with all the hate and the longing for love, why can't you let your self be?"

Her voice was small and somewhat dead as she replied, "I could . . . if only I could just get in control of myself . . . then I could let myself be."

"O.K.," I said, my voice dying too, "let's see what we can do about it."

3

EVOLUTION

Then the Lord God said, "Behold, the man
has become like one of us, knowing good and
evil; and now, lest he put forth his hand and
take also from the tree of life, and eat, and
live forever . . ."—therefore the Lord God sent him
forth from the Garden of Eden, to till the
ground from which he was taken.

Genesis

It has not always been this way. Human beings have not
always felt that their selves were objects. There was a time
when people were not concerned about the self. It was a time
of simply being. It was the time after life became aware of living, but before the human will became drunk with power. In
those days human beings felt nothing special about being
human. Newborn people entered the world with no more fanfare than accompanied the hatching of a bird's egg or the
sprouting of a flower. And when someone died it was no different than a leaf falling from a tree. Nothing special.

Picture a scene, around a water hole in some warm Medi-
terranean land, where prehistoric men and women quenched
their thirst. There are hoofprints and pawprints in the mud.
Among them are the prints of human feet. There is heavy

21

green vegetation around the mud. The sky is clear and the breeze is warm. It is morning.

A hunched, hairy figure emerges from behind a tree and hesitates. In his hand he holds a stick, something he found in his wanderings. He sniffs and turns his eyes left and right. Sharp, clear eyes, missing nothing. Glittering eyes, open to his surroundings. Then he moves toward the water, squats beside it, cups his hands, and drinks. What can we presume is going on in his mind? Nothing special. No great thoughts. Probably no thoughts at all. Probably just crude awareness. An awareness that entertains only sights and sounds and smells and touch sensations. And the taste of the water. An awareness uncomplicated by names and judgements and plans. This human being is aware of very much. He is even aware of awareness. But he is not thinking about it at all. He is life which has simply become aware of living.

He is a gatherer, a forager, and a hunter. When hungry, he finds berries or leaves, and he eats. Or he may club an animal to death and consume its flesh. But there is no thought of eating. He may offer some of his food-discoveries to others of his kind, but there is no thought of sharing. When attacked by some predator, he may fight back. But there is no thought of defense. He senses going to sleep and waking up, but he does not label them. When something happens, it simply happens. He is not concerned with why or when or how it happens, or if it will happen again. When he does something, it is done, and there is no analysis of motivation or efficiency. He has a sense of being, but no thought of "I am."

Stand by the water hole as time passes. Perhaps tens of thousands of years. The water has dried up and come again, repeatedly. There are fewer footprints now, and the vegetation is quite different. Now it is in fairly orderly rows. At one side of the water hole is a path, leading to a small hut made of sticks and dried mud. This is the house of a farmer.

Somewhere during those tens of thousands of years people

learned that they could plant seeds to raise food rather than simply forage for it. A kind of willfulness has emerged. Humans have become able to do things intentionally to the world in order to satisfy themselves. And they have also learned to talk. No longer do they simply sense. Now the things they sense have names. And the combination of will-to-do and language has created still another sense. The sense that there is some*one* willing and doing. That some*one* is "I."

Watch now as the farmer emerges from his hut. He is less hairy and he stands more straightly than his predecessor. And though he seems to walk with more confidence, he is less acutely aware. He has less need to be, for he has now defined this land as his territory and intruders are few. But even if he needed to be as acutely aware, he could not. For now there are thoughts in his mind, and they occupy much of his attention. He is less alert, and there are some furrows in his forehead. Perhaps he has been wondering whether his crop will get enough water. He is less attentive to changes in the wind and movements in the distance. He is more secure, but his eyes are not so clear.

As he moves toward the water he thinks, "I see the water." As he bends down, "I drink . . . good." Then he takes a gourd and fills it. In his mind, "For later." As he stands to leave, he hears a sound from the other side of the water. Another human being. They look at each other, muscles tense. Thoughts follow one another quickly. "Stranger . . . attack . . . run away . . . what will he do?" But the intruder turns and leaves. The farmer's heart is pounding. "Will he come back? Are there others with him?" He stands still, straining to see and hear. For a long time. Nothing happens and slowly he calms down. He heads toward his hut.

Just before he gets there he stops and looks back. Nothing on the horizon. Nothing moving in the trees. The sun is on the water, and the farmer thinks again, "I see the water." In his simple memory he reviews what has happened. "I see the

water. I drink. I fill gourd. I see stranger. Stranger goes. I see the water now. My water."

His heart is no longer pounding, but there is uneasiness in his thinking. The water is his, and he may have to protect it. It is something others want. He can't rest too easily. He is worried. But deeper than this, more insidious than this, and far more disquieting than this is a creeping horrible sense in his mind as he looks at the water. "I see the water. I am seeing the water. I drink and protect it. *I am not the water. The water is different from me.*" He feels now the pain of a basic wound. The wound of the first discrimination. The wound that was left when human thought sliced self from other. A wound which has not healed to this very day.

Already he has bought the delusion. Already he has accepted insanity. Already he carries the burden of the human predicament. To feel separate and autonomous. He feels a moment of longing, a distant memory of a time when he shared his consciousness with the water and there was no difference. No thought-discrimation.

But then he remembers he has work to do, and he must get busy or the night will catch him unprepared. So he pushes the longing, nagging emptiness out of his mind and goes about his business. He has learned to bury his sanity. Even in his simple mind the delusion is too strong, and sanity too weak.

Delusion, according to modern psychiatric definition, is a fixed mistaken belief. Something unreal which seems very real. This is what has happened to the farmer. He now feels that he is a self, separated from the rest of the world. But is he really separate? When his forebears learned to impose their wills upon the earth, when they began to think in words and sense a difference between self and other, did they really *become* separate? Did humankind really step outside the process and flow of nature, or did it just begin to feel that way?

Nothing *really* changed. There was no *real* sword which

severed humanity from the world. But it does indeed feel that way. Thoughts can sometimes seem very real.

It must have seemed to that farmer that he had once been in Eden and had now been cast out. But he didn't really leave. He wasn't really cast anywhere. Eden was, and is. He just can't believe it. Then, in moments when he notices the sunlight on the water, and when he feels a longing for reunion, he simply cannot comprehend. His sanity cries out, "Exist. Be. You are no stranger to the water. You are brothers. Simply be." But he can no longer understand. So he buries the voice. Back to work. Back to willful doing. Back to the delusion of separateness. Because now delusion seems more real than reality.

Stand by the water hole while another few thousand years pass. More people have gathered around the water, and a village has been built. More discriminations have been made. Speech is becoming refined. More things have labels. And people have become more sophisticated in willfully making and doing things. A small irrigation project has begun, plows have been made, and animals trained to pull them. Willfulness and power, becoming more sophisticated, have tended to pull the consciousness of people further into the delusion of separateness. But at this precise moment, in this precise village, an answer has been found for the nagging voice of sanity. For the time being, the people in this village are listening to their sanity.

The answer has come in the form of religion. Out of the pain of separation caused by their discriminating minds, people have made another discrimination which has a quality of healing. It is the idea of a creation. A beginning in which were fashioned, all together, the earth, the sky, water, animals and people. For a while now people can remember that they are brothers and sisters to the rest of the world. This is the pristine dawn of religion, before it became superstitious.

As we watch, a woman comes from one of the dwellings,

carrying a bowl to get some water. Her movements are slow, and she seems to be sensing the breeze as it blows across her skin. Hers is not precisely the sharp clear awareness of that first hairy creature we saw, but it is somehow more immediately sensitive than the worried confidence of the farmer. As she bends to get the water, she seems to be going through a kind of ritual. Her eyes close for a moment, and she makes some slight movements of her hands. Then she looks at the water intensely, almost devotedly, as if she were worshipping it. She gathers it up and returns to her house, careful not to spill a drop.

Her little ritual and her reverence for the water and the wind are ways of remembering her roots. She is reminding herself that she is a child of the same origins as the water, and she appreciates. Religion is born, and it serves to call the consciousness of people home. For a while, sanity is heard.

Several thousand more years pass. The water hole has dried up, and the water has not returned. Someone has dug a well. Whoever it was had been thinking, "There is something wrong here, that the water has not come back. We will fix the situation. We will dig a well and pull the water from beneath the ground." The well has produced great quantities of clear water and the village has grown. The farms now stretch for nearly a mile around. The people gather together more frequently. As we watch, we see what has happened to religion and to the voice of sanity. It is sunset.

A large number of people are gathering at the well. They are costumed and painted. In their midst, by the well, there is one man who stands out from the rest. Clothed in an animal skin, a mask on his face, he is muttering a monotone chant which neither we nor the people can understand. The people sit in an attitude of reverence. Someone lights a fire and a drum begins to beat. The man in the middle starts to dance, twirling and leaping through the smoke. As the sun goes below

the horizon many of the people join the dance, and a frenzy begins to build. It lasts all night. When the sun rises again, a small animal is brought into the circle, bathed in water from the well, killed and thrown into the fire. Finally the people return to their dwellings.

Religion has changed. What had been a way of calling people's consciousness back to their roots has now become a way of trying to insure a good harvest. The idea of creation has moved to the idea of creators, powerful gods who rule over the things people cannot control. Unable to exert their will upon the wind and rains, people have invented gods who can. And now the people try to control the gods, through sacrifice and homage. Religion, once a way of listening to the voice of sanity, has fallen prey to the insatiable will of human beings to do and to control. Religion has been transformed into superstition.

If we stand by the well a few hours longer, we can see some more of the discriminations which have been made. After the nightlong ritual one man has remained by the well. All the others have returned to their houses, but this one has stayed, sitting still, like a rock. And he is staring at the sun. Later in the day, people come to the well and see him sitting there. They are puzzled by his behavior. No one else has ever acted this way. They have learned to discriminate between normal and abnormal behavior.

After a while, the medicine man is called. He approaches cautiously, walking around the sitting man, looking him over very carefully. The medicine man is thinking, "There is something wrong with this person. There is something very wrong and I am expected to do something about it. I must appease the gods when the rains do not come. I must cast out the evil spirits when illness strikes. Now I must do something to remedy this man's problem." So the medicine man begins another incantation, and he dances around the man who is staring at the sun, and after a while the man gets up and walks away.

The medicine man thinks, "I have helped this man. I have fixed what was wrong." Psychotherapy is born.

Psychotherapy was born out of the same need for control and self-assertion that changed man's wholeness into separation and religion into superstition. When the water hole dried up, something was wrong and needed to be fixed. And so people dug a well, and fixed the water problem. When the rains didn't come, people tried to influence gods who could fix the problem. And when something went wrong with some*body*, in body or in mind, someone would try to fix it. The Will of Humankind was forging its mark on the face of the earth, toward ever-increasing power, accomplishment, achievement and improvement. The world became compartmentalized into *things*, things to be handled, altered and fixed. And people became some of those things.

The small voice of sanity was heard from time to time saying, "Rest from all this struggle. Simply be." Most of the time it was ignored. On the rare occasions when it was heard, it was perceived as another problem that needed to be taken care of. Another thing to fix. And everything that was done about it helped to bury it. It could not be heard clearly and allowed to bloom because it would demand the sacrifice of delusion, and people have not been prepared to give up their insanity. No matter how painful it may be, no matter what deep suffering it may cause, the human delusion of separateness is clenched in sweating fists, gripped with white knuckles, as if it were the dearest possible possession.

This is simply the way any delusion is held. If you have a delusion that someone is plotting against you, following you with murderous intent, you will suffer continually. Perhaps you will never be able to rest, always fearing that they will be waiting around the next corner, ready to kill you. Perhaps the delusion tears your mind and destroys your spirit and makes you rather kill yourself than let them do it, but you will not

give up the belief. Because as awful as the delusion is, it serves a purpose. It keeps you from perceiving something that you fear even more.

The fearsome thing we feel we must avoid by clinging to the delusion of separate selfhood is *being*. *Just* being. Being *without* the idea of self-determining willful control of destiny. Being *without* self-definition. That seems like death. It seems that to cease defining the self would be like nonexistence.

It feels like death. But it's not. Self-definition is simply an idea; a discrimination wound made by the sword of a thinking mind. If self-definition dies, it is no more than the passing of a thought. We fear the death of a figment.

When people do give up a delusion, if they happen to find out what it was they were afraid of underneath, they are likely to say "It was just a figment of my imagination." Precisely.

We could return to that water hole once more, in present times. There's a city there now, and the discriminations have become so numerous and complex they could not be listed. Delusion has become so deeply entrenched that sanity is seldom heard. People living in this city now laugh in scorn at primitive humanity's superstitious dances and rituals. But they're only laughing at methods. They do not laugh at primitive humanity's grinding, agonizing belief that in one way or another one can willfully control one's own destiny. They do not laugh at the idea that human beings can learn enough and do enough and fix themselves and improve upon themselves enough so that finally they will be happy. They do not laugh at the delusion. For it is their delusion as well, and ours.

But there are cracks in the streets of the city. And despair whips the corners of the buildings each morning. The people are tired. They have been searching for a way to wholeness for thousands upon thousands of years, and they are tired. They are tired of fixing and improving, and it may be that they will soon give up. Then it is possible that sanity will again be

allowed to bloom. When self-definition has burned itself out.

But for the time being, the delusion goes on. And it is re-established, reaffirmed and reenacted in the growth of each child born into the human race.

4

CHILDREN

The sublimest song to be heard on earth
is the lisping of the human soul on the
lips of children.

Victor Hugo, *Les Miserables*

On occasion, and usually by accident, science creates poetry. I learned the phrase "Ontogeny recapitulates phylogeny" in freshman biology, and it has always seemed poetic to me. Even its meaning is poetic. It means that in the growth of each individual organism, the entire development of the species is reenacted. Each developing baby plays out in microcosm the centuries of evolution which have preceded it.

A human embryo begins as a single vibrant cell, much like an amoeba. This one cell grows into many, and soon the freshly forming creature sprouts a set of gills, just like a fish. Then a bit later the embryo begins to look like a salamander, complete with tail. The gills recede, turning into ears and throat muscles, the fetus grows into its tail and begins to look more human. Then a coat of downy fur grows, soft; warm, mammalian. Finally most of the fur is shed and a fully human infant is born.

This is recapitulation. The playing out of all evolution in one single human baby. But the recapitulation does not stop

31

with physical attributes. Watching the growth of children we can see the recapitulation of consciousness as well. We can see control, self and will develop in a manner strikingly similar to that which occurred with primitive man over a period of hundreds of thousands of years. We can also watch our children learning to be crazy. Developing ways of stifling sanity. Learning to make objects of themselves. Becoming intoxicated with the morphine of self-improvement.

What is specifically human about awareness is that we are aware of being aware. I'm not sure exactly when this kind of awareness happens in the development of a baby, but I'm certain it occurs well before there is thought, and long before there is any idea of a "self" which *has* awareness or a will which controls awareness.

Some kind of awareness is present before birth. An unborn baby responds definitively to sudden movements and loud sounds. It has periods of waking and sleeping, when its awareness changes from one state to another. At birth, the infant's awareness is obvious. The baby is flooded with sights and sounds, temperature changes, pressure and pain. And it is very responsive.

Control is also present at the moment of birth. It may be hard to think of control in an infant who has yet to develop a sense of self, but nonetheless control is there. Just as it is in animals. Animals have desire for food when they are hungry, and they will control things to get food. They will control where they go, how they move and what they do in order to eat. Most of this is instinctual, but it is all a form of control in order to respond to desire. The same is true of the infant human being.

I was in the delivery room at the time of our first child's birth. Through an overhead mirror my wife and I watched the baby being born. The doctor said, "Push now, the head is coming." With the next contraction, a small, purplish, ugly, lovely

head emerged. The doctor smiled. "One more contraction and we'll know whether it's a boy or a girl." We could see the baby's face in the mirror, eyes closed, expressionless. While waiting for the next contraction, the doctor took a rubber-bulb syringe and sucked some fluid from one of the baby's nostrils. The face winced. Then the doctor tried to insert the syringe into the other nostril, but the little face grimaced and the head turned to avoid the syringe. Betty and I were awestruck. Here was our child, not yet completely born and already *learning*. It was as if the baby were saying, "You got me once with that thing Doc, but you'll have trouble getting me again." With only his head born, our son was learning to exert control. In an instant, in the midst of being born, he learned that something going in the nose is unpleasant, and he tried to avoid it. Long before any idea of self or will. Long before any idea of anything.

In the hours and days immediately after the birth of any baby, control becomes much more sophisticated. A newborn infant reflexively responds to pain, hunger and cold by wriggling and crying, but soon it learns that wriggling in one direction helps more than wriggling in another. It learns that certain sounds and sights are associated with good feelings, and others with bad. It learns that crying often brings help. It begins to associate that help with a certain form, usually that of the mother. Within a few weeks the baby has learned to discriminate between stimuli, to excercise its control more efficiently, and even to some extent to distinguish its mother. Still there is no thought of this or that, no idea of self or other, no concept of desire or control.

As time goes on, the infant responds more to mother than to other people. It may cry even when nothing is wrong, just to get mother to come. It learns to mimic smiles and sounds, and to sense its own constancy while other things change. It learns that it can control its own body more than it can control other

things. It learns to interact with its environment very well. And still there is no thought.

Thus far, there has been little difference between the consciousness of the human baby and the consciousness of animals. But then *words* happen. Things start to get labeled. Ideas and thoughts erupt, and the human infant begins to follow a path no other animal has trod.

With much help from parents, things start to be given names. First the "other" things. Mama, Dada, ball, toy. Then things about "me." My name, tummy, hand, toe. Then the quality of things. Nice, pretty, cold.

As the child becomes mobile, crawling around the floor, it learns an especially important word. "No." "No" seems important because it is usually associated with emphatic action on the part of the parents. A stern voice or perhaps a slap on the hand. At first, "no" is another label. This is a ball. That is a puppy. That is a no-no. But soon "no" becomes much more than a label. It becomes the very ground out of which springs the concept of self-determination. When parents simply said "No," behavior simply responded. But when parents start saying "Don't *do* that," the child begins to sense that he or she *is* somebody who should *do* the controlling of behavior. This is the beginning of a truly human self-concept.

Nearly all the messages which children get about themselves are couched in terms of what they are *doing* and how well or poorly they are controlling themselves. "You're a good girl." "You ate all your dinner." "Don't do that again." "Go to sleep now." The emerging self-image is intimately, deeply associated with doing and control. There even comes a point where the child defines itself only in terms of what it can control. And whatever seems beyond control is seen as not-self. Tripping over a toy, the child may say, "The floor bumped me." Having had an excretory accident the child may announce, "My pants wetted themselves." After sneaking a candy

from the kitchen, the child may explain, "I didn't do it. My hand did."

But parents won't put up with this confusion of self-responsibility for long. They make it very clear that the child is responsible for controlling the things it does. From this point on, the child is very close to insanity. It is ready to accept the following sequence of ideas:

1. Behavior must be controlled. (True enough.)
2. There is something behind both behavior and control which is the self. (Questionable.)
3. It is that self which should *do* the controlling. (Even more questionable.)
4. If control of behavior is inadequate, then the self needs to control the self to make the self control behavior in a better way. (Absolutely crazy.)

There are times when parents sense the pain this process is causing in their children. They try to ease the little one's struggles by emphasizing behavior control rather than self-control. "I'm a bad boy," the child says. "No you're not," respond the parents. "You're a *good* boy. You just did a bad thing." But these attempts are usually weak and in vain. The child continues to equate the value of its self with the ability to control its self. The child has already gone overboard, and is well on the way to a life of self-determination.

Review for a moment how far human children have come from the animals. Desire, control, and discrimination are all present and operative in the animal world. So is learning. But without words or concepts with which to label things, a self-image never occurs. Though a rabbit may distinguish itself from a fox by running away, the rabbit never has any idea of a self which initiates or determines that behavior. Though a mother bear may exert control over her cubs by cuffing them when they

stray toward danger, and though the cubs learn to control their wanderings as a result of being cuffed, there is no image of any self which is *doing* the controlling or learning. The mother bear never says "you" to her cubs. She never asks them to explain their behavior. And she never tells them to control themselves.

This is not to say that there is anything inherently better about animals not having a sense of self. Nor is it to say that human beings are flawed because they do have such a concept. There is nothing wrong with a concept of self. The problems begin when the idea of self *becomes mistaken for reality*. When the sense of self seems to become *substantial*. When it begins to seem like a *thing*. And true insanity sets in with the feeling that one should build, fix, improve upon, or otherwise control that thing.

As the image of self is developing, another concept is being formed. The concept of will. Will is another idea which begins to take on a substance of its own. The idea of will begins as soon as a child learns that it can choose to control or not control itself. A child grasps the rudiments of will from the "No's" it has heard from its parents, and from having said "No" to itself. But full and definite establishment of will finally occurs when the child says "No" to others. In saying, "No, I won't eat my dinner," or "No, I will not go potty," the child is proving how well it has learned the parental teaching that it is *somebody*. The child is decidedly and emphatically underscoring the difference between self and other, and stating in no uncertain terms that it will determine its self.

Saying "No" can be a lot of fun. Very powerful. After two years of almost total dependency and being controlled by others, the child feels fresh and liberated when he or she can say "No" *to* those others. But for the parents, it can be a bit of a rough time. In continuing to tell the child that he or she is responsible for himself or herself, the parents have made their point. Sometimes when the child is about two or three, the

parents may wonder if they have not made their point too well. By this time, the question is not so much what should be controlled, but who is controlling whom.

Throughout the rest of childhood, the faculties of discrimination, control and self-determination become refined and elaborated. In adolescence, when sex hormones begin to flow and parental ties begin to break, the self takes on far more substance and importance. And a drive for self-exploration becomes evident. At times this may appear very self-*centered* and self-*ish*. At other times it may seem very altruistic and loving. But what the adolescent is doing is making a dynamic attempt to discover what the substance of this mysterious self really is.

People may ask of the adolescent "What are you going to be when you grow up?" The adolescent asks of himself, "Who am I?" Between these two questions a sort of friction erupts which makes for a very lively dance with identity. The words "What are you going to be" speak for delusion. They imply that the person is a "what," to be defined by doing. But sanity proclaims the person as a "who," evident in being.

Delusion and sanity rub against each other in adolescence, and a colorful series of experiences results. One day, identity may seem very solid and stable. On the next, the adolescent may walk about in a daze. On the following day, there may be a religious conversion, bordering on fanatacism. And on the day following that, apathy.

Delusion and sanity are at war over the self. The one wanting to grasp and determine it, the other wanting to free it to be what it will be. The one fearful of losing the self, the other willing to give it up.

Toward the end of adolescence, the battle ebbs. Dust clears from the field. Usually, delusion is the victor. Identity has been found, and sanity loses yet another battle. It loses because it has very little cultural support. Language does not give it good weapons with which to fight. Values do not hold it in high esteem, for the values of culture are often the secret

agents of delusion. They say one should make something of one's self. Make some thing of your self. But most of all, sanity loses because it is not a killer. It can destroy nothing. Its only real weapon is love, and its only strategy is affirmation. And so sanity once again is covered, buried beneath the carnage of the battlefield. There it remains, constant, unchanging, incredibly simple.

Through the entire process of human identity formation, through birth and childhood and adolescence, the child is carefully watched. By educators and psychotherapists, but most of all by parents. Sometimes parents watch with awe, sensing the intricate beauty of their children's growth. Sometimes parents watch with fear, unable to know what to give their children, how to direct them. Not realizing the possibility of fully, freely being with their children, parents wonder *how* to be with their children. What is the proper technique? What is the best method? Caught in this dilemma, it is not unusual for parents to turn to psychotherapy for help. For guidance in the proper methods of raising children. And psychotherapy, it seems, always has something to say.

In its many forms, psychotherapy has offered a veritable smorgasbord of guidelines as to how children should be raised. A host of suggestions, almost all of which take the form of methods and techniques.

There was a time when psychotherapists advocated strictness, hard work and solid rules. Then, in an almost universal misinterpretation of Freud, permissiveness became the way. More recently, parents have been told that the best child-raising involves listening to feelings and straight communication. All are methods. Whether a specific method works well or not is unimportant. What is important is that parents have an insatiable hunger for methods, and psychotherapists have an unending supply. When the method is what counts, the child is lost. For methods are not used for being. Methods are used for building.

Of all the questions I've been asked as a psychiatrist, the most common and disturbing ones have been about how to raise children. It has always seemed rather strange that people can expect psychiatric training to create an authority on child-raising. It would make much more sense to search out a grandmother whose offspring are living fully and beautifully, and ask *her* about it all. But parents seem to want methods, and psychotherapy is where the methods are to be found. Complex, sophisticated methods. Grandmothers usually have only a few methods. And they're usually very simple. Grandmothers often say things like, "Well, I just did the best I could, taught 'em right and trusted in God. And I always made sure they washed behind their ears." Sane as those words may be, they're just too simple to satisfy most modern parents' appetite for techniques. Grandmothers like to see children grow. Method-hungry parents want to see children built.

The more methods we get, the more we feel like we are building our children. And the more we feel like builders, the more methods we want. Even if we use words like "raising" or "growing" rather than "building," we still feel we are doing the raising. Persisting in the belief that we are growing or raising our children, we shall continue to feel separate from them. They will remain objects for our manipulation. We will be managing their growth process rather than participating in it.

If I could now answer all the questions I've been asked about how to raise children, I'd say "I really don't know. I honestly don't know whether it's better for you to be strict or permissive, demanding or acquiescent, whether you should spank or restrict or understand. I simply do not know. Not as a psychiatrist, and not as a parent. But whatever you do, please continue to do the best you can. Just please do it in the sense of participation in growth. Watch with awe as your children's petals unfold. Marvel at the growing. Be with them in it, as fully as you can."

One of the saddest results of the "help" psychotherapy

has given to child-raising is that parents are encouraged to manipulate themselves *more* in order to manipulate their children *less*. Young mothers and fathers can be amazingly masochistic about this. Almost invariably feeling ill prepared for the job of growing children, they seek advice. From doctors and psychotherapists. Or from books by doctors and psychotherapists. Finding some specific recommendation, they often proceed to follow it even if it feels deeply wrong.

I've seen mothers crying in agony, stifling their desire to hold their screaming child because some "authority" said infants should be held for no more than an hour a day. I have seen fathers stand back while their hearts ached to respond to a child, because they'd been taught that the mother should take care of the emotional stuff. I've seen parents driven to near hysteria by the screaming tyranny of their toddler because someone had said they shouldn't lose their temper with the child. And driven to exhaustion because they felt they should never "reject" a child by saying, "Leave me alone for a while, I'm tired."

All done in love. All done with the best of intentions. Done to prevent the child from getting, God forbid, a complex. But at such a price. The price of parents interfering with themselves, of stifling who they are, of giving complexes to the *parents*, so that at some future time they might be able to say, "I did a good job raising my children." We might get a raise for doing a good job building cars in Detroit. But for doing a good job building our kids we get deeper into our delusion of separation. And the children, what do they get out of it? What do they learn by watching their parents?

I am very grateful that psychotherapy has *not* been able to come up with a sure-fire mistake-proof guaranteed child-raising method. If there were such a method, I fear we'd lose all

hope of being with our children in their growing. On the other hand, I'm glad we're concerned enough about our children to worry about them. It is a big responsibility, and one has to do one's best. We have to worry about our children, and we have to suffer with them, and we have to hope for them. With all of this, it seems only fair that we allow ourselves the wonder of being with them in growth. Too often, this most precious reward is sacrificed. We sacrifice it now in the hopes of some fantasied future reward of being able to say we did a good job. Grandmothers, far more than psychotherapists, know the folly of this.

The natural growth process in children will occur. It will occur, in most cases, in spite of us. Almost no matter what we do, it will happen. We seldom kill our children by trying to grow them. What we do kill is our simple awareness of the natural growth process. Being so interested in taking credit for the growth and carrying the burden of it, we fail to see its wonder.

In those moments when we do see it—and we all have those moments, now and then, happening to glance into his room when he's sleeping, or seeing her eyes at Christmas—we can listen to sanity. In those moments we can be who we are with our children as they are. Maybe that means we'll be strict. Or lenient. Or sentimental-sweet. Or understanding. Or rejecting. It probably means that we'll be doing the very best we can in the best way we know. But we won't feel like it's all our doing. Seeing it, marveling at it, we can at the same time be an integral, active part of it.

5

THE FIX

Drink iron from rare springs;
    follow the sun;
Go far
To get the beam of some
    medicinal star;
Or in your anguish run
The gauntlet of all zones to an
    ultimate one.
Fever and chill
Punish you still,
Earth has no zone to work against
    your will.

Genevieve Taggard

By the time they reach age 21, most everyone has gone crazy a
few times and most everyone has gone sane a few times.
Enough to know the difference. But many will have decided
that crazy is the way to be, and they will be trying very hard to
make some thing of themselves.

Some will find identity by giving their lives to a company.
They will receive a gold watch at the end of twenty years and
then look around themselves and say, "Well, this is what I
worked for. Financial security. Status. Respect. But somehow
it doesn't seem as wonderful as it should."

Others will pledge their lives to the raising of healthy, well-adjusted children. Then the children will grow up and go off to raise children of their own. And there will be a time of empty loneliness. "I've worked long and given much. I'm glad my children are doing well, but what now is left for me?"

Still others will fail at what they had determined to make of themselves. They'll flunk out of school or lose the "good job" or mess up "what could have been a good marriage." Then perhaps they will try something else. If they have the energy. But it won't be precisely what they wanted, and despair will settle in.

Some of these people, the "successful" ones as well as the "failures," will just quietly stifle their doubts, make do with whatever they have achieved, and resign themselves to living through a number of remaining barren years. Others will turn about in their despair, searching for ways to regain some sense of self-control and self-determination. They may try to learn something new, take a course, seek out a new experience. Or they may find a group or a cause to which they can pledge allegiance, something with which they can identify themselves.

Or perhaps they will enter psychotherapy, seeking to find some fresh insight, understanding or encouragement which will renew their energy for self-determination. For many, this will work.

But when psychotherapy "works" in this way, it simply stifles sanity again. To a person who is approaching the point of possible giving up psychotherapy says, "Now don't give up. There are still many ways to get back in control of yourself and of your destiny. Let me help you." Saying this, psychotherapy fans the dying embers of delusion, promising renewed vigor, new opportunity. It is deaf to the voice of sanity which is pleading, "Allow me to give up. Let me sacrifice the struggle. Allow me to accept and be, simply, who I am."

Acting as the good child of civilization's craziness, psychotherapy will recharge batteries for self-manipulation and open

new doors to mastery. It will work. For a while. Until fatigue sets in again. Or until all the new doors have been entered and nothing of ultimate worth has been found behind them.

With or without the "help" of psychotherapy, some people will come to a time of ending. Having exhausted all the visible avenues toward peace and completion, being exhausted themselves, having seen every promise of fulfillment broken, some will assert the final attempt at self-mastery. The ultimate target of delusion. The ominpotence of suicide.

Most people see suicide as giving up, but in fact suicide is the antithesis of giving up. It is the final assertiveness of self attempting to control self. The ultimate challenge to being. Mastery. As abhorrent as suicide is to society, it pays the final homage to society's delusion. It is in fact the logical culmination of a life which is lived in accordance with society's belief in self-mastery.

I have said before that there are many forms of suicide. Alcohol and drugs as well as guns and pills. Slow, insidious as well as quick and definite. In attempting to destroy a self which cannot be found, suicide winds up attacking one or more *attributes* of that self. Least common but most obvious is the attack upon one's body. A more subtle but more frequent target is one's will. The will can be "killed" through immersion in passivity, subjugation to drugs, or subjugation to other people.

But suicide's most common target is awareness. The awareness which lets us know we exist. To kill awareness, to murder or drug or daze the awareness of being which is our only link with our living, is no different from murdering the "self." To kill immediate present awareness is to be dead for a while. And this is something that nearly everyone does, thousands of times a day.

Immediate awareness is killed in countless ways; in work, in play, in human relationships, in food, in worry, in racing toward success. It is no accident that one says "I lost myself,"

to describe the drowning of awareness in activity. Dulled, robotic, moving through life oblivious to being, we awaken to immediate living only now and then. And most of those precious waking moments become caught up in evaluation of the past or worry about the future. But it is not really our "self" which is lost in the daze of doing. It is awareness. Awareness is killed. Whatever the motivation—to rest or to get beyond the agony of self-concern—we kill the precious awareness which informs us of being. This is the way in which countless mini-suicides are committed daily.

To wake up from the daze, to come home to consciousness again, to live brightly and fully with awareness clear as winter air—this sounds wonderful. But it also sounds like a fantasy. It appears as a dream beyond human capacity. It sounds like something which would require an incredible amount of doing and an unimaginable degree of fixing. It sounds this way because we have come to associate awareness so intimately with control that it is almost impossible to conceive of one existing without the other. Being so used to evaluating and fixing ourselves every time awareness occurs, it seems difficult to conceive of being-in-that-awareness and resting at the same time. But it is not so difficult. It is no fantasy. And it takes no special fixing. It doesn't even take doing. It takes perhaps some kind of allowing, allowing oneself to give up. But not suicide. It takes allowing of relaxation, but not lethargy. It takes acceptance, but not passivity. It takes simply being. But even that seems difficult. To simply be, to fully, dynamically, energetically be, and not *do* anything about it. It seems perhaps that the delusion is too firmly entrenched and sanity too incomprehensible. Sometimes it seems impossible.

Still, there is always room for great hope. For at every level of despair there is the possibility of giving up. In the midst of every dimension of delusion there are sparkles of sanity.

For one thing, the story I have told about human growth-

into-delusion does not apply to everyone. There are many people who are born with grace into this life and never accept the delusion. They never come to feel separate, and they are spared the agony of feeling that they have strayed from their roots. These people are often not very outspoken. Usually quiet and unassuming, they seldom come to public light. It is easy to forget that they exist. Still, they are many in number and can be found in the most unlikely places. In a factory in a small Michigan town, I once came upon a woman whose eyes were so clear that I could not help but feel awed in her presence. She seemed not to know this, and only smiled gently at me. On a Pennsylvania farm, an old grandfather laughed lovingly as I spoke of understanding life. He twinkled, but said no words in response to me. Instead, he invited me to help with the milking of the cows. A suburban housewife heard me discussing the difficulties of being immediately aware. "Why is it so hard," she said, "when you *are?*"

There are people like this everywhere. They simply have no great reason to announce themselves. They have no need to write, speak, teach or learn about awareness or being. Because they simply are, and their simple being says more than words ever could. These are the people whom William James called the "once born" of religion. For them, religion and living are synonymous. Being and awareness are unified. Worship and living life are one and the same thing. For them, the only "special" religious activities, the only "special" dances they perform with life, are celebration and thanksgiving. They live as best they can and accept their being at that. They do not try to do more than their best. Their behavior is responsible, but they assume neither credit nor blame. There is no need for them to try to live, for they are immersed in the process of living.

The rest of us are in James's category of the "twice born." Feeling that we have somehow come away from the essence of

our being, that we have travelled somewhere off from our roots, it seems that we must *do* something to come home. Somehow we must work our way forwards or backwards to being rather than simply be. Trying to live rather than living. Fixing rather than healing. Building rather than growing. For the twice-born, religion, learning, psychotherapy and all other forms of doing are possible vehicles *to* nature. Ways of coming home.

For us, the twice born, there is great hope. At each point along the paths we follow, giving up is possible. Every footstep on the road to self-mastery represents a possibility for quitting the struggle. At the age of two or at the age of eighty, and at every point in between, giving up may happen.

In the early years of life, giving up usually takes the form of faith. A leaping forward into a belief that one is loved, accepted, forgiven and redeemed just as one is, with nothing special needing to be done. In later years, giving up more often comes from despair. From the wisdom of realizing that no amount of continuing effort, no amount of fixing, will enable one to "get it all together." Despair then is forever a doorway to life.

It must be an act of grace, or of something beyond the individual will, which enables certain people to give up at certain times. Whether the giving up occurs gradually or swiftly, with great fanfare or absolute stillness, giving up is not something that can willfully be done. It can be allowed or it can be resisted, but it cannot be done. And that is where hope lies. Not hope in continuing effort, but hope for some kind of mercy. Hope that today or next month, or five years from now there will come a time when the struggle will be sacrificed.

It seems that psychotherapy could help people realize this. It seems that therapy could be an opportunity for recognizing the possibilities for sanity in each moment of life; that it could provide space for giving up, when giving up is ready to hap-

pen. But instead psychotherapy says, "Keep trying. You can do it."

A troubled person enters a therapist's office, falls into a chair and sighs, "I'm so tired. Life is such hard work. I feel like giving up." How loving and beautiful it might be if the therapist could say, "That doesn't sound like a bad idea at all." But the chances of a therapist saying anything of the kind are a thousand to one. The therapist will panic at such a statement. He or she will have visions of suicide. And suicide would be a mark of the therapist's failure as well as the client's. So the therapist will feel, "We can't have this kind of attitude. We must do something about this." And then, the therapist will offer a fix.

There's nothing really special or out of the ordinary about the psychotherapeutic fix. There are fixes for everything in this life.

In one day's bounty of television commercials, fixes are offered for every conceivable human defect. Fixes for constipation. And for diarrhea. For runny noses, stuffy noses, ugly noses and pimply noses. For insomnia. For drowsiness. If you're bored, there's something exciting to fix your boredom. If you're ignorant, there's always something to learn. If you're not attractive enough, there's a beauty fix. There are fixes to make you smell good. There are even fixes to make you smell natural. And to make your hair curly if it's straight and straight if it's curly.

In all kinds of advertising, from the blatant affront of TV commercials to the subtleties of word-of-mouth, nothing can escape the fix. And it's not just that fixes are *offered*. The message also is that one "ought" to be fixed. That if perchance one should pass a certain fix by, not partake of its wondrous possibilities, one really isn't being very responsible for one's self.

Our attitudes toward this fix-pitch are very interesting. On the one hand, there is a strong desire to be fixed. On the other,

there is a feeling of being insulted by the suggestion that we *ought* to be fixed. It is not too difficult to accept that one's house, automobile, clothes or sewing machine need to be fixed or improved upon. And it is without great discontent that one might learn that there are better ways of washing dishes, laundering clothes or fertilizing the lawn. But it becomes more irritating to be told that one should fix the way one's body smells, the way one wears one's hair, the form and substance of one's breasts, the configuration of one's hemorrhoids or the water level in one's sinuses. As the suggestion of fixes approaches closer and closer to one's sense of "self," one tends to become more insulted. Suggestions as to how one should behave, or feel, or what one should aspire to, come as more of an affront to human dignity. But in spite of the insult there is always a market for the fix.

Pills, liquids, understanding, knowledge, do your body this way or that. Change your food, change of scenery, change behavior. If the child is hyperactive—energy fix. If lethargic—stimulation fix. When worried, do an anxiety fix. When depressed, a happy fix. Having marital problems? Marriage fix. Sexual difficulties? Sex fix. Too shy and self-conscious? A confidence fix. Can't say no and stand up for your self? Assertive fix. Feel weak, vulnerable, abused in life? Power fix. Poor? There's a way to get money. Feel a gap between yourself and your children? Communication fix. Understanding fix. Alienated? Meaningless? Wondering what it's all worth? Spirit fix. Religion fix. Buy this belief. That technique. This prophet. That guru. And be happy. Obsessed? Entranced? Hallucinating? Preoccupied, impulsive, confused, despairing, suicidal, want to kill somebody? Mind fix. Be well adjusted. Analyze, free-associate, express feelings, get in touch, reenact, work it through, understand, relate, scream it out, live it out, act it out, transcend, integrate and become whole.

From ghettos to pollution and from impotence to domina-

tion there is a fix for everything. Why then, one might ask, is humankind still so troubled? The usual answer to this question would be that we just haven't found quite the *right* fix yet. Or that we haven't been fixed quite *enough* yet. Or that not quite enough people *want* to be fixed yet. Always the problem seems to be somewhere in the method. Yet there's nothing especially wrong about the methods. Except that they are seen as fixes.

Looking back over history, it seems there may be another reason why all the fixes haven't been able to fix us to our satisfaction. It appears that the more fixes that are discovered, the more there is to be fixed. With each improvement the more there is to be improved upon. The unending river of fixes continues to branch and branch, forming countless tributaries, innumerable swamps, but never reaching the ocean. You can make your own analogies between this and the fix of the drug addict. Sometime, at some point, sanity will have to ask, "How long will this go on?"

Learning teaches us only how ignorant we are. Which would be beautiful if ignorance could be accepted. Power teaches us only how weak we are, which would be fine if weakness could be affirmed. The discovery of new fixes teaches us only how much in us is imperfect. Which would be superb if only imperfection could be loved. If only imperfection did not always have to be fixed.

There is a tree outside my window. One half of it is full and green. The other half was struck by lightning many years ago. The gnarled, empty branches of this half frame the spring leaves of the other. Do I call it deformed, inadequate, in need of surgery because it is not perfectly round and full? Its imperfection is its beauty. Its imperfection is its perfection.

Human beings might recognize the beauty of an imperfect tree. But human beings can no longer see themselves as natural and beautiful in their own imperfections. Not when fixing offers perfection. It is easy to love imperfection in nature,

but not in ourselves. Fix we must, and the fixing requires more fixing . . . .

To say that this leads to alienation is mild. It leads to much more. Alienation is a wandering emptiness, dry, lifeless, barren. There is a quality of quiet to the despair of alienation. But modern society is dynamic, driven, relentlessly striving, very noisy. There is more than alienation in this. There is a deep propulsion to *do* something about the human condition; a chasing and racing after something somewhere which will make it all better. A challenge to conquer alienation. To master despair. People are propelled by the belief that continually increasing effort, more and more sweat, more and more noise, will finally bring peace.

It is beyond this agonizing struggle for self-improvement, beneath the endless fatigue, that alienation turns malignant. With the feeling that people are unnatural. All living things grow, heal, develop, and do what needs to be done to live. But human beings are the only creatures who try to improve upon their very selves. And this leads to a pervasive sense that anything created by humankind is somehow artificial and contrived.

Sensing the choiceless insanity of their compulsive attempts at fixing, people look upon "nature" as very distant from themselves. The more we continue to wreak havoc upon the ecology of nature, the more we ache with nostalgia at the thought of wilderness untouched by people. On the one hand there is compulsive driving to improve upon nature, and on the other a deep sense that what is natural is better than what is manmade. The illogic of this is to be expected, and its humor is not surprising.

In the midst of fixing and improving upon nature we long for untouched wilderness. There seems to be an air of pristine purity about something which has been "untouched by human hands." As if our hands were dirty. There is a quality of fresh-

ness about a place "where no man has set foot." As if our feet inflict wounds upon the ground. We speak of "virgin forests" as if a kind of rape took place with the entrance of humankind. Looking at the untouched beauty of newfallen snow, one sometimes wishes human footprints would never mar its surface. But the prints of animals seem only to add to its beauty. So at times we feel like interlopers on the planet earth. And very often, we feel like strangers in our own homes.

Untouched forests and newfallen snow are, according to human discrimination, part of the nature which is *outside* us. But we have also come to feel distanced from the nature *within* us. There is a sense of being-ness deep inside which often seems very far away. Whenever one speaks of wanting to "just be" or to "relax and be myself," that is an expression of longing for *inner* nature. The desire for a way of being which is as pristine and fresh as new snow. It lies, we feel, somewhere beyond or beneath all the self-manipulation and improvement. The dilemma is that it always seems to be somewhere other than here, sometime other than now. It is perhaps Eden, the garden from which we were cast because of our knowledge. But there is no distance between the time or place of Eden and our immediate consciousness. Eden is. One need not travel to get there. One need not do anything to get there. But that is very hard to do.

6

DISCUSSIONS
WITH
TWO PEOPLE

We are healed of a suffering only
by experiencing it to the full.

Marcel Proust

CARLA

Carla was, and is what is known as a "facilitator." A leader of
human growth groups in which people build and fix themselves. One day she spoke to me of feelings. She had learned,
she thought, that in order to be whole one should express one's
feelings. So every time she had a feeling she would express it.
And it would be "worked through," understood, and integrated.

"God, I'm tired," she said. She explained that her marriage, her family and her friendships had become so complicated and out of control that she felt about to collapse. She said,
"This morning I asked my husband a question, and he turned
his back on me. I thought he was shutting me out, and I told
him how it made me feel. But he just exploded. He said he
only wanted to get something out of the refrigerator and why
did I have to take everything so personally. Then we got into
this big fight. Ah, we eventually got it worked through, but
. . . you know I just wonder if we'll ever get enough worked
through, so we can just be together."

I asked a simple question. No special insight intended. Just curious. "Why did you need to tell him how you felt?"

She looked at me, surprised. She opened her mouth as if to say, "What do you mean? How can I have a feeling and *not* express it?" But the words never came. Her mouth just stayed open, for a long time, and then she started to cry. Great heaving sobs, her shoulders shaking in spasms.

I had no idea what was happening at first. After a while, she stopped crying, looked at me and very quietly, slowly said "I thought . . . so long . . . that I *had* to, *must* tell people what I felt. Like I'd be dishonest if I didn't . . . or I'd be repressing something . . . it never occurred to me just not to say something I felt."

She went on to say that as a child she *had* stifled the expression of many of her feelings. She *had* been repressing them, and there were many times when she *had* been dishonest about them. Then she had some therapy and began work in the human potential movement. Encounter groups, sensitivity training. In this process, she felt, she had fixed herself. She learned to stop repressing and to start expressing. And she felt liberated. For a while. Until the expression began to create more problems than the repression had. The fixing had created more things that needed fixing. That was how she came into therapy with me. Of course the therapy was more fixing.

I hadn't meant, when I asked about her expression of feelings, that she needed more fixing. But after her learning, healing, calming realization that everything did not have to be expressed, she did begin to see another fix on the horizon.

She said, "I need to learn *not* to express so much. That would be such a relief." By then I was caught in the fixing too, for I agreed with her. But in my heart was the question, "O.K., when we get that fixed, what will be next?"

There came a time in Carla's life when she began to take it easier on her self. For a long while, she saw this as the final

fixing she had always needed. But slowly she began to give up even that idea. I don't know whether it was from fatigue or realization, but she began to give up. There was no great insight. No breakthrough in therapy. But she seemed less interested in improving upon herself and more excited with the process of living. Once she said to me, "It's not really that important . . . I mean the way I live my life is not really that important if I just do the best I can . . ." And then she started to laugh. Big hearty guffaws. "It's the most important thing in the world, how I live, but it really doesn't matter! Because I'm going to do my best at living, and I couldn't do more than that anyway, could I? I mean, I've put all this effort into making my best better. That's crazy. How can I do that? Popeye said it right. Popeye has it all together. 'I am what I am and that's all that I am,' that's what Popeye says." We both collapsed in laughter. Somehow she had been able to begin giving up, and I was privileged to share her celebration. A celebration of a just-beginning restfulness.

JOE

Joe was, and is, a therapist. He'd had a lot of therapy himself, and he didn't come to me for "help" with any problems— we were simply friends sharing our thoughts and hopes. Joe has a strong sense of the religious aspect of his life, and he has a deep belief that there is a creator with whom communication can take place and in whom everyone's being is given meaning.

One day Joe told me, "My faith in God makes things tolerable. Sometimes even beautiful. It's helped me make it through lots of rough times . . . when I'm sure I would have crumbled without it. But my faith should let me rest. I mean it should be a way of knowing, underneath, that things are basi-

cally all right. I should be able to rest in that, but I can't. All
my faith does is tantalize me . . . tease me with the possibility
that somehow . . . you know, sometime, someday *maybe* I'll
be able to really relax."

He went on to describe himself as a "workaholic" who
could never quite relax as long as there was some need left to
be filled, some knowledge left to be learned. He compared his
need-to-do with hunger. "I'm stuffed. I feel stuffed . . . but
I'm still hungry. Like I've crammed myself full of doing and
responding to things and learning things and coping with
things. Like I gobble up every challenge that comes along. I'm
stuffed, but I'm still eating everything in sight. Maybe someday I'll explode."

For him, work and achievement really were like eating.
He had a feeling that maybe the next job he ate, the next task
he chewed up, the next knowledge he digested would finally
satisfy him. But it never did. And the more he ate, the more
things there were to be eaten. And he never knew which one
would finally satisfy his hunger and let him rest.

"I have a friend," he said, "who used to be just like me.
Going, going, looking for the big thing to do to fulfill himself.
He had a heart attack. I went to see him in the hospital. He
was lying there and he had this peaceful smile on his face. He
told me, 'Now I can rest, Joe. I have to. I don't have any
choice.' Now he's fully recovered and he's doing just fine. You
know, he's still doing a lot. He's still a real dynamic, energetic
guy. And he's still very successful . . . but somehow he's also
resting. Underneath. Like though he keeps doing a lot, the
doing isn't so important to him. It isn't *everything* to him. He's
not all caught up in it. He's just being himself, and he seems
very peaceful about it. Now how come *I* can't do that? While I
still have a choice? What do I have to do, stuff myself to death
before I can rest?"

As I remember it, our discussion ended there on that day.

Both of us had the feeling that we wanted to move ahead and try to come up with something he could do to ease his dilemma. But in the same moment we also knew that anything we might suggest would just be another thing to do. Another fix. Another piece of work-food for him to cram into his already bloated being. So we were silent. We sat right through the desire to say something or suggest something or even hope something. And toward the end, just before we got up to leave, we both felt a little peace. Just a hint. Too delicate, it seemed, even to express it.

On another day, Joe told me the following story. "I had to give a talk on behavior therapy to the professional association last night. You know what happened? I'd really been worried about the talk. Like how well I'd do, and whether they'd be interested in what I had to say and stuff. I stewed about it like I stew about most everything. I started to sit down and write the whole thing out, get it prepared just right, but I got to feeling just sick of it. I said 'To hell with it. I'm not going to bust my back over this one. There's too many other things to worry about. If I do O.K., I do O.K. If I don't, I don't. It's not life or death.' So I just relaxed. And I went in there with about three sentences written down and I spoke off the cuff and it was the best damned speech I ever gave. Even *I* was spellbound by it."

Even though he was speaking about something which had gone very well for him, he seemed sort of angry as he talked. As if he were feeling the injustice of all his needless struggling, angry with himself for knowing the value of letting be, even knowing how, but being able to "do" it only on rare occasions.

He continued, "It all went just beautifully. They all said how good the speech was, and afterwards I was driving home, feeling really good and peaceful. That's when it happened. Things started to change. I watched it this time and I know just what happened. I had this good, warm feeling. And then a thought came. Like 'Boy, I sure handled that well.' See, that

was a kind of pride or something. Which would be O.K. except it wasn't anything I really could take credit for. I mean, if I just relax and let be, I can't really take credit for the good stuff that happens, can I? I can feel good about it, sort of celebrate it, but I can't really take credit. Anyway, I *did* start to feel proud about it. And that set me up. I can see just exactly how it happened. The first thought was 'I did a good job.' Then the next thought, right on its heels, was 'Yeah, and I hope I can do as good a job tomorrow . . . when I have that important interview or something.' You see? And then all the peace and celebration just evaporated and I was stewing again."

Joe said he knew, intellectually, that he both functioned better and felt better when he could relax and let himself be, but for some reason these letting-be times occurred only frequently enough to tantalize him. He couldn't put it into continuing practice. Of course that's because it can't be *put* into anything. It can't willfully be *done*. But Joe tried.

One way he tried was to say "To hell with it" more often. But pretty soon he found himself getting lazy that way. It didn't work. He realized that saying "To hell with it" wasn't letting himself be. It was stifling that part of himself which needed to work and achieve. No matter what he *tried* to do, he couldn't let himself be. He was always pulling on one side of himself and pushing on another. He became very frustrated. Letting himself be had become another task to tackle. Another thing to be mastered. And this was one he couldn't pull off.

Finally he sighed and said, "I've always known I was obsessive-compulsive. I thought I'd gotten rid of most of that in therapy, but I guess I haven't. I'm just a compulsive nut." He smiled a little as he said this, but the smile was not humor. I knew what he was thinking. He was wondering if he needed more therapy. And he was feeling very tired. He began to cry then, and I did too. We both knew that therapy too would be just another thing to do. But tired as he was, Joe couldn't

shake the feeling that there was something wrong in him, and that he needed fixing, and that the fixing would take a lot of work.

I told Joe how I shared the very same kind of pain. We spoke of how millions of people share it, having such great difficulty in letting themselves fully and simply be who they are. How men and women all over the world are caught up in trying to improve themselves, make themselves different or better than they are. How the bionic man is the hero of our times, the man who was rebuilt, made better than he was.

Finally Joe said, "If I could only draw a line somewhere. If I could say, 'sure I need to do this well, and sure I have responsibilities, and sure I can improve things about myself,' but if I could just draw a line somewhere between improving things *about* myself and improving my *self*. If I could just finally say, 'I will work very hard on this and that, but here is me and me I will let be.' If I could just draw that line, I think I would be able to rest."

Joe never sought out more psychotherapy, and he didn't have a heart attack either. But he is more relaxed now. There was no great illuminating realization—no breakthrough into being. But somehow, perhaps through repeatedly seeing the crazy humor of his bind, he gradually began to relax.

The most significant realization he had was that in order to relax he had to allow himself to be tense. In other words, he recognized that he was a tense, driven person, and as long as he was trying hard to relax he was just increasing his tension. He finally found himself saying "O.K., I'm tense. That's part of who I am right now. So I'll just let me be." And almost in the very saying of this, in the simple act of giving himself permission to be who he was, he would begin to relax.

As the months passed, Joe continued to get caught up by worries and struggles and striving. But there was a difference. He'd found a sort of "place" from which to view it all, laugh

gently at it, and give it permission to be. So that underneath the tension, he was beginning to relax.

When we talked recently, Joe still described himself as being "a long way" from his ideal concept of how he should be. But he could see himself growing and healing, and he was willing to let that process take place at its own rate. He put it this way. "My body still gets tense. My mind still gets obsessed with needs to do things right. My emotions still get hooked by success and failure. But *I* am relaxed."

As he saw it, there were two levels in his being. One was the rather hectic day-to-day level of necessity and accomplishment. In this level he needed to respond to the world around him in an energetic way. There were mouths to be fed, people who needed help, a society needing his full participation, and a world he hoped would be somewhat better because of his presence. But underneath all of this, Joe felt there was another level, one he called "existential." It was a level in which he could appreciate his being. He could be anxious and driven in the day-to-day level, but still relax at the existential level. That's what he meant when he said, "Underneath it all, I can still relax."

When I asked Joe about what was happening to his religious faith, he paused for a long time. Finally he said, "It's still there. More so than ever, I guess. But I'm not *using* it so much. As I think about it, I guess I had been using it as a way of coping with stress. It was a kind of tool to help me live. That's changing now. I can't quite put my finger on it, but it's like . . . well . . . I'm not leaning on it so much. It's becoming stronger but more diffuse at the same time. I feel its presence more and more . . . but it's harder to describe what it is. Sometimes I feel as if it's sort of replacing me somewhere down deep. And that scares me a little. But at the same time I trust it. I don't know . . ."

I suppose that this is just the very beginning of healing for

Joe. It is just a tentative budding of sanity. He still clings to a solid image of a "me" somewhere behind all the attributes of himself. And he still is compartmentalizing his being into different dimensions and levels. But that's just fine. No doubt his sanity will be quite different from my perception of it. But mainly he has quit trying to fix himself. Whatever that "me" behind everything is, he's letting it be. He'll let it be what it is, even if it does turn out to be nothing at all. He's realized that whatever the "me" is, it is beyond his power to catch it and mold it. So he can relax. And as he relaxes, "me" becomes less important. Joe is healing, I think. Not healing himself. Not being healed by anybody else. Joe is simply healing.

7

PSYCHOTHERAPY

Within my earthly temple there's a crowd.
There's one of us that's humble; one that's proud.
There's one that's broken-hearted for his sins,
And one who, unrepentant, sits and grins.
There's one who loves his neighbor as himself,
And one who cares for naught but fame and pelf.
From much corroding care would I be free
If once I could determine which is Me.

Edward Sandford Martin, *Mixed*

Throughout this book I have used psychotherapy as an example of the fixing-delusion which now pervades nearly all of our civilization. Carla and Joe are examples of psychotherapists, but they are also simply people. People who like thousands of others are suffering the pain of dying into sanity.

Psychotherapy as an art and science has been suffering the very same kind of agony. It too is in the process of dying-to-be-reborn. Its very identity as the mind-fix of mankind is gasping what appears to be the last breaths of life.

The mortal wound of psychotherapy occurred when it made objects-to-be-fixed of the people it was trying to help. Exactly when this occurred is lost in history, but for generation upon generation psychotherapy has been caught in a self-im-

posed maze. Feeling that it must fix something, it has been endlessly searching to specify exactly what that thing is. In the 1800s, psychotherapy tried to fix the brain. Early in the 1900s, it tried to fix the mind. More recently it has gone after behavior, relationships and consciousness. Even the human soul. Trying to step back into the role of the priesthood, psychotherapy may have completed its life cycle. Attempting to objectify the human soul may have been psychotherapy's suicide.

An elderly man once told me, "Watch who is the hero in popular jokes and cartoons, Jerry. You'll see that they're all about who seems to hold the greatest hope for mankind. When people feel their hope is in religion, the jokes will be about priests. When psychotherapists promise salvation, *they'll* start appearing as the heros of jokes and cartoons."

Sure enough, when I was a youngster in the 1940s, many of the popular jokes were about clergymen. This was the age of the "Did you hear the one about the priest and the rabbi?" jokes. Then in the 1950s, the hero began to change. Slowly the priest disappeared from the cartoons, to be replaced by the psychoanalyst. The clerical collar was gone, to be replaced by a beard, a Viennese accent and a couch. Then people were asking each other, "Did you hear the one about the guy who walked into the psychiatrist's office?"

In the '60s, the clergy began to feel that psychotherapy was perhaps the only way to offer "real help" for people. Many of the clergy were feeling that the church wasn't accomplishing much. So they left. In droves. Some to immerse themselves in social action. Many to chase the hopeful star of psychotherapy.

As all this was happening, I was training to be a psychotherapist. When I started practice, directing a drug abuse program in a small Pennsylvania town, there were many clergypersons around who were busy learning psychotherapy. I helped teach them. But at the same time I was also learning

that my psychotherapy wasn't really helping my clients. They'd solve their neuroses. They'd fix their personality problems. But underneath all the improvement they still seemed empty.

Many of those who were addicted to drugs remained addicted, even though it appeared that their "psychological" problems were getting resolved. Those who did go on to a drug-free life, a life filled with meaning, were candid enough to let me know that their transformation had little or nothing to do with my therapy. They explained that what had made the difference for them was some kind of deep spiritual, existential experience. An experience which went far beyond their bodies and minds and somehow got them more interested in being and less interested in *how* to be. I recognized the spiritual basis of these kinds of transformations, so I asked my clergy colleagues for help in understanding it.

But by then my clergy colleagues were immersed in psychotherapy and their answers came straight from Freud. "Well, maybe it's a change in cathexis, a primary narcissistic experience, or perhaps some displacement of Oedipal feelings," they'd say. Then it began to dawn. Here I was, a psychotherapist suddenly wanting to become a priest, in the midst of priests who wanted to become psychotherapists. There's a lesson here, and it goes deeper than that the grass is always greener. The lesson is that an accurate perception of reality lies beyond *both* traditional psychotherapy *and* traditional religion.

The same kind of paradox can now be seen in the newest field of psychotherapy: transpersonal psychology. The transpersonal school has grown out of psychotherapy's chronic inability to go beyond a person's autonomous ego, to a deeper, more spiritual level. Transpersonal psychology is the up and coming thing in psychotherapy right now and it relies heavily on mysticism and Oriental thought. As a matter of fact, Ameri-

can culture as a whole has become very interested in the mystical secrets of the Orient. See who seems to offer hope for humankind now. See who's in the cartoons now. The Guru. The Yogi. The Swami. But the relationship between West and East is strikingly similar to the relationship between clergy and psychotherapists. Americans, tired of technology, scientific productivity and materialistic leisure are turning to the Orient, seeking the key to a peaceful spirit. And what is the Orient doing in return? Gobbling up the technology and scientific productivity of the West, seeking the key to materialistic leisure. Again, the lesson here is deeper than that the grass is always greener on the other side of the Pacific. *Neither* East nor West has the answer. Because the answer is not something anyone can possess.

Once more I must underscore that the defects or changes we can identify in psychotherapy are not the special *fault* of psychotherapy. They are simply reflections of culture. And not even just Western culture. It doesn't seem to be anybody's special fault. It's more like a huge cosmic joke being played on all humanity. I cannot help but understand Robert Frost's prayer that if God would forgive the many little tricks "I've played on Thee, then I'll forgive Your great big one on me."

It is indeed humorous to see psychotherapy in its recent history, chasing the elusive self across the wilderness of human experience. Trying to find it, hold it, study and fix it. In the eighteenth century, psychotherapy tried to catch the self by ordering it to bow to the commands of God's morality. ". . . the affectations of the heart . . . must spring from a chaste mind and . . . Christian piety" (from an 1801 description of Burton's *Anatomy of Melancholy*). In the nineteenth century, neurologists moved in upon the brain. The pineal body, a little nubbin at the base of the brain, was felt for generations to be "the seat of the soul."

Around the turn of the twentieth century, Sigmund Freud

pulled psychotherapy away from both religion and neurology and focused on the *functions* of the human mind. Freud saw religious activity as mere displacement of sexual and aggressive instincts and he tended to feel rather threatened by things bordering on the mystical. Thus though Freud kept a healthy respect for the field of neurology, he turned his back on religion.

It seemed to Freud that the self could be examined in terms of how it functioned and the energy it used. In the 1920s, he came up with his famous "Structural Hypothesis" of id, ego and superego. While claiming that these "Structures" were concepts and not real things, Freud and his followers nevertheless began to relate to them as if they *were* real. They spoke of something being *in* the ego, or energy coming *from* the id. In this, the Freudians simply bought the age-old human delusion of seeing the self as an object. They just gave it a different name.

The tributaries of Freud's great knowledge went on to try more clearly to define the human mind and self. Adler conceptualized the self as a unity of personality and stated that infants start from a position of inferiority and strive for superiority and "self-realization." Rank emphasized the importance of the human will in separating self from other. Sullivan saw the self as a "system," a technique for avoiding anxiety. Horney spoke of a triple concept of self, including "actual" self, "real" self, and "idealized" self. Assagioli spoke of a personal self and a higher self. People started distinguishing between the self with the little "s" and the Self with the capital "S." Phrases like "self-realization," "self-actualization" and "self-awareness" became very popular. The idea sprang forth that one could be separated and alienated from one's self. (Without great consideration of who it is that is alienated.) And it was assumed that one should look somewhere to find one's self. (Without great consideration of who it is that is looking.)

There were real selves and false selves, good selves and bad selves, unfulfilled selves and completed selves, solid selves and diffuse selves.

In the midst of this gaggle of selves, behavior therapists labeled the self as a repertoire of behaviors and then gently set the whole idea aside. They should be commended for this, for of all the schools of psychotherapy, the behaviorists are perhaps the least likely to try to meddle with one's soul. The existentialists also set the idea of self aside, in the name of phenomenology. No preconceived ideas. They did go ahead and try to meddle with it but at least they admitted having no way of knowing what it was they were meddling with. Scanning the pages of twentieth century psychotherapy, one gets the impression that there are little selves running all over the place. Yet each remains incredibly elusive. Nowhere has the self really been found.

There is great value in all this work on self. It is a probing into delusion and it carries the merit of negative findings in research. One can learn as much from what is *not* found in a scientific investigation as from what *is* discovered. What has not been found is the self.

Perhaps there are bodies, senses, behaviors, thoughts, feelings, memories and hopes which can be willfully modified. But it looks as if psychotherapy will not find a self to modify. If a self exists, it is lying somewhere beyond our touch, unknown, incomprehensible, indefinable. Perhaps it is as ineffable as God, as inexplicable as the cosmos. And if it is to be fixed in any sense, perhaps it will have to be God or the cosmos that will do the fixing.

One might have hoped that this realization was what accounted for the new transpersonal school of psychotherapy. But I fear this may not be the case. Some of the giants of psychotherapy, often toward the ends of their careers, have alluded to the need to go beyond objectivity and self-fixing. Jung

was especially notable in this and many transpersonalists try hard to follow in Jung's footsteps. But all too much of transpersonal psychology reeks of being simply another wave of delusion. Rather than to fix brain or mind or even self, much of transpersonal psychology wants to fix consciousness. Again, I fear these are simply new names and new techniques for the same old insanity.

I remember the day I became a transpersonal psychotherapist. I was approached by a young psychologist who had heard of my interest in meditation, spiritual awareness and such. He asked me to speak at a symposium as a representative of "my field" of transpersonal psychology. This struck me as interesting and a bit reassuring. There had been a time when I was "Freudian" and then I was "eclectic" for a while and then "sort of an existentialist." But after my experience with trying to treat drug-addicted people, I hadn't been at all certain what I was. So for a while I became a transpersonalist. Problems began immediately. I was expected to present transpersonal ways of fixing people's difficulties. To lay out the great transpersonal smorgasbord of meditation, psychedelics, biofeedback, Eastern mysticism and assorted condiments, each with its specific goals and techniques.

I should have known better, but the temptation was too great. I should have realized that in defining myself as *anything* I could not help but objectify myself, the people with whom I worked and the ways in which we worked together. There is a seductive security in identity-making, just as there is security in any delusion. But there is also despair. I am no longer a transpersonalist. One sometimes wonders how many identities will have to die.

Psychotherapy now faces the very same dilemma that every individual human being has faced throughout history. It must die to be reborn. It must lose itself in order to find itself. It must be willing to sacrifice its entire identity if it is to follow

the path toward sanity. It must be willing, as must each person, to sacrifice power, self-definition, self-manipulation, and self-determination. Psychotherapy must sacrifice any idea that it does healing. And since this is its basic identity, psychotherapy, as we know it, will die.

The time seems right for this death and resurrection, but it might not come to pass quite yet. It may well be that the possibilities which transpersonal psychology has to offer will be turned toward greater and greater self-power. To more fixing. This has already happened in many spheres. How many people use meditation as a way of increasing their private efficiency and success? How many seek contact with other planes of consciousness in order to have some experience or develop some ability which will make them special? How many therapists use meditation, biofeedback or psychedelic drugs to fix, improve upon or otherwise "alter" the consciousness of their clients?

All these things are happening. It is to be expected. But what is unknown is whether that is *all* that will happen. Whether the wealth of mysticism will *only* be turned to the self-fix. Or whether at some point psychotherapy will finally give up. Again, the situation of psychotherapy is the same as yours and mine. It is possible that giving up will happen. Some way, sometime and perhaps soon, it just may happen.

8

TRUE GROWTH
AND
HEALING

Nothing prevents our being natural
so much as the desire to appear so.

Francois, Duc de la Rochefoucauld

If psychotherapy as fixing does die, perhaps the rebirth of
sanity will reflect a realization of what true growth and healing
really are. Delusion leads one to assume that growth is building and that healing is fixing, but what really is the nature of
growth and healing?

It will be difficult to specify this, for to do so will tend to
make objects of growth and healing, and they are not objects.
It may also make growth and healing appear as things-to-be-
achieved, and they are not. Still it is perhaps worthwhile to try
to describe some of the aspects of true growth and healing. It
might help us to recognize them, and perhaps appreciate
them, when they occur.

Basically true growth and healing are neither events nor
interventions. They are processes. Processes that happen. Look
at growth first.

GROWTH

True growth is a process which one allows to happen rather

than causes to happen. A seed grows into a plant because it is its nature to do so, not because you or I *do* it. If a seed finds itself in rich earth, with reasonable quantities of water and sunlight, growth will happen. If we sprinkle the ground with fertilizer, water it regularly and keep pests away, we become involved in the growth process, and growth may be stronger and richer. We are participating in the growth, but we are still not doing it.

But if we were to be displeased with the speed of growth, and if we were to dig up the seed, pry it apart and attempt to pull the young sprout forth before its time, we shall have gone too far. In trying hard to do the growing, we can actually interfere with the process. Then perhaps the seed will die.

In tending and nurturing a flower, we may be participating harmoniously with the rest of nature in the flower's growth. But if we try to pull the petals apart, we overstep. In the one way, we are participating in the process of growth. In the other, we are trying to *make* something. It is in this trying to *make* that one begins to feel separate. The thing being made becomes an object, different and distanced from the maker. Then perhaps the maker will begin to feel unnatural.

More than what one does, it is one's basic attitude about the doing which determines what is natural and what is not. If the attitude in planting and nurturing a flower is such that one *feels* participation in the natural flow of things, then one does not add to the delusion of separateness. But if one truly feels that he or she is actually *doing* the growing of the plant, even if one never touches it, a sense of separation will occur. Many of us who love to have plants around, who enjoy being with the green things, still use phrases like, "I am growing tulips in the front yard." There is no harm meant in this, but the words do reflect that subtle separation-sense which creeps in repeatedly, reflecting that one is more a manager than a participant.

Children are growing "things" too, and parents are, so to speak, the gardeners. What is our attitude toward the growth

of our children? We cannot deny that again and again we feel that we are growing them at best, building them at worst. "I tried to raise my children the best way I could." I tried to raise. As was the case with plants, this attitude is bound to make objects of the children, and to keep us separate from them.

It is quite possible to move into an attitude of participation in growth, but such a transformation requires something which feels like sacrifice. One of course would sacrifice the feeling of being in control of things. There is some threat in this, but it really doesn't go too deep. A careful, honest scrutiny of the situation reveals that one really isn't very much in control of things anyway. So all that is sacrificed here is a wistful delusion.

Perhaps a greater sacrifice is that one cannot take credit for the growing. One can marvel, celebrate, enjoy, revere and honor the growing of plants and children, but one cannot take credit for doing it. Awesome, joyful participation is a part of growing. But pride really doesn't have a place.

There is a flip side to this question of pride, which requires an even deeper sacrifice. If one cannot take ultimate credit for the growing process, one also cannot assume ultimate blame if the process "fails" in one way or another. This point is easily misunderstood, but it must remain.

Parents and gardeners generally do the best they can at any given point. If they do their best at participating in growth, credit and blame are meaningless. If the child or the plant should wither in one way or another, there is room for sadness and grief, but not for blame. The only time when personal guilt and blame are justified is when through conscious, malicious, manipulative intent, one has done one's worst instead of one's best. Within the attitude of *doing* the growing or *killing* the growing, there is plenty of room for credit and blame. But in the attitude of participation, both must be sacrificed.

There is no doubt that this is a very real sacrifice. Feeling somehow as if one *must* be motivated by desire for credit or fear of blame, what is to be expected if one were suddenly to be liberated from both? The spaciousness of this possibility is awesome.

Perception of true growth means to realize that one is not doing the growth. To fully recognize that the parent is not inside the child, causing cells to multiply, blood to circulate or vitamins to be digested. To perceive that neither parent nor child is doing that. But that it is simply, wonderfully happening.

In delusion, the verb "to grow" is transitive. It has a subject and an object. "I grow you." In sanity, "to grow" is intransitive. One can only say "You are growing." But perhaps even this is inaccurate. Perhaps "growing" is really almost a noun. "Growing is happening."

HEALING

All that has been said of growing can be said of healing. Too often one thinks of the physician or psychotherapist as "one who heals," but *nobody ever heals anybody else.* No one person ever heals another. Nor does any one person heal himself or herself. Like growth, healing is a natural process, as much as ongoing part of us as the beating of our hearts.

If you cut your skin, you bleed for a while, and then the blood clots. *Who* or *what does* that? A scab forms and if you don't pick at it too much, the cells of your skin multiply, rejoining, covering the broken spot. Who or what does that? At this level, the healing process is almost identical to the growth process; a multiplication and refinement of cells and function. It happens. You don't do it; at least not with any will. And most decidedly the doctor does not do it. As with growth, one can only say "Healing is happening." No subject. No object.

This is true for all healing, whether physical or psychological. If I have a bad cut, the doctor will bring the skin edges together with stitches. Hopefully the doctor will do his or her best, and I will be grateful. But this is not healing. Any more than sprinkling fertilizer on plants or giving vitamins to children is growing. What the doctor does is bring the skin back into a more natural state, line it up, cleanse it and put on a bandage; all so that healing *can occur* with a minimum of pain and disfigurement. If I break a bone, the doctor will set it straight and put it in a cast. But this is not healing. It is helping healing, hopefully participating in healing, but it *is* not healing. It is making things more natural and giving the bone a rest so that the healing process can occur more fully.

Whatever the illness or injury, the role of the physician is relegated to three primary activities:

1. To bring the diseased or injured part back into a more natural state.
2. To cleanse and purify.
3. To provide rest.

All that these procedures do is make the setting more convient for the natural healing process to take place. With infections, the role of antibiotics is to purify and cleanse. The same is true of surgery for appendicitis.

Without the physician, sometimes healing will not occur. Sometimes the injury or illness is too great, and death happens whether or not the physician is present. But sometimes the presence of the physician makes the difference between life and death. Even so, this does not mean that the physician does the healing. The physician simply plays a part, just as my white blood cells play a part in fighting infection. Sometimes the part of the physician is necessary to the healing process. But without the rest of the healing process, the physician could do nothing but autopsies.

It is not too difficult to realize the natural healing process when one is talking about the body. But sometimes the natural healing process is more difficult to see functioning in the human mind. Yet every psychotherapist has seen it, time and time again. When psychotherapy *is* helpful in terms of a specific psychological problem, it is because therapy has presented a clearer vision of reality, which constitutes "a bringing of the diseased part into a more natural state." And because therapy has seen the eradication of irrational fears, obsessions and worries, which amounts to *purification and cleansing*. And it has encouraged self-acceptance and minimized anxiety, thus *giving rest*. But these factors alone mean nothing. There is something else that happens in a troubled mind. Something which results in integration, renewed functioning, and a wholesome, meaningful approach to life. That something has not been "done" by either therapist or client. That something is healing.

Just as there is a need for someone to plough the field or plant the seed or parent the child or suture the cut, there is often a need for someone to participate in the healing process of the mind. Someone to help foster the conditions of naturalness, cleanliness and rest, so that healing can occur more fully. But in the same regard, just as alienation is compounded by the gardener's feeling that he or she is doing the growing, or the parent the raising, or the physician the healing, it perpetuates insanity to feel that either psychotherapist or client is doing the healing of the mind. And it is blatant insanity to feel that either is *fixing* the mind.

There is nothing radical about this idea. Physicians and psychotherapists, off duty and over cocktails, would be the first to admit that all they really do is plough the ground for healing. But in the office, or in the operating room, or in the psychiatric ward, it all seems to change. Then, in the midst of all the *doing*, both therapist and "patient" dive back into the delusion that one is to be fixed and the other is the fixer. All too often. They go crazy together.

The dichotomy between an attitude of participation in healing and an attitude of *doing* the healing occurs everywhere. It is not confined to the doctor's office. One can see it clearly in the way one approaches one's own mind. If some psychological problem occurs, some fear or ambivalence or worry, one naturally does one's best with it. Usually this involves some attempt to bring things back to normal, to cleanse, and to rest. But often people don't stop at that. They don't allow the natural healing to occur. They keep picking at the emotional scab, rewrapping the psychological bandage, reopening the mental wound. Checking to see if it's doing all right. Applying this technique or that method. Picking at it again and again. All the time feeling that they are trying to heal themselves.

With this kind of picking at one's mind, healing may find it difficult to happen. The attempts to make things more natural wind up making things more contrived and artificial. The attempts to cleanse wind up adding more and more contaminants. And the attempts to give rest wind up making greater and greater demands. I laugh at myself in this repeatedly. "Don't bother me," I say to my family. "I've had a rough day and I'm trying to rest." Trying very hard to rest. Working at it, even.

But if one simply did one's best, did what one could do to respond to a problem, and then allowed room for healing— gave space and light and air for healing to happen—that's when healing *can* happen. When it's allowed. This seems to require an element of trust. That with one's fingers *out* of the wound, resting instead of meddling, healing just might happen. Or it requires despair. Realizing that no amount of additional meddling will make the healing any better anyway, so that one might as well rest. Either trust or despair is necessary. And either one will permit the healing to happen.

9

THE LESSONS
OF
SANITY

And starting fresh as from a second birth,
Man in the sunshine of the world's new spring
Shall walk transparant like some holy thing!

Thomas Moore

If the delusion of separation and thingness and fixing dies, and
if sanity is finally allowed to be free, what will sanity tell us
about growing and healing and living?

Being far from sane myself, it is presumptuous of me to
predict. But like most psychotherapists, I do have something to
say about it.

It would be better to attend to the words of those who are
truly sane. Those whose being prompted the great religions of
the world, for example, have clearly spoken a truth that rever-
berates in thousands of hearts. But of course they have also
been misunderstood.

In the midst of delusion, it is difficult to discern the
whereabouts of those who speak the truth. And once found, it
is hard to know whether we understand them. To whom
should one listen? And in what ways should one try to understand?

Knowing all too well the inadequacy of intellect in "figuring out" the truth, perhaps it would be best to listen with

the heart as well as with the mind. To trust, or at least begin to trust, that what is true will resonate with the unborn sanity within us and that what is false will not. In the last analysis, one has no other test of truth anyway. There really is no other choice.

It is in this way that I have compiled the material which follows. Listening to teachers and looking into quietness, these ideas have resonated with me. Keeping in mind that I claim no special authority here, it would be well for you to ask your own intuition about these ideas. If they fail to "connect" with you, let them pass. If they do resonate with your own deep sense of truth, simply listen to the harmony. They imply no special action. *Nothing needs to be done about them.*

I. ATTITUDE TOWARD MIND

People characteristically think of mind as a thing. Or in more sophisticated terms, a process. Sanity of course does not see mind as a thing. But it goes on to ask if mind is a process, who is having that process and what is being processed? Perhaps the mind is like the seasons of the year, changing, having impact, but never to be caught or frozen into something solid. One can experience autumn, be in the midst of it, sense it. But one can not hold it; not without robbing it of its life. Mind is the same way. It is not possible to catch a thought and hold it.

So mind cannot fully be understood by objective analysis. One cannot deduce the basic function of mind or describe "its" nature. Mind cannot be figured out. But this does not mean one cannot know and understand mind fully and deeply. It is possible to see mind happening, closely, immediately. Thoughts can be seen arising in consciousness, taking form and passing on. Emotions can be seen erupting like sudden rainstorms, building with great energy and ending in absolute

stillness. But this way of knowing mind is not deductive or analytical. It is very intimate and direct. One can learn something *about* a rainstorm by studying meteorology. But to fully know, one must feel the rain upon one's face.

When we *do* learn something about the mind, we always want to *use* that learning. To put the knowledge to good use. As if value lay only in use. Who is it that wants to use this knowledge, and for what ends? Perhaps knowledge is like fertilizer, heaped about the roots of a tree. Must one then try to push the fertilizer into the roots? Pull it up through the cells of the trunk? Drive it into the leaves and instruct it to turn green?

Sometimes it is obvious that the agony within one's mind is caused by one's own hands. That suffering and complexity are created by the presence of one's own fingers, pulling and pushing, directing and redirecting, picking and manipulating. Even realizing this, one tends to think that *more* such activity will bring peace. It is helpful to remember that hands can stroke gently in order to appreciate texture. And that they can spread wide in awe. And that they can fold quietly in reverence. Or open in love.

You probably wish to love your mind. You can, but remember that loving something does not mean making it the way you want it to be. Remember that loving something means allowing it to fully, freely be exactly what it is.

You also probably wish to trust your mind. You can, if you would give it a chance to be trusted. Resting for a moment in one's attempts to *make* the mind trustworthy, one will see the mind *becoming* trustworthy. This need not be accepted on faith. To so do would require that one kill one's fears, and that of course would be simply more manipulation. But slowly, if the mind is given a chance now and then, quietly, you may *discover* that it can be trusted.

Rather than learning how to make mind trustworthy, perhaps we need to learn how to leave our minds alone. For it is

only then that we will discover how reliable they truly are.

II. *CONSCIOUSNESS*

Most people, most of the time, are concerned with the *contents* of consciousness. Perhaps it is more valuable to watch consciousness itself. Preoccupied with the sounds one hears, perhaps one misses the silence from which they come. Watching clouds, does one neglect the sky?

We tend to feel consciousness is a creation of the brain, but where is it when one sleeps or dreams? And we tend to feel that consciousness is our possession. Sanity asks us to consider, at least for a moment, that we may be the possessions of consciousness.

There is a habitual assumption that one must do something about every thing that enters consciousness. That one must somehow manage it all. And this takes tremendous energy, causing us to block many things out of awareness so that a few things can be managed well. Sanity asks why this must be so. Why does one feel one must judge every stimulus, evaluate each sensation, respond with desire or fear to every idea, or at barest minimum, label what one sees? To be able to do these things is wonderful. But to *have* to do them is slavery.

Everyone has experienced the indescribable beauty of clearly seeing a flower and never once calling it "flower." Sanity simply asks that this be remembered.

III. *PAYING ATTENTION*

Having to label, judge and respond to everything which enters consciousness, one comes to feel one can be aware of

only a few things at once. What do we do with the rest? We shut out millions upon millions of stimuli, saving only those which seem "important." We erect barriers against perception, barriers that take a lot of work to keep up.

The barrier against internal stimuli is called "repression." The barrier against external stimuli is called "paying attention." Paying attention means to block out many things so that one or two can be dealt with. But paying attention makes nothing more clear. It simply shuts out what one feels is "irrelevant." Paying attention is what keeps you from hearing that sound in the background, and from feeling the book in your hands as you read. Paying attention takes much effort, and one becomes tired afterwards.

Sanity questions whether paying attention to something is always necessary. It hints that it is possible to relax the barriers against perception, allowing countless things to come fully into awareness, and not have to pay attention to any one. And that it is also possible to be acutely aware of one thing without shutting anything else out. And even that it is possible to pay absolute attention to nothing at all. Whether one *should* do this or not is something which can be learned from experience and exploration. But that one *can* do it is something one should know.

IV. *BEING AWARE*

Immediate awareness is a gift, the purpose of which is to see living. But most of the time we want awareness to be a tool. Becoming immediately aware of living, we *use* that awareness to evaluate the living. To think *about* living. And as soon as this happens, awareness is gone again. Kidnapped. Immediate awareness has assumed the quality of a judging

parent, asking "Should I be doing this?" or "How well am I doing this?" and in the process awareness becomes uncomfortable.

So, much of the time, one goes about living unaware. Eyes blinded to the wonder of the immediate moment, consciousness glued to a task or lost in fantasy. As if one feels it is more comfortable to be a robot than a harassed little child.

Sanity proclaims that immediate awareness is simply a state of appreciation. One need do *nothing, nothing at all* with it. It is a gift, freely given. Immediate awareness is the clear clean air without which healing and growth are stunted. The question is whether one can receive this gift as freely and gently as it is given. Whether one can allow space for one's being to breathe.

V. *DESIRE*

Most of the time we assume we are motivated by desire. That without being driven by desire or repulsion we would cease to act. And so we hold desire and fear, clinging to them as if they were our very source of energy. But perhaps one would not stagnate without them. Perhaps motivation could come from beyond them. From the simple situation at hand.

You are standing on a corner with your child. He steps into the street and you quickly pull him back. Must it be said that you did this because you desired to keep him alive, or because you feared for his safety? Is it not possible that you pulled him back because he stepped into the street?

Consider that desire and fear might simply be the salt and pepper of life. Serving to help you savor your being. That rather than determining behavior, they simply give it color and interest.

One may try to overcome desire. And yet one knows that

fighting desire makes it stronger than before. Waging war against it makes it an enemy. Is it not possible for there to be space between desire and behavior, killing neither, appreciating both?

VI. *NEUROSIS*

One assumes that neurosis is a defective way of living. Inexorable habits, insurmountable fears, undying thoughts and feelings. A burden weighing down the shoulders of one's life. And so we struggle with the pieces of neurosis. Experiencing a neurotic fear, one tries to work it through, understand it, express it, suppress it, counteract it or bypass it. All of which are designed to get rid of it.

But everything one does to get rid of neurosis makes it seem more real. More important. More like something to be rid of. And if a piece of it is destroyed, something else inevitably comes to take its place.

Perhaps one must recognize that there is no way out. It is possible to adjust neurosis, restructure it, make it more socially acceptable and temporarily more comfortable, but there is no way out. For in trying to get out, one continues to make credible that from which one is fleeing. It cannot be done. In one blink of the eyes another reality can be seen, the freely being immediate present, where neither self nor neurosis continues to be defined, but one cannot "get there."

But perhaps healing could be allowed. Treating your self with gentleness, accepting fully, seeing clearly, being fully as you are, *being* as neurotic as you are, healing might happen. Healing occurs when awareness is open and when acceptance is total. But the acceptance must be so complete that it even includes love for all one's attempts to fix one's self.

VII. *PSYCHOSIS*

There is an assumption that psychosis comes when one goes beyond one's self. That the worst insanity arises when ego crumbles and dissolves. And therefore we tend to uphold the worth of ego strength, fortifying and bolstering it until self determines all.

But consider that psychosis may be the result of struggling to *regain* ego. That the symptoms of insanity are the clutching fingers of a mind trying to regain control, unwilling or unable to give up.

If one becomes psychotic, perhaps it is because one has touched the face of God and could not relinquish the importance of self. Considering this, one cannot help but find compassion.

VIII. *ACCEPTANCE*

Always there is a desire to accept some things and reject others. Who is making this choice, and with what wisdom? Does one accept what feels good and reject what does not? And where does the acceptance come from? Figuring out the strategies of acceptance, one walks into a jungle in which the paths branch and branch until irrevocable blindness is finally realized.

Acceptance of this or of that is jungle exploration, and beautiful as such. But as a way out of the jungle it does not work. If you feel *you* must choose to accept or not to accept, then realize that you might choose to accept *everything*. Total, complete acceptance is a very real possibility. It involves accepting beauty and ugliness. And accepting responsibility and laziness, both, completely. It even means accepting one's own inability to accept.

Perhaps this sounds like nothing. Like nothing happening at all. But in accepting everything, one cannot help but let one's self be. What is the quality of *this* kind of nothing?

IX. *RESPONSIBILITY*

Behavior needs to be responsible. But who is responsible *for* that behavior? If *you* choose between this and that, then *you* are responsible. To conceive that there may be no substantial "you" behind behavior is no excuse for avoiding responsibility. For conception and realization are not the same. As long as one still believes in one's sense of self, one is responsible.

It is only when self-importance truly ceases that all behavior springs with inherent responsibility from the siuation at hand, and yet there is no one there being responsible. This may be absolutely true, but it is at the same time a pipe dream. Can two realities be perceived at once? Perhaps it is not so important, because the fact is that as long as one *does* feel responsible, one is.

Thus it is possible to affirm responsibility, and even self-determination. But remember that responsibility is the road which travels between guilt and pride. And that guilt and pride both serve the sense of self. Remember that responsibility is the bridge between credit and blame. Which are also servants of one's image of one's self.

To strive for pride and credit at the expense of guilt and blame is both human and delightful. But to rail against the pain one feels in this struggle is but a temper tantrum. Pride cannot be without guilt, nor credit without blame. Just as happiness cannot be without sadness. Biting into the completeness of this life, appreciating its flavor, one can live richly. But always both sides must be tasted equally.

And if one side is sacrificed, so must the other be. To go

beyond the polarities of responsibility, all must be affirmed equally, or all must be denied equally. Transcendence does not play favorites. Neither is transcendence something which can be done, for any attempt to *do* transcendence must come from desire for happiness or for release from pain. Recognizing this, it is possible to rest *in* responsibility, not *from* it.

X. *LOVE*

We think of loving someone. As if love were something one could create, give or receive. Often we even feel that love is something one "should" do. And then one may begin to wonder if one is capable of loving.

Who does the loving? Consider that loving cannot be "done" by anyone. When love is recognized, it is already there. Happening. It can be discovered, its presence can be recognized, but it can never be manufactured. And though love may be buried from awareness, it cannot be killed. So there really is no question as to whether one is capable of loving. The only question is whether one is capable of seeing the love which is already there.

We tend to think of love as attachment, binding, bonding and committing. But love is only free. Love accepts and allows totally. Because there is oneness in love, there is no giving and no taking. There is not even relationship. What does it really mean to *be in* love? Not that I have love for you, but that you and I are *in* love? We exist, as one, immersed in love, more deeply than in the air we breathe.

And this "self" which creeps in upon freely being time and time again. Can it be loved? It certainly need not be hated. Only love will free it to be what it will be, while hatred can but force it into more and more rigid, frozen postures. Discover then, the love that is there for your self and for your predicament.

Searching beneath anxiety, one will find fear. And beneath fear hurt will be discovered. Beneath the hurt will be guilt. Beneath the guilt lie rage and hatred. But do not stop with this, for beneath the rage lies frustrated desire. Finally, beneath and beyond desire, is love. In every feeling, look deeply. Explore without ceasing. At bottom, love is. Realizing this, need one do anything about the anxiety one feels?

XI. WORK

Work is generally thought of as pushing against something. Overcoming a resistance. Force. And we assume that something not requiring work is of little value. But where is the work of being alive? Does life have greater value if one works at living? Or does perhaps work have value because one *is* living?

Perhaps true work involves overcoming no resistances, but rather learning to relax in such a way that no resistances exist. Lifting a brick to build a wall, you see your hand moving the brick. But in one blink of the eyes, you can see hand and brick moving together.

The difference between work and play is only a matter of attitude. Work, fully done, is play. When the body works, it is dancing. When the mind works, it is dreaming. Appreciating the joys and sadnesses of both, one moves within the process of life.

XII. SUFFERING

One nearly always seeks to avoid pain. And one nearly always struggles with pain when it comes. Must one manage one's self away from pain? If your hand touches a flame, must

you pull it away? Or does your hand simply pull away, because of the pain?

It is helpful to look at the difference between pain and suffering. Pain is a stimulus, like cold or green. There will be a response. But suffering is you or I struggling against our pain. Pain can exist freely, without suffering, as when you pinch your skin or stretch very hard before relaxing.

Suffering is the effort one puts against one's pain, beyond response, beyond healing. Suffering is what one heaps on top of pain, the second-guessing of pain, the raging against what is, the refusal to accept what is happening.

Consider that one can allow one's pain to be cared for, through one's own natural responses, without any special management. Then where there was suffering is only space.

XIII. *LIVING*

We feel we have life right now, but really life has us for this moment. Therefore there is no need to try to live. Even in the extremities of crisis, there is no need for any special attempt to live. For living, in and of itself, will struggle to go on.

One can choose to live or die, but again one must ask who does the choosing. One can choose this again and again, and perhaps this could make one feel powerful. But the role of choice in life most deeply is simply to determine whether one will be *aware* of living or not. Whether one goes through the motions of living like a sleepwalker, or whether one awakens to the process now. Too often in searching for a richer life, a fuller life, one's eyes become blinded to the immediate wonder of the life that is. Sometimes we pray, "If I should die before I wake . . ." But perhaps a deeper prayer would be "If I should wake before I die . . ."

If one can discover love for one's search for a better

life, without attempting to destroy it, and if one can find compassion for the striving, then the beauty of this very moment will not be missed.

We often feel that "To be or not to be" is the question.

"To be or to try to be," that is more the question.

10

FREELY
BEING
RESPONSIBLE

I am the captain of my soul;
 I rule it with stern joy;
And yet I think I had more fun
 When I was a cabin boy.

Keith Preston, *An Awful Responsibility*

Sanity, at least as I have pictured it, seems to be telling us to allow ourselves to be what we are, fully, dynamically and without any great extra meddling. To simply, freely be. It is saying that peace and fullness lie in giving up the struggle to master one's self.

This is a very tantalizing possibility. But it is also easily misunderstood and abused. Words like acceptance, allowing, giving up and letting be can encourage passivity and irresponsibility. Sometimes it seems very difficult to walk the line between arrogant self-responsibility and passive lethargy. I think the answer is to be found by stepping into a different dimension of self-perception. Getting back away from the laziness-arrogance polarity and seeing more of the totality of any given situation. Then, moving *into* the situation, what needs to be done will become clear. And the complexities of figuring out what is responsible and what is not become irrelevant. One winds up simply doing what needs to be done.

It may be of help to look at the story of one man's struggle with responsibility and freely being. This man happens to have been a drug addict. If this should make it a bit difficult for you to identify with him, it might be valuable for you to consider your own addictions. Everyone has addictions. Any "bad" habit which we find ourselves wanting to "overcome" is an addiction. Whether it is to drugs, alcohol, food, tobacco, sex, television, sports, self-importance, power or work, the basic quality is the same. One does something because it makes one feel good now. Later on there may be a price to pay, but now it feels good. And the more we do it, the more desire there is to do it again. As with popcorn or potato chips, it's hard to stop at just one. An understanding of one's own addictions makes it a bit easier to understand those of people who are labeled as "junkies" or "alcoholics."

When I first met John he was twenty-three years old and addicted to heroin. He was short, skinny and pale, but his eyes were deep and lively. He came to the clinic for "help" with his drug problem, but his motivation was not the most pure. Like many other clients of the clinic he came under duress. He'd been apprehended in an attempt to steal money from the office of the construction company where he worked, and the court had given him the choice of getting help or going to jail.

In our first interview it was obvious that John was intelligent, but his intelligence had been of little help to him. Coming from a lower-middle-class family, with alcoholic parents who separated when he was very young, he had never quite been able to find a direction in life. It had seemed to him that his school teachers, his bosses on the job, and the public authorities were all harassing him rather than helping, and he had essentially given up on life. At least that's the way he described it.

"Every time I'd get some idea about doing something constructive with my life, I'd get shot down. I wanted to be a

musician, but the school didn't have music lessons. I tried to write, but the teachers always gave me Ds and Fs because of my bad grammar. They never saw what I was trying to say. There was nobody at home I could talk to—Mom was always tired trying to take care of us five kids. So anyway, I started smoking some dope with friends and it made me feel O.K. You know . . . like there wasn't anything to worry about. Then I just started doing harder drugs. I still want to make something of myself, but now I'm addicted and I gotta get some help."

Most psychotherapists would see, from these few words, that John is immature, that he has some problems with authority figures, and that he tends to blame others for his problems rather than taking responsibility for himself. Also that he's probably more interested in getting out of trouble than in really bettering himself. All these insights would be essentially true, but there's another dimension which has to be investigated. I asked John how he felt about himself as a person in this world, what he thought about the meaning of life.

"It's a crummy world, and there's no sense fighting it. I just gotta get along the best I can. If I could get some real big money, like those dudes in Washington [politicians] I'd be as good as anybody. But they keep you down. I'm as good as the next guy, but I never had a chance."

I asked about any religious feelings he had.

"I used to go to church with my mother. She used to make us go. I couldn't stand it. All them hypocrites acting holier-than-thou, and then going out and knifing people in the back to get money. They talk about love and they run around on their wives. They look down on junkies like me while they're drinking their martinis. It makes me want to barf."

At the beginning of the interview John had been passive, uninvolved, apathetic. But now he was showing some steam. He really seemed angry. I asked him about God.

"You're gonna think this is crazy, but LSD is God. God's

supposed to make you feel all right in this world. He's supposed to love you, right? Well the only time I feel at home in this world is when I'm tripping on acid. That's God. And don't try to lay anything on me about getting high on God without drugs. I've heard that before and it's a lot of bull. Those Jesus freaks are worse than junkies. They're cop-outs just as much as drugs. Only they think they're better than anyone else."

"What are they copping out from?" I asked.

"You know, when they want something they sit around and pray for it. Me, I go out and get it. And when they got problems they smile and say, 'God will take care of it.' Me, I shoot up some good heroin and any problems I got are taken care of."

"Until you come down."

"Right. But they're no better'n me. They live in a fantasy world. I live in a drug world. It's no different. They take their hassles to God. I take mine to dope. We're all copping out."

"What wouldn't be a cop-out?"

"To go right in and handle the problems you got. Get busy and do something about 'em. Get a job, get married, raise a family, do your thing. That's why I wanna get off this dope. I want to get straight, make some money and start a life for myself. I'm sick and tired of copping out."

Thus far, John's feelings have been about the same as thousands of other drug-addicted persons who walk into clinics for help. And the course he followed for the next couple of months was also typical. There was an attempt to kick the narcotic habit, but he couldn't do it. He was drug free for several days, but then he got into an argument with his boss and walked off the job, bought some heroin and started "shooting up" again.

"I couldn't make it. You can't kick dope this way. I want to get on the methadone program."

At first, John blamed his getting back on drugs to the se-

verity of his craving. But when I pressed him about it he said he really felt O.K. without the drugs, until he got into the fight with his boss. Then he started feeling an old feeling.

"It's like you can't win. Every time things start to go right there's someone around to hassle you. My boss wouldn't trust me with the keys to the office. He said he was afraid I'd steal something. He said I should be grateful that he took me back on the job at all, after I stole from him the first time. I guess I can understand his not trusting me, but how you going to get anywhere if nobody gives you a chance? Man, I still want to get out there and do good, but it seems like there's no hope."

John went into a second phase of his "treatment." He took the drug methadone which stopped his physical craving for dope, and the therapy that went along with the methadone was geared toward helping him realize that he was responsible for himself. He agreed that he was responsible for himself. He said he knew that all along. And he'd show everyone how responsible he was if he were just given the chance.

The "chance" came when he got a promotion on the job after several months of good work. He said he was making enough money to get married. He'd already bought a car and had enough for a deposit on an apartment. He was very bright and hopeful. The entire clinic celebrated his marriage. His wife was very young but very much in love with him. Two weeks later she ran off with another man.

John immediately left his job, left the clinic, and went back to street drugs. He was admitted to the hospital a few weeks later after an overdose of heroin.

"O.K., you don't have to tell me," he said, "I did it myself. I should have handled it differently. I'm responsible for getting back on drugs. I'm just too weak. I copped out again."

After John got out of the hospital and back into the clinic program, we started talking more about his sense of responsibility. It rapidly became clear that though his behavior and

words were often irresponsible, he had always felt *very* responsible. *I* want this and *I'm* going to get it. Those guys are
always hassling me so *I'm* going to quit trying. Even in blaming others for his own failures, he still felt responsible *for letting "them" win.* He felt weak and impotent, and to feel weak
and impotent is to feel very responsible. He told me of a fantasy which occurred in various forms: in dreams, daydreams,
and under LSD.

"I'm walking down this city street and I'm very small.
About the size of a pea. All the people are huge. The buildings
are mammoth. I'm scared by my smallness. Weak. Helpless.
But I have this magic phrase I say. 'Snow go, snow go, snow
go.' And then it starts to snow, and as it snows on me I get bigger and bigger, like a giant snowman, and everybody gets
scared of me."

In street jargon, heroin is often called "snow." But the importance of this fantasy is deeper than the idea that heroin
compensates for feelings of inferiority. The important thing is
that he wants to be big and powerful, and he *does* something
to make this happen. He wants to loom over other people
rather than have them loom over him, and he *makes* it happen.
He chants his magic words and it begins to snow and he gets
big. The important thing is that he did it. He's responsible for
it.

At another time he described his feelings when he'd insert
a needle into a vein to inject heroin. He really liked doing that.
"I don't know why, it just feels good." He, like many other
people addicted to narcotics, said, "I could get high off of just
shooting up, even if it were water." The good feeling here is
that *he is doing something to himself* which will have a powerful impact. A sense of effectiveness upon himself. A sense of
responsibility. *I* did it. *I'm* effective.

In a distorted way, John was a very responsible person. A
real self-determiner. He felt very badly about himself and

often got depressed when things didn't go well, but he never wanted to let go of his sense of responsibility.

In this light it can be seen that in blaming others for his own faults, John was really trying to hold on to a sense of responsibility. To admit that he had failed, through his own fault only, would mean that he was a nobody. That he was incapable of responsibility. But in blaming others he could say, "I'm responsible for my actions. I want to do right. They're just too big and powerful for me. They beat me every time."

A lot of rage goes with this. Anger against himself for being weak, and anger against others for being strong. So his reaction was usually to do something he could see as assertive and responsible. Destructive, but still assertive and responsible. Like walking off the job. "I ain't going to let them treat me that way." Or stealing from "them." Or shooting dope.

Irresponsibility in our society is usually taken to mean a free-wheeling, do-what-feels-good, thoughtless, motiveless attitude. This is just a superficial interpretation. What looks like irresponsibility is usually very powerful. There are usually heavy, grinding motives. John, for example, was at war. He was waging battle after battle to protect his own sense of power and responsibility.

John described this process in some detail when he discussed getting fired from his job.

"I went to work that day with the best of intentions. No drugs for several days. I was going to do a good job and I even thought I might ask the boss for a raise that day or the next. I was supposed to get some papers from the office, and that's when he said he couldn't trust me with the keys."

I asked him what he felt, immediately, right then.

"Shocked. Then that changed to anger. Ah, in between the shock and anger I guess I was hurt. He didn't trust me to be responsible. Yeah, and then I thought 'Well he doesn't have any reason to trust me—I did try to rob him.' But there wasn't

anything I could do about that. *That's* what really made me angry. I was feeling angry with him, but I was really angry because there wasn't anything I could *do*. So I walked off the job. Like *that* was something I could do. Keep my pride. But when I got home I was so depressed about losing my temper and losing the job. I felt powerless again. So that's when I shot up."

In this sequence John never once let go of seeing himself as responsible. As the determiner of himself. Is it possible that John's problem is too much sense of responsibility rather than not enough? Or is it just that his sense of responsibility is different from the rest of society's?

This question can be carried further by looking at what happened to John as he began to overcome his addiction. The first step was to finally admit that the drug was more powerful than he. That his habit was irrevocably beyond his control. That there was no way he really could be responsible for it. Not that anyone else was responsible. Just that he was powerless to do anything about it himself. This didn't happen until he'd been addicted for many years, and had tried to quit many times. Until he'd struggled in every way he knew and had no choice but to give up. At this point his pattern changed. Always before when he'd given up, he'd done so with anger and willfulness. "To hell with it," he'd say, and turn to something else, equally destructive.

But at this time of giving up, he couldn't be angry anymore. He couldn't have any real feeling, for there was nothing else to turn to and nothing to be angry with. All he could do was give up and live. This was a kind of ultimate admission of *irresponsibility*. "I can't do it." With this, he started to heal. Alcoholics Anonymous knows how important this admission of powerlessness is if healing is to happen, but John had to find out for himself. He also discovered another basic tenet of AA's philosophy; take it a day at a time. John just naturally started

living his life one day at a time, because there wasn't any other way to do it. He didn't really fight his urges to use dope. He simply didn't shoot up. He didn't *overcome* the urges. He just didn't respond to them in any way.

Then there came a time when he started to think again. "I've been off drugs for several months now." And there was a bit of pride in his voice. His hunger for responsibility had reoccurred. "I did it. I kicked the habit!" And he began to get excited. Dreams of powerful self-determination arose again. And with the hunger for responsibility came a renewed hunger for heroin. The two had gone together for him for so long that when one returned, the other did too. And with a mind-trick so subtle that only addicts can appreciate it, he said, "I can handle it now. I'll prove it to myself by shooting up just once." And he was off again, off and running and addicted.

The treacherous thing about responsibility is that it so easily becomes hooked to pride, power and self-importance. As long as it is *behavior* which needs to be responsible there is no problem. **One** does what one needs to do. What is right, appropriate and good. But when responsibility gets hooked to saying powerfully, "*I* can do this. *I* can control my behavior. *I am* responsible," then treachery is close.

Responsible *behavior* and enterprising *action* are necessary, dynamic and beautiful. Responsible behavior and enterprising action are generated by the situation at hand. They spring from all the factors combined in the present situation. From what needs to be done. From the individual's sense of right and wrong. From desires and hopes, impulses and values. All these things go to produce responsible behavior and enterprising action.

But too often, in the individual's internal mental world, responsible behavior and enterprising action are clouded under the thought "I am being responsible," or "I am enterprising." Then what becomes important is not the need of the situation

but the significance and power of the "I AM." Then responsibility becomes a useless adornment. An energy-sapping accoutrement which serves only to clutter the situation.

There is one more significant chapter in John's story. After his "slip," he did encounter another time of giving up. This time he was more savvy to the treachery of his sense of responsibility. Or at least he thought so. He recognized that giving up meant giving up. And that there was no room for personal power in any true healing process that might occur in him. So he became quite comfortable with letting himself be.

At first, his letting himself be was very gentle and helpful. It was a natural part of giving up. It meant to accept himself totally, as he found himself at any given time. He described it one day like this:

"I was sitting on the bus, riding to work. All of a sudden I had this surge of laziness. Like 'I don't want to go to work today. I'd rather sleep.' In the past I would have struggled with that—trying to put the feeling out of my mind. And I would have failed, probably. And the struggle would have created more struggles and pretty soon I would have been all knotted up about it. Probably would have taken some dope. But this time I just said to myself, 'O.K., you got a lazy feeling. That's O.K. And you're here on the bus riding to work and that's O.K. too.' And then the impulse wasn't there anymore."

So he'd begun to learn to accept himself and let himself be, and he was doing fine. He was growing into a rewarding, peaceful, dynamic life. But his acceptance wasn't really total, and it began to get him in trouble.

"I'd gone to this party and I was having a good time. There was a girl that I really liked and we hit it off real well. Then somebody started passing around some marijuana. I really wanted to smoke some but I knew it might get me back into the drug scene. So I held off. I realized I was struggling with whether or not to smoke it so I real quick got into letting

myself be. I said to myself, 'You really want to have a smoke and you're fighting yourself, so relax and do what comes naturally.' I relaxed, and what came naturally was to have a smoke. Now I've been smoking more. No hard stuff, but it's got me worried."

The power-responsibility thing came in again here when he told himself to stop struggling. But what really got him in trouble was that he couldn't accept himself totally. He thought he was letting himself fully be, but he'd really been very selective. When he tuned in to his feelings he was struggling with himself. There were two armies at war in him. One was saying "I want a smoke." The other was saying "It'll get you in trouble." If he'd *really* let himself be, he would have accepted both sides. Just as he had on the bus. He would have accepted the struggle. But instead, he took sides.

He didn't want to be struggling so he stifled that part of himself. He didn't want to be manipulating so he said, "I'll do what comes naturally." In retrospect, this was clearly another mind-trick. Doing what comes naturally really meant going ahead and smoking. So he'd stifled his conscience. In attempting to let himself be, he'd rather skillfully managed to get what his impulses wanted. This is a very subtle but very common abuse of self-acceptance and of letting one's self be. It so easily becomes a cop-out. A way of avoiding a necessary struggle.

If John had to think all this through every time a decision was to be made, he'd be almost paralyzed by the subtleties and complexities of it all. But eventually he found that the way was indeed very simple.

"When I've got to make a decision, I don't have to do anything special. Or *not* do anything special. All I need to do is accept what's going on in my mind. The only thing is it's got to be *total* acceptance. If I've got a struggle going on between an urge and my common sense, I got to accept it *all*, the urge, my common sense, *and* the struggle. Then it gets worked out

the best way I can. I haven't taken sides or killed anything or added anything. I find I go ahead and do the best I can, and it usually works out fine."

There is wisdom, fear and sacrifice in this way of self-acceptance. The wisdom is in John's realization that he can't really *add* anything of value to his struggle anyway. All he has to work with are his impulses and his common sense, and he might as well let them work it out. By getting involved in the battle in any way other than accepting it, he's only going to cloud the picture and distort the outcome.

The fear is that he's been so used to being responsible *for* himself, he's afraid to let himself *be* responsible. He's afraid it won't work somehow. Hopefully though, the wisdom overshadows the fear and he'll be able to accept and allow himself to be.

The sacrifice is really twofold. The first is a potential sacrifice. If he lets himself work out the conflict between impulse and control, he always runs the risk of not getting what he wants. Or getting what he doesn't want. He may have to do without. If that's the outcome, he'll just have to accept it.

The second sacrifice is that he can't take credit for the outcome. He can't indulge in self-pride or a sense of having "been responsible." His mind and his body worked out the problem within the situation at hand and he can't take credit for it. All he can do is watch. Perhaps he could be permitted some awe, or wonder, or appreciation. Maybe even gratitude for the process which worked through him. But no credit.

All he can do is watch. But the watching is really the important part of it all. Most of the time, especially while he was addicted, John did not watch. His eyes were closed to his being-in-the-present-moment. He went around acting and reacting, waking up only when some strong feeling came along. Some desire or fear or guilt or anger or hope. The rest of the time he was quite unaware of being. And while he was un-

aware, all sorts of things went on unconsciously. Rage got directed in very destructive ways. Warm, loving impulses got killed. Fear ruled.

But with his eyes open, accepting all, the various forces inside and outside could dance together, freely, dynamically, and the being of John was given space to emerge.

The importance of awareness then is not so that we can better control ourselves. It is not so that we can analyze and interpret our minds or bodies or the world around us. To use awareness as a tool for self-manipulation only leads to treachery. Awareness is a space giver. An open window, letting the fresh air in. It unties the knots and loosens the tension. Awareness with full acceptance is like pure sunlight shining into a cellar, making it possible for healing to happen and growth to take place. One has to do nothing *with* it.

11

GENTLE
MEDDLING

Force is no remedy.

John Bright, *On the Irish Troubles*

Sanity speaks clearly when it says, "Be who you are, completely." Recognizing that at core this natural process of being is
beyond control, it is tempting to relax totally. But as John
found out with his addiction, one cannot fully be if one stifles
the desire for change and improvement. So we are left with a
dilemma. Sanity lies in just simply being, but for most of us
just simply being *includes* some desire to change the way we
experience life. The dilemma sounds complex from a rational
point of view, but the answer is really quite simple. One simply moves in the direction of accepting one's self more and
more completely. Then in the process of this acceptance, sanity
simply begins to emerge.

So, recognizing and accepting some continuing need to
change, what *does* one *do*? Simply be who you are, completely.
Better yet, just realize that you *are* being who you are, right
now, completely. That's all.

There are times when that *is* all. When this awareness just
happens, easily, naturally. These times are gifts, and all one
has to do is accept them, move into them, allow them to be.

But there are many other times when the will to meddle with one's self comes on very strong. Then one cannot "simply" be. One cannot kill one's will to meddle. That must be accepted too. In those times perhaps one *must* meddle with one's self. Then there are perhaps some ways of meddling more gently. Ways which are tender and not severe, open and not grasping, quiet and not noisy. This chapter will present some possibilities for gentle meddling.

But once more let me say that if you can be yourself without feeling that you are meddling, or if you can be relaxed and accepting *of* your meddling, there is no need to do anything extra. The ideas and suggestions in this chapter are for those times when it seems one *must* meddle, and when one cannot even help but meddle with the meddling. These ideas and suggestions are *not* techniques to achieve "just being." They are only touches of gentleness, at best a practice. Perhaps they may ease one's acceptance of just being, but they do not, and never can, produce just being. Just being simply is.

There may occur a tendency to use some of these ways of meddling as escapes from discomfort and difficulty. This warrants close scrutiny, for to escape is to remove or kill a part of one's experience, thus limiting the fullness of life. We all tend to strive for happiness at the expense of sadness; that is naturally human. But to try to *use* freely being to promote one side of life over the other will always be an abuse. So these ideas and suggestions are not ways to bliss without pain. They are simply ways of meddling that one might hope would help clarify one's perception and appreciation of *both* bliss and pain.

At the beginning of Chapter 9 I gave a caution about my own presumptuousness in relating what I felt to be the messages of sanity. This same caution should apply here, along with the major overriding danger flag against using these suggestions as ways of greater rather than less self-manipulation.

I. *GENERAL ATTITUDES*

In all things, above all, be gentle with yourself. Not especially weak, nor especially passive. Just gentle. Nothing should be destroyed, nothing denied, nothing stifled. All goes on, as it will, and hopefully one can be wide awake, deeply within it all.

There should be no detachment or distancing from life, yet there can be a sense of freedom and space within the process of living.

There need be no special activity or passivity. No more or less than is naturally there within you. You are who you are, but there is no need to decide or determine who you are. You do what you do, but there is no need to be actively hooking that doing to an idea of what you ought to do or should do. Such hooking will occur, spontaneously, if allowed. There is no need to manage it. You are who you are no matter what you do, so there is no need to try to be.

II. *SELF-IMAGE*

Forget worrying about who you are. Hold on to no idea of identity. But neither try to destroy any sense of identity that is there. Allow the sense of identity to come and go. No grasping for it. No attack upon it. No clinging to it. No freezing of it.

Evaluate your self only to the point that is natural for you. To the point that feels right and comfortable at the time. Neither add nor subtract anything special. Don't add any extra "I'm proud," or "I'm bad" or "The heck with it" or anything. Simply accept your self-evaluation as it is and then quit.

Whenever and wherever you encounter your self, an image of self, an evaluation of self, a fear for self, a desire for self, self-consciousness, pride or guilt or whatever, don't kill it. There is no need for battle. One needs do nothing special *with*

it. Just back off from it a little, see it and take a deep breath. Let it be and its energy will, in time, be free.

Manipulation and fixing of self is like a ladder, each rung building on the one before it. One manipulates, and then manipulates the manipulation. One alters, then alters the alteration. Fixes, and then fixes the fixing. One does need to know when to stop. Without awareness, this can become an endless ladder to despair. But with awareness and humor, the ladder has a final rung. Where rest is possible. So watch your ladder of self-manipulation, and grin.

Let your self be. Totally. Without a single iota of equivocation. Let it all exist, as awful or wonderful as it may seem. Permit it absolutely. If there is a desire to kill something within yourself, ask forthrightly, "Who is killing whom?" And be exceedingly gentle. To struggle with yourself will make you very important.

Self-importance is a trap, but it is not something one can attack directly. If one makes a frontal attack on self-importance, success or failure will foster pride or guilt. And these in turn will make the self even *more* important. So it is foolish to try to stop being interested in one's self. It is much wiser to nurture interest in other "things." In awareness of the immediate present. In whatever work needs to be done. In the sun and the wind. And in other people. It is wise to be with others, in friendship, teamwork and community. For if one can be interested in others, openly, with no cultism or competition, the importance of private-selfhood just might be forgotten for a while. In giving without hope of receiving anything in return, not even the pride of "I am being good," being can become unfettered. Sanity can never be a completely private matter.

III. *LOOSENING AND OPENING*

Search within both mind and body for anything that is tight, and allow it to loosen. Look for anything which is being

held and relax that holding, as if you were slowly opening your hands and letting go. Whatever is being held, one can ease one's grip.

In the midst of any situation, no matter how tense or pressing, it is possible to relax. First the body, just easing the muscles and allowing the limbs to become flexible. Then the mind, in the same way, relaxing. Not avoiding the tension of the moment, it is possible to relax *into* it. Deeply.

Wherever one finds oneself managing, stifling, killing, controlling, grasping, holding, craving or struggling, and where one cannot accept these things going on, it is possible to slip their bonds. In any given moment, you can simply step aside from this tightness, as if you were slipping out of an old overcoat and gently walking away. Perhaps in the next moment the tightness will return. But then relaxation can happen again. Permanence is a myth at any rate. One may think about life in terms of days and years. But one may live it only in this very instant.

There are knots, tight places, in every aspect of living. Body, mind, moving, talking, thinking, seeing, eating, loving, everything has its knots. Whenever a knot is found, it can be allowed to loosen and perhaps unravel completely. Never by picking at the knot itself, but rather by easing the tension upon it. It is helpful here to take a deep breath and let it out, allowing the tension to go with it.

IV. TRUSTING MIND

Practice trusting your mind. For a few minutes every day, give your mind a chance to be. If you have regular prayer or meditation times, you can do this too. Or you can set aside a special time. Or simply do it whenever it seems right.

1. Sit down, or lie down, and take a few minutes to get physically comfortable.

2. Take a few deep breaths to relax. Brightly waking up as you breathe in, relaxing your body as you breathe out.

3. Relax your face, your shoulders, your stomach, and your breathing.

4. Then, for a few minutes, just be. Allow your mind to do what it wants. Have no expectations for it, ask nothing of it, just let it be. If it wishes to be noisy, let it be noisy. If it wishes to be quiet, let it be quiet. If it wants to go off on a fantasy, O.K. If it wants to be bored or blissful, scared or angry, let it be.

5. For these few minutes, don't try to do anything special. And don't try not to do anything special. Just be.

V. *EXPECTATIONS*

Expectations are the long arm of desire, reaching forward in time and attempting to force reality to produce what one wants. If expectations are satisfied, a sense of power may evolve. If they are not satisfied, one may become disappointed with life. Expectations are bound to happen, but they do not have to be taken too seriously. If expectations are not held too strongly, they will rise and fall of their own accord, adding nothing but color to the process of living. They become accoutrements of life rather than the reasons for living. Underneath, it is possible to move toward an attitude of expecting absolutely nothing. Nothing.

Then one can move into life with openness. It is as if one says to the world, and to life, and to one's self, and to God, "Surprise me!" In marriage for example, this simple shift of attitude can make the difference between boredom and beauty. One awakens in the morning to find one's spouse is still there! The children gather for breakfast! How marvelous!

VI. *DESIRES*

Once one has discovered that desire is not the primary motivation for living, an entirely new approach to life is possible. In the process it is tempting to want to overcome some of one's desires. This can be very freeing, but it can also become a trap of tenseness. If desire is to be given up, one must also give up the desire to be desireless. So perhaps it is better simply to loosen one's grip on desire. Take it less seriously. See it clearly rather than engage it in a taut battle. Watching any desire closely and immediately, it is often surprising to see that the desire lasts for only a few moments. It may return again soon. But each time its tenure is very brief. There is some release in this. And one experiences a tendency to laugh.

Recognizing this coming and going of desire, it becomes evident that any prolonged wanting comes more from an *idea* of desiring than from the impulse itself. Then it is possible to let go of any idea of wanting, and the entire sphere of desire becomes open, spacious.

If you do decide to limit your pleasure directly, it is wise to do so only to the extent that feels like lightness, openness and freedom. If it becomes heavy and serious, this is a signal that sacrifice is being overdone. And probably one is *wanting* very much to be without desire. Perhaps it is better not to initiate too many extra sacrifices. But when the opportunity for sacrifice comes along, be willing to accept it. This way, one is not so much in the business of choosing and managing one's own sacrifices.

VII. *ACCEPTANCE*

Things are as they are whether one accepts them or not.

So they may as well be accepted. If one can accept everything, just as it is, totally, one simply can be. But *total* acceptance is very rare. There can be no exceptions if acceptance is total. Nothing withheld. If this kind of acceptance sounds passive, then it is incomplete. One has forgotten to accept one's desire to change things. If one can accept each situation just as it is, and also accept one's own reaction to that situation, just as it is, there is nothing left but wonder.

Acceptance of one's self is often more difficult than acceptance of a situation. But anywhere, any time, it is possible to do the best one can and then say something like, "I accept," or "Thy will be done," or "I offer everything else to the universe."

Likewise in looking at one's self, it is possible to judge, fix and evaluate only to the extent that is normal and usual, and then say "I accept," or "Thy will be done," or "I offer everything else to the universe."

And if you find dissatisfaction with your own ability to be freely, try this:

1. Accept your craziness—completely.
2. Accept your dissatisfaction with being crazy—completely.
3. Accept your attempts to do something about it—completely.
4. Accept your inability to accept whatever you cannot accept—completely.

VIII. *ATTENTIVENESS*

Awareness is the nutrient field in which sanity will grow. Sometimes it is possible to encourage free awareness by being attentive. Attentiveness is different from paying attention. In

paying attention some things are blocked out so that awareness can be focused on one thing. In attentiveness, nothing is blocked. One is open to all that is.

One can try to keep as sharply aware as possible, in all the things one does—not so that one can be in better control, but just to *see*. In order to nurture this attentiveness, one must find a way of being relaxed and alert simultaneously. At times this may seem like going against old habits, in which relaxation means dullness and alertness means tension. But relaxing with bright awareness can happen. And one might do well to encourage it.

Become aware of *now*. Bring awareness gently into the full immediate present. Whenever tension occurs, whenever some fantasy or worry has carried your attention "away," simply blink your eyes and see what is, right here, right now. Be sharp, clear, bright. Do nothing which will dull awareness.

Sometimes with immediate awareness, a judging parental quality will develop. It will evaluate and label, worry and plan. And it will capture awareness again, kidnapping it from the here and now. When this happens it seldom can be fought. But if one can take one more step back and *see* the judging happening, awareness will then remain bright and present. No matter what is going on, it is possible to be aware, right now.

In all things, be aware now. Watch your movements, how they flow from one to the next. Watch your hands move. Eating, talking, working, see it all happening in that very moment. In the middle of a busy day, listen to your breathing. Be aware of the beating of your heart. When any sound stops, listen to the silence. In listening to music, let your breathing go with it.

Try keeping a thought, word, image or prayer going somewhere in your mind all the time. Listen to it whenever you can. And if you must pay attention, pay attention to your immediate being, to the consciousness you share with all creation.

IX. SPACE

Sense space. Sense openness. Find spaciousness in every situation. Begin perhaps with sensing the physical space around you, between you and someone else. Then sense space between you and your feelings and experiences. But then allow the idea of you to pass away. Then only spaciousness, in and through and around everything, remains.

X. TIME

Let each moment, as it strikes you, be totally fresh and new. Make no extra connections of yourself with past or future. In planning or remembering, simply see that it's occuring now. There is no need to struggle into an awareness of now. No need to get into the immediate moment. You are already there, and all it takes is relaxing to realize it.

XI. LEARNING

Learning springs from being. One does not learn to be. The making of concepts is like a work of art, an attempt to express or describe experience. Concepts should never dictate experience. They should only reflect it. Thus approach life without conception, totally open to what may be.

If you should move to sacrifice concepts, be sure to sacrifice the concept of being without concepts.

If you learn from books or teachings, reading the Bible or the Talmud, the Sutras or the Gita, let the words flow into you as if they were raindrops to nourish your soul. You need not pull the words into yourself. Simply let your spirit drink. And when you speak, to teach others or to paint a word picture of

being, you need not push the words out. Let them flow forth from you as from a spring.

XII. *COMPASSION*

Remember to look for compassion rather than make it. Find love rather than build it. When you discover it, simply watch.

In your doing, do compassionate things. Do loving acts. But do not confuse this with love.

XIII. *PRAYER*

If you do pray:

1. Pray
2. Do the best you can
3. Accept the whole situation
4. Watch with awe

If you don't pray:

1. Do the best you can
2. Accept the whole situation
3. Watch with awe

If you can't pray:

1. Do the best you can
2. Accept the whole situation
3. Watch with awe
4. Be still and listen

If prayer happens, watch who's praying. Sometimes it seems like you praying, and sometimes it doesn't. Listen to noisy prayer. And listen to quiet prayer. And if there's no prayer at all, listen to that.

XIV. *HUMOR*

If you don't try to make light of things but simply find the humor which is there, self-importance is eased without pain. It is helpful to seek out the humor in everything you do—perhaps even to write down the most heroic, tragic, painful, nostalgic, meaningful, important things in your life and look for their funniness.

XV. *WAITING*

Practice the deep, quiet art of waiting. In making decisions, if a direction seems right, follow it. But if nothing seems right, wait. Wait for rightness. If there is no time to wait, move ahead to do whatever is the best you can do. *Then* wait.

And in living, do not rush your sanity. Do the best you can. Then wait.

12

THE FEAR
OF
SANITY

Death in itself is nothing; but we fear
To be we know not what, we know not where.

John Dryden, *Aurengzebe*

Sanity does not come without a price. Or at least a feeling of a price. The price itself is the death of delusion, and the direct experience of the price is fear.

There is a strange fearsomeness about giving up into life, going beyond self-control, listening to sanity. It is not quite like any other fear that humans can experience. In it, all the opposites of life are swirled together: living and dying, belonging and abandonment, power and impotence, joy and dread. This is a fear worth seeing very closely.

The fear of freely sanely being is made up of a series of layers. For most people the outer layers all have to do with losing control. At first the fear of losing control may take on a rather fleeting psychological flavor. "If I let my mind be—my feelings—my fantasies, maybe I'll find out that I'm basically crazy." Or perhaps there is fear of experiencing some feelings one does not wish to have. Scary feelings. Petty jealousies. Revenge. Rage. Fanatacism. Or, worse yet, mediocrity. But soon one realizes that in accepting one's own awful qualities, one can also accept their natural suppression, and relaxation can

happen again. It may even turn out that one's insides are not as horrible as they had seemed.

One of the fears associated with loss of control, then, is of self-discovery. Or more precisely of discovering certain *qualities* of self. Finding out the true attributes of who one is and perhaps discovering that they're not very nice. Going beyond self-control means to confront one's images of one's self very directly. To relax the barriers against perception and to be open to what is. There are times when to do this begins to feel like great unpleasantness.

Another layer of fear is that of disappointment and unintended sacrifice. Giving up control of self means that perhaps one will not get what one wants. Or that perhaps one will get what one doesn't want. Perhaps one will not have any fun. There is a sense of risk-taking here. It is not a very deep or heavy fear, but it plays its part in making people defensive against sanity.

Then a deeper layer of fear is encountered. "If I give up control and allow myself to be, will someone or something take over? Who or what will it be? And can it be trusted?"

This fear is born in the delusional idea that in order for there to be control, one must somehow do the controlling. A friend of mine named Bill described this rather graphically. "I was sitting quietly, letting my whole being relax. Things became superbly quiet. It was wonderful. I became aware that the only thing left which I could identify as 'me' was a little observer, just passively watching everything. The peace was incredible, and there was great beauty there, beyond all words. But there was another feeling as well. A deep, creeping dread. Here was my life, JUST GOING ON! Breathing happening, heart beating, birds outside singing, sounds of traffic in the background, and it was all SIMPLY TAKING PLACE! I got this idea that someone else, somewhere else, just had to be *doing* all that. And I got so scared I started to shake, and

before I could identify what was happening the peace just evaporated. I became very conscious of myself again, and then I wasn't scared anymore. But the beauty was gone."

Bill realized, intellectually, that his fear was both natural and unfounded at the same time. He recognized that what he had experienced was the "fear and trembling" so often described by those who have perceived the sense of some universal process. He said "It's just that I've been so used to holding the reins of my life. I feel naked if I ease my grip at all." But he'd also had the feeling that someone or something else was taking over, and that was somehow even more terrifying. "Maybe if I knew it was God," he said, "if I could name it God and believe in its benevolence, it wouldn't be so frightening. But I don't know what God is. And what if it's not God? What if it's evil?"

This is the fear of ultimate vulnerability. People usually deal with this fear in one of three ways. First, they may become so frightened that they retreat with great haste to the more comfortable and familiar world of managing their own destinies. But if they realize that in the process of managing their own lives they still cannot be certain about good and evil, they may seek out a faith. If this faith is fairly strong, they can enter into sanity with a simple prayer. Even without a clear sense of to whom they're praying, they can say, "Thy will be done." But if the faith is not so strong, their trust in benevolence not so great, they may enter sanity through the doorway of despair. "I know I can't manage it all. And I don't know who's going to. Still, there is no choice but for me to give up to what is. Whatever it is. I can hope it will be good, but good or bad, I shall have to accept it."

The fear of whether control will be assumed by something good or evil is understandable enough, but beneath this question lies another terror. What if there's nobody there at all? Can things simply take place, happen, *be*, without anyone

doing it at all? Can it all just go on, like some cosmic perpetual motion machine, just happening, all by itself?

This is the next layer: a fear of aloneness. Of abandonment. A woman described it to me this way. "It was like I was an astronaut in outer space, and my lifeline had just broken. I was drifting deeper and deeper into emptiness, free, swirling voidness, totally silent. I was so terribly, terribly alone. I was afraid I'd just drift out there and never get back. Just stay there, nowhere, forever. I don't think I've ever been so scared. Still, it was so beautiful."

Many of these fears have a very familiar ring to many people. In one way or another, to a greater or lesser extent, nearly everyone has experienced them. So these are very natural fears. Yet they all come from delusion. They are all basically unfounded. The fear of vulnerability to evil, for example, is a myth because if one simply sacrifices one's attempts to control the self, one in no way kills one's own inner sense of rightness and wrongness. One simply allows whatever sense of good and evil one has, to be there. And thus one remains as capable of distinguishing right from wrong as ever. One simply ceases the struggle of continually trying to improve upon this ability. In allowing one's self to be, one cannot cast discretion to the winds. One simply allows it to be what it is.

And the feeling of abandonment is also mythical. It means that one is convinced that one is somebody distinct and irrevocably separated from the rest of the world, and thus capable of *being* abandoned. Sanity itself would be reassuring. If heard, it would be saying, "You are at one with the world. You always have been and always shall be. How then can you be abandoned?"

And the image of drifting helplessly into a void is also just as crazy. The woman who described this experience had in fact been sitting in a meditation group when it happened. She was in a real room full of real people. And she wasn't really drifting

anywhere. She was right there all the time. The experience she had was just a projection of her fear. Simply an image of her fear of losing a sense of self-in-relation-to-others.

But to hear that these fears are unfounded, to recognize their unreality with one's intellect, does not at all mean that the fears will cease. All this knowledge does is allow one to perceive the fear with a sense of space. To see the fear more for what it is as it occurs, rather than being totally captured by it.

Each person has his or her own configuration of fear-layers. For some, loss of control is most prominent. For others, loneliness and abandonment. But for all of us, the fears have times of seeming very, very real. And they cannot be bypassed. Moving through one's own layers of fear is a sort of purification, the sacrifice of pieces of delusion. It is this which accounts for the strange quality with which fear of sanity is imbued. It is this which makes fear of sanity unlike any other kind of fear. The fear of sanity is always associated with beauty. None of its terror occurs without a background of great wonder, and never does one experience its dread without an aura of peace. Thus it is a sweet sort of panic that one experiences as the layers of fear are peeled away and the voice of sanity is heard more clearly.

As one comes closer to the center of these layers, it becomes evident that all the fears are simple manifestations of a single basic dread. This is the core-anxiety: Nonbeing. Death. One realizes that each of the layers of fear has been one aspect of the sense of self screaming for survival. Delusion sensing the threat of direct scrutiny and pleading for its life.

One may have habitually associated the sense of self with control, or with management, or with relationship, or with the satisfaction of desire. These predilections will determine which of the specific fears are most terrifying to the individual. But since nearly everyone has come to associate self with *being*, the loss of delusion always seems like death at core. The final ac-

ceptance of sanity requires a realization that being simply is. That there need be no separate "one" who is *doing* the process of being. To lose one's self in order to find one's self, to die in order to be reborn; these are not empty propositions. They are not simple platitudes. There are times for everyone when they feel very real.

Those times, when death looms most realistically, ironically occur when life is most fully perceived. It is in deeply sensing our existence that we most completely fear death. Looking deeply into the immediate functioning of one's mind, watching thoughts rise and fall, or acutely sensing emotion, or breathing beauty deeply, this is when one is most likely to sense, "I AM." And the more vibrantly one senses "I AM," the more vivid is the awareness that "I MIGHT NOT BE."

A colleague of mine, after experiencing some considerable fear in watching his mind at work, had a memory. "I remember having this kind of fear when I was a little kid. Maybe about five or so. When I first realized that I was thinking. And I suddenly became aware that I *was*. And right then—immediately, came this tremendous fear. 'If I *am*, then it's possible that I might *not be*.'"

It is in fully perceiving life that one comes to fear death the most. This is, of course, the brink of sanity. One more step and life is no longer perceived as by an observer, but lived, by a participant. And at that point self is no longer defined. Death of self-image has occurred. But of course nothing has really died. Just a mistaken idea, replaced by the truth.

If it is in fully perceiving life that one most vividly fears death, it is no wonder that humankind tends to kill awareness of being in so many ways. It is no wonder why we walk dazedly through so much of life. And why full appreciation of being is reserved for moments now and then. Moments we have come to call "peak experiences." This continual suppression of awareness is simply one of many defenses humankind uses

against the fear of sanity. It is a form of repression, more deep and pervasive than any of the private psychological repressions described by Freud and his followers.

The story of humanity's attempts to avoid sanity does in fact read like a psychological case history. Humankind went crazy in its youth and now fights to preserve delusion in its maturity. Great energy is expended to avoid the fear of fully being. It is as if sanity were a driving force within mankind, like sex or aggression. More gentle perhaps, but even more powerful and threatening.

Psychotherapists are familiar with the threats of sexuality and aggression, and with the defense mechanisms people use to counteract these threats. But seldom has psychotherapy identified the threat of sanity and the defenses used against it. People *repress* sanity repeatedly by shoving it totally out of their consciousness, diving into the depths of delusion in order to avoid fear. And they *displace* sanity, seeking union, meaning, fulfillment in every conceivable way *except* in fully freely being. And they *project* their fear of sanity onto other people, labeling as "fanatic" anyone who proclaims to have experienced deeply living. And they *isolate* sanity, separating ideas *about* it from the experience *of* it, spending their efforts talking and writing about life rather than living it.

As a matter of fact, fully freely being has been more repressed and distorted than either sexuality or aggression. It has been, in recent generations, a taboo more pervasive than the taboo of sexuality in the Victorian era. The deep openness of life, the meaning of being, the experience of God were things one simply did not speak about openly. They were considered more private and personal than one's bedroom. It is only recently that America has begun to emerge from this age of spiritual Victorianism and has started to affirm, however tentatively, the personal search for being completely alive.

Now, as one might expect, people are beginning to talk

excessively about it. About consciousness and being, awareness and transcendence, spirituality and mysticism. As usual, the pendulum will probably swing too far. It *is* better sometimes to keep quiet about these things. But not out of fear. Simply out of the realization that words don't work. And that words are dangerous. For as we know so well by now, words often get substituted for the reality they attempt so poorly to describe.

There is one other aspect of defensiveness against sanity which should be mentioned. It has to do with a kind of self-determining "backlash." Several months ago I was participating in a retreat with a group of people who, like myself, were busily trying to freely be. Of course we didn't get very far with it because we were trying so hard to do it. But there were times. Times of open acceptance of what is. Times when the trying stopped and being started. Several weeks later, one of the participants told me of his experience. "While I was on the retreat I felt wonderful. I really felt like I was able to let myself be. More than ever before. I thought it was a great experience. But now I'm not so sure. Because as soon as the retreat was over I found I was trying to commandeer my life more than ever. It seemed like I was worse off than when I started. I don't know what to make of it."

As we talked, it became clear that even though he'd felt no great fear consciously during the retreat, his sense of self apparently had been threatened considerably by the experience of freely being. And in his response after the retreat, it seemed that his sense of self was making up for lost time by demonstrating how very powerful it could be.

Part of the problem here may have been that he had pushed himself a bit much on the retreat. The usual mistake of trying hard to "just be." And he had later paid a price for his hard-pushing of himself. But the other factor was that there were times when he really did relax, and he really did begin to ease his grip on the controls over himself, and that resulted in a backlash. Sometimes, after an experience of just being, the

pendulum swings back and life seems more controlled than ever.

With this understanding, it might be possible to find a bit of compassion for self-centeredness and egocentrism in oneself and others when it occurs. For example, it had always been a mystery to me that certain people who proclaimed to be on a "spiritual" path sometimes appeared to be extremely self-concerned. Where I presumed they "ought" to be interested in selfless giving to others, they appeared far more interested in their own personal image. I used to react with rage when I encountered this. It seemed so hypocritical. But perhaps this self-centeredness is simply the backlash of a very threatened ego. Perhaps it is something those people needed to go through. Perhaps it is something that *can* be gone through, for any of us.

At this point, I feel it is necessary to repeat a warning. As I indicated at the very outset, one of the most destructive tendencies in the human condition is that as soon as one identifies an imperfection, one wants to fix it. And the fixing requires more fixing. Having just proclaimed that people all over the world are busily distorting and repressing sanity, I now fear that there will be a desire to do something to remedy the situation. Nothing is more likely to lead one away from awareness of being. Let us simply be aware of the way things are, the good and the bad, and allow that awareness to move through us toward healing. Nothing special need be done. And nothing special need not be done.

The fear of sanity creates a lively process for discovery of being. The fact that the fear is not founded in reality does not in the least detract from its energy. At times it is easy to take this fear very seriously. And, in the sense of delusion, it is serious. It really does mean death of one's sense of substantial and important self. But in the sense of sanity, there is some delightful humor in our struggle against dying.

Suddenly discovering that one is experiencing a "peak" of

being, a union, a peace beyond words, there occurs a recognition. "Wow, this is beautiful. This is a great experience." And as suddenly as it came, the experience slips away. Why? Because the sense of self has been deeply threatened and it becomes very sneaky. It says, "This is such a wonderful, blissful experience, I want to keep it forever." In the guise of "wanting to keep it," one very subtly gets back in control. And of course the experience is destroyed. There is truly marvelous humor in this treachery.

Or in simply watching one's self trying to stop trying or working at relaxing, it becomes very difficult not to giggle. And if a giggle is permitted, a guffaw is usually close on its heels. And if *that* is permitted, being may become free in spite of oneself.

13

FAITH, PRAYER AND TRUST

Know you what it is to be a child? It is to
be something very different from the man of
today. It is to have a spirit yet streaming
from the waters of baptism; it is to believe
in love, to believe in loveliness, to believe
in belief . . .

Francis Thompson

Fear of losing control, of vulnerability, and of abandonment
rest like cloaks over the basic anxiety of nonbeing. Taken together these fears are simply too fierce for most people to handle unarmed and undefended. It is a heroic image to think of
facing self-loss nakedly, with total vulnerability. But of course
heroism is very seductive. One is tempted to feel "I am being
heroic in my holiness. I have faced the ultimate fear of nonbeing. My soul is on the mountain, whipped by universal winds,
alone, triumphant I have met the universe and lived!" And of
course this simply helps to reestablish the importance of one's
image of one's self.

So for most people it is both humble and necessary to
think that when they give up control of self there is someone or
something to give up *to*. It is only from the deepest despair
that one can give up totally to nothing at all. Most people have
a real need to say "Thy will be done."

Even though this approach raises interminable questions about who or what takes control, and whether the new controller is basically benevolent or sinister, it still seems more comfortable to give up to something than simply to cast one's self to the winds of a chaotic void.

This is where a concept of God becomes important. To be sure, all concepts about God are wrong. Just as one's concepts of other people can never substitute for the people themselves. In deep meeting with other people, one senses that no concept, no matter how wise, could ever capture their essence. And of course the same is true of a concept of God.

But the fallibility of a God-concept does not lessen people's *need* for such a concept. Nor does it keep people from treating a concept as the real thing for a while. If one is deeply frightened, deeply pained and in great need of reassurance, one has neither the time nor the energy to cogitate about the fallibility of concepts. One simply grabs hold of a concept and uses it the best way one can. And sometimes it is just as necessary to have someone or something to thank when life has been especially beautiful. If one needs to say "Help" or "Thank you," one simply needs to say it, and often one needs a sense of someone or something to say it to. If one needs to pray, it often seems that a concept will do, in lieu of the "real thing."

It's a kind of idolatry to worship or pray to a concept. But sometimes, especially during the process of giving up self-control, concept-idolatry becomes imperative. The feeling may be, "Here I go, slipping, falling under, losing my grip, opening up, allowing, and I'm *scared*." Then words seem to come. "Dear God, protect me." "Holy Mary, Mother of God." "Lord Krishna, guide me." "Allah protect me." "Our Father who art in heaven . . ." Voices speaking the concept-names of God in fear. The fact that the words themselves are determined by culture is unimportant. The feeling is that one needs help and needs it *now*.

Faith plays a very important role here, for up to a point the stronger one's faith is, the easier it is to let go. Up to the point of letting go of faith itself and allowing it to grow into trust. But since faith is as much a gift as love, it matters little to know that faith can ease fear. One "has" only as much faith as one is aware of. Like love, more faith cannot willfully be manufactured.

It is usually assumed that people need faith in order to pray. But this is not necessarily true. For many people, both faith and prayer seem immature, weak, childish. And faith is willfully disavowed. But prayer keeps popping up. Like sanity, it is almost never totally repressible. It may be disguised and distorted, but it keeps slipping out. And sometimes prayer without faith can really be what nurtures sanity into fruition.

A young man named Michael gave his account. "My family was pretty religious, and I used to pray a lot as a kid. But after I got into college I began to realize that faith was a crutch and prayer was just evidence of being immature—not being able to stand up for yourself. So I canned the whole business. I just shucked all the religious stuff and set about to live as fully and constructively as I could. Now and then, when I was really scared, or when I wanted something very badly, a stupid little prayer would squeak out. Like I'd find myself whispering, "Dear God . . ." But I'd squelch it quick, because it embarrassed me. Nobody heard it, but I was still embarrassed. It didn't fit my image of myself.

"Then several years ago I got into meditation. It started out as a trip. I just wanted to see what it was like. But after a while, I began to sense something—like a different way of being that might be possible. I can't really describe it, but I got more serious about meditating. As that happened, I started going 'deeper,' letting myself go more fully, opening up and letting be. And I got more and more frightened. I'd feel my controls loosening, my image of myself just slipping away.

Then one day the fear got so bad it literally forced words of prayer out of me. Since I had no viable concept of God, the first prayers were very sophisticated, like 'Oh universe, all your chaotic tumbling randomness, help me. Let the chips fall where they may, but I hope the chips fall in such a way that I won't be destroyed.' "

He chuckled as he said this, aware of the great lengths to which he'd gone in order to avoid anything sounding the least bit religious.

"Then after a while, it seemed like it just took too much energy to come up with all the big words, so the 'prayer' shortened itself to 'Power of the cosmos, protect me,' or 'Sequence of events, be kind.' " He grinned as he continued. "Finally I just gave up and the prayer became, 'O.K., God, whoever or whatever you are, thy will be done.' See it had dawned on me that my talking to the universe was no different from talking to God. I was just using different words. I remembered times when I had silently thanked a tree for being beautiful or silently asked a girl to fall in love with me. It was all the same. I'd been praying all the time anyway. Just without any concept of God. Anyway, with this realization I was able to let prayer happen and not be ashamed of it. I had no faith about it. It just happened. After this, prayer came more freely. Not like I was *doing* it, but rather that I'd given it permission to happen. Prayer kept happening when I was afraid, and there was something about it that eased the fear just a little. But I also found myself praying when I wasn't afraid—when I was happy or sort of celebrating.

"I used to think people made up God out of their fear. Now I don't think that's quite right. Maybe fear makes the concepts of God, and maybe fear can propel prayer into your consciousness, but it's more like prayer was there all the time. It was just a part of who I was, and I wasn't aware of it. And the concepts of God are just tools or ways of making it easier.

But the source of prayer and the nature of God are basically beyond any doing or labeling that I can accomplish. If I need a certain concept of God from time to time, that's O.K. I can use it—maybe even treat it as absolute when it's necessary. But all along, underneath, I can know it's really beyond me. Somehow with that approach I'm not embarrassed by prayer anymore. I don't feel I'm copping out. I'm just letting me be."

As Michael discovered, concepts of God or of a universal process can act as a kind of bridge between total in-control self-determination and total openness and acceptance of what is. Any kind of faith can be a bridge in this way. A help in transition. Something to mediate a transformation, so that one does not have to leap from delusion into sanity with no handholds at all. So that one need not go totally naked into the awesome openness of sanity. So that one does not necessarily have to endure the treachery of heroism.

When Michael was in college he saw faith and prayer as crutches and he cast them off. Now he may still see faith as a crutch, but he recognizes that there are times, for him, when such a crutch may be necessary. There is a place for crutches. When one looks across a lake on a bright summer day, one shields one's eyes from the sun. This is using a crutch. Climbing up a steep hill, one grasps at branches and rocks to keep from slipping. This is also a crutch. Yet one does not feel guilty or embarrassed about it. There is no special credit to be gained by *not* shielding one's eyes from the sun or grasping handholds on a hill.

But a crutch is always used in transition. It helps one travel from one place to another, or to change from one perception to another, and there comes a time when the crutch is no longer necessary. In the transition between delusion and sanity, the crutch of faith becomes transformed. Faith turns into trust. Trust based on the solid experience of having repeatedly allowed one's self to be. Then there is less frantic grasping for

concepts and more calm acceptance of what is. No need to invent beliefs. No need to cling to one's faith. No need to prepare concepts with which to face the experience of living.

As the experience of God deepens, there is less need for a concept of God. As reality is met more closely, ideas *about* reality can be relinquished. As life is more openly accepted, there is less need to think about living. And as one moves more intimately into the fear of nonbeing, self-protection can be eased. Then concepts fall back into their more natural place. Rather than being idols substituting for reality, concepts become works of art, attempts to communicate reality rather than prescribe it.

At this point, the disputes between one concept and another seem petty and irrelevant. This faith or that, science or religion, spirit or psyche are meaningless. To struggle with religion or faith or prayer or God becomes a waste of energy. The realization dawns that sanity is spiritual. It simply is. Like the primeval man's unity with nature, there is no question about it. No need to figure it out, explain it or defend it in any way.

It all, just simply, is.

ABOUT THE AUTHOR

CHRISTINE A. LARSON is an adjunct faculty member in the University of Kentucky system with twelve years of business development experience for Fortune 500 firms in healthcare and financial services. Her doctoral research focuses on evidence-based medicine in women's health. Her objective is to ensure good science drives both diagnosis and treatment in healthcare.